Applications of Artificial Intelligence in Pharmaceuticals

Anandhavalli Muniasamy
King Khalid University, Saudi Arabia

Gauthaman Karunakaran
Government Pharmacy College, India

IGI Global
Scientific Publishing
Publishing Tomorrow's Research Today

Vice President of Editorial — Melissa Wagner
Director of Acquisitions — Mikaela Felty
Director of Book Development — Jocelynn Hessler
Production Manager — Mike Brehm
Cover Design — Jose Rosado

Published in the United States of America by
IGI Global Scientific Publishing
701 East Chocolate Avenue
Hershey, PA, 17033, USA
Tel: 717-533-8845
Fax: 717-533-7115
Website: https://www.igi-global.com E-mail: cust@igi-global.com

Library of Congress Cataloging-in-Publication Data

Names: Muniasamy, M. Anandhavalli editor
http://id.loc.gov/authorities/names/n2025011069
http://id.loc.gov/rwo/agents/n2025011069 | Karunakaran, Gauthaman, 1972-
editor http://id.loc.gov/authorities/names/n2025026384
http://id.loc.gov/rwo/agents/n2025026384
Title: Applications of artificial intelligence in pharmaceuticals / edited by Anandhavalli Muniasamy, Gauthaman Karunakaran.
Description: Hershey, PA : IGI Global Scientific Publishing, [2026] | Includes bibliographical references and index. | Summary: "This book offers a comprehensive exploration of how AI is revolutionizing every facet of the pharmaceutical industry, from drug discovery to hospital administration. This book is designed for professionals, researchers, and enthusiasts seeking to understand the transformative power of AI in healthcare"-- Provided by publisher.
Identifiers: LCCN 2025007453 (print) | LCCN 2025007454 (ebook) | ISBN 9798337320434 hardcover | ISBN 9798337320441 paperback | ISBN 9798337320458 ebook
Subjects: LCSH: Pharmacy--Data processing
http://id.loc.gov/authorities/subjects/sh2010011246 | Artificial intelligence--Medical applications
http://id.loc.gov/authorities/subjects/sh88003000
Classification: LCC RS122.2 .A67 2025 (print) | LCC RS122.2 (ebook) | DDC 615.10285--dc23/eng/20250618
LC record available at https://lccn.loc.gov/2025007453
LC ebook record available at https://lccn.loc.gov/2025007454

British Cataloguing in Publication Data
A Cataloguing in Publication record for this book is available from the British Library.

Table of Contents

Preface xvii

Acknowledgment xx

Chapter 1
Current Challenges in the Pharmaceutical Industry and AI's Role in Addressing Them 1
Shruthi A. Gauthaman, Faculty of Medicine, Mahsa University, Malaysia
Sakthynathan S. Magesh Kumar, Faculty of Medicine, Mahsa University, Malaysia
Riyazdeen Kamaldheen, Faculty of Medicine, Mahsa University, Malaysia
Kaurish Murugesan, Faculty of Medicine, Mahsa University, Malaysia
Mukesh Kumar Viswanathan, Faculty of Medicine, Mahsa University, Malaysia
Harini Devendran, Faculty of Medicine, Mahsa University, Malaysia
Anandhavalli Muniasamy, College of Computer Science, King Khalid University, Saudi Arabia

Chapter 2
Innovative Implementation, Ethical Challenges, and Future Prospects of Artificial Intelligence in Pharmaceuticals 27
Reshma S., Department of Artificial Intelligence and Machine Learning, Dayananda Sagar College of Engineering, Bangalore, India
Jigar Rupani, School of Business and Management, Christ University, Bangalore, India
M. Lalitha, Department of Humanities and Sciences, CVR College of Engineering, Rangareddy, India
K. Gowri, Department of Pharmacology, SRM College of Pharmacy, SRM Institute of Science and Technology, Chengalpattu, India
M. Sambathkumar, Department of Mechanical Engineering, Kongu Engineering College, Erode, India
M. Suresh , KPR Institute of Engineering and Technology IT, Kovai, India

Chapter 3
Quantum Computing in Drug Discovery: Revolutionizing Pharmaceutical Research 59
Anandhavalli Muniasamy, Department of Informatics and Computer Systems, College of Computer Science, King Khalid University, Saudi Arabia

Chapter 4
Implementation of Neuro-Pharmaceutical Innovation in Eco-Friendly Drug Manufacturing 97
Shwetha G. K., Department of Computer Science and Engineering, Vidyavardhaka College of Engineering, Mysuru, India
Rajesh Vyankatesh Argiddi, Department of Computer Science and Engineering, Walchand Institute of Technology, Solapur, India
Ashish Avasthi, Faculty of Computer Science, Poornima University, Jaipur, India
Lovely Jacob A., Department of Chemistry, Little Flower College, Guruvayur, India
Reshma S., Department of Artificial Intelligence and Machine Learning, Dayananda Sagar College of Engineering, Bangalore, India
Ravy Kannan, KPR Institute of Engineering and Technology, India

Chapter 5
The Potential of Generative AI in Drug Development 125
Deepak Gupta, Institute of Technology and Management, Gwalior, India
R. Sudhakar, Madanapalle Institute of Technology and Science, India
Sofiya S. Mujawar, D.Y. Patil University Ambi, India
Rita Kadam, D.Y. Patil University Ambi, India
Vivek Patil, D.Y. Patil University Ambi, India
Anurag Kumar, D.Y. Patil University Ambi, Pune, India
Prashant Ahire, Symbiosis Institute of Technology, Pune, India
Kapil Gupta, Amity Institute of Pharmacy, Gwalior, India

Chapter 6
AI-Driven Smart Manufacturing and Automation in Pharmaceutical Production 157
Arshi Naim, Business Management, European Global Institute of Innovation and Technology, Malta
Anandhavalli Muniasamy, Department of Informatics and Computer Systems, College of Computer Science, King Khalid University, Saudi Arabia
Mohammad Ibrahim Khan, International Medical University, Malyasia
Mohammad Faiz Khan, Ministry of Interiors, Security Forces Hospital, Saudi Arabia

Chapter 7
Supply Chain Optimization-based Drug Polymer Analysis Using AI Model for Synthesis and Characterization 195
Lubin Balasubramanian, SRM Institute of Science and Technology, India
G. Balamurugan, SRM Institute of Science and Technology, India
Nagamany Abirami, Sri Venkateshwaraa College of Engineering and Technology, India
U. Muruganantham, Manakula Vinayagar Institute of Technology, India
S. Magesh, Dr. M. G. R Educational and Research Institute, India
R. Manikandan, SASTRA University, India

Chapter 8
AI in Hospital Administration and Formulary Design: Optimizing Resource Allocation and Patient Flow........ 215
Kanagaraj Rengaramanujam, Verland Foundation, USA
Anandhavalli Muniasamy, College of Computer Science, King Khalid University, Saudi Arabia

Chapter 9
Electronic Health Records Unleashed: Strategies for Leveraging Big Data in Healthcare Research........ 247
Komal Bhardwaj, Maharishi Markandeshwar Institute of Management, Maharishi Markandeshwar University, Mullana, India
Aishwarya Tipara, Upgrad, Hyderabad, India
Garima, Maharishi Markandeshwar Institute of Management, Maharishi Markandeshwar University, Mullana, India

Chapter 10
Attention-Driven Sparse Graph Convolutional Networks for Early Detection of Liver Disorders From Medical Data 273
Shahnazeer C.K., Pondicherry University, Karaikal, India
Sureshkumar G., Pondicherry University, Karaikal, India

Chapter 11
Artificial Intelligence Enabled Dynamic Drug Overdose Response System 297
Sachin Sharma, Amity University, Mohali, India
Kumar Mayank, Graphic Era University, Dehradun, India
Prachi Pandey, Graphic Era University, Dehradun, India

Chapter 12
Investigation on Data Driven Modelling and Estimation of Concentrations in Three-Compartment Model for the Benchmark Pharmacokinetic System 333
V. Sujatha, SRM Institute of Science and Technology, India

Chapter 13
AI Driven Pharmacovigilance Case Study: Predicting Adverse Effects of Drugs Using NLP and Patient Feedback 357
Ruchi Jakhmola Mani, Amity University, Noida, India
Barsha Rani Bora, Amity University, Noida, India
Nureen Amin, Amity University, Noida, India
Manan Garg, Amity University, Noida, India
Kusala Vanam, Amity University, Noida, India
Snigdha Debashis Bhattacharjee, Vivekanand Education Society Institute of Technology, Mumbai, India

Chapter 14
Building a Knowledge Network of Drug-Drug Interactions Using Natural Language Processing and Graph Databases: Drug-Drug Interaction and Graph Networks 389
Ruchi Jakhmola Mani, Amity University, Noida, India
Harsh Lalwani, Amity University, Noida, India
Angamba Meetei Potshangbam, Discovery Boulevard, Imphal, India
Shikha Rani, Discovery Boulevard, Imphal, India
Kriti Katare, Discovery Boulevard, Imphal, India
Abhishek Chauhan, Chaudhary Charan Singh University, Meerut, India

Compilation of References 423

About the Contributors 465

Index 473

Detailed Table of Contents

Preface xvii

Acknowledgment xx

Chapter 1
Current Challenges in the Pharmaceutical Industry and AI's Role in Addressing Them 1
Shruthi A. Gauthaman, Faculty of Medicine, Mahsa University, Malaysia
Sakthynathan S. Magesh Kumar, Faculty of Medicine, Mahsa University, Malaysia
Riyazdeen Kamaldheen, Faculty of Medicine, Mahsa University, Malaysia
Kaurish Murugesan, Faculty of Medicine, Mahsa University, Malaysia
Mukesh Kumar Viswanathan, Faculty of Medicine, Mahsa University, Malaysia
Harini Devendran, Faculty of Medicine, Mahsa University, Malaysia
Anandhavalli Muniasamy, College of Computer Science, King Khalid University, Saudi Arabia

The pharmaceutical industry is facing a range of challenges, including skyrocketing drug development costs, inefficiencies in clinical trials, supply chain disruptions, stringent quality control standards, and the complex world of marketing and sales. This is where artificial intelligence (AI) steps in, acting as a game-changer by addressing these hurdles with cutting-edge tools like computer-assisted drug design (CADD), predictive modeling, and data analytics. This chapter delves into how AI-driven solutions are boosting the speed, accuracy, and efficiency of pharmaceutical operations, while also recognizing the hurdles posed by inconsistent data, intellectual property issues, and ethical concerns. A thorough look at AI's role in pharmaceutical companies reveals its benefits, drawbacks, and future possibilities, all while stressing the importance of ethical considerations and the need for regulatory flexibility to fully harness AI's groundbreaking potential.

Chapter 2
Innovative Implementation, Ethical Challenges, and Future Prospects of Artificial Intelligence in Pharmaceuticals 27
Reshma S., Department of Artificial Intelligence and Machine Learning, Dayananda Sagar College of Engineering, Bangalore, India
Jigar Rupani, School of Business and Management, Christ University, Bangalore, India
M. Lalitha, Department of Humanities and Sciences, CVR College of Engineering, Rangareddy, India
K. Gowri, Department of Pharmacology, SRM College of Pharmacy, SRM Institute of Science and Technology, Chengalpattu, India
M. Sambathkumar, Department of Mechanical Engineering, Kongu Engineering College, Erode, India
M. Suresh , KPR Institute of Engineering and Technology IT, Kovai, India

Incorporation of pharmaceutical industry and artificial intelligence (AI) is revolutionizing patient care, drug development, and discovery. Drug interactions have been predicted using machine learning techniques, optimal molecular structures have been designed, and clinical trial lengths have been reduced. Ethical problems including violations of data privacy, biassed algorithms, and unequal access to AI-informed treatments have been highlighted in the face of these technologies Reacting to these problems, regulatory models have been debated and passed. It is well known that artificial intelligence can drive therapeutic developments and customize medicine. One expects continuous innovations in artificial intelligence technologies to change the pharmaceutical industry. Ethical standards must be reinforced and openness kept if artificial intelligence is to be fully embraced. Innovation must guide newly developing projects.

Chapter 3
Quantum Computing in Drug Discovery: Revolutionizing Pharmaceutical Research 59
Anandhavalli Muniasamy, Department of Informatics and Computer Systems, College of Computer Science, King Khalid University, Saudi Arabia

The integration of quantum computing in drug discovery has the potential to revolutionize pharmaceutical research by significantly enhancing molecular simulations, drug screening, and optimization processes. Traditional computational methods often struggle with the complexity of molecular interactions, leading to high costs and extended timelines in drug development. Quantum computing, with its ability to process complex calculations exponentially faster than classical computers, offers innovative solutions to these challenges. This chapter explores the fundamentals of quantum computing, its application in pharmaceutical research, and real-world case studies from leading organizations. It also discusses existing challenges, potential solutions, and future directions for adopting quantum computing in drug discovery. By addressing key technical, ethical, and regulatory aspects, this chapter provides a comprehensive analysis of how quantum technologies can accelerate and optimize the drug discovery pipeline.

Chapter 4
Implementation of Neuro-Pharmaceutical Innovation in Eco-Friendly Drug Manufacturing 97

Shwetha G. K., Department of Computer Science and Engineering, Vidyavardhaka College of Engineering, Mysuru, India
Rajesh Vyankatesh Argiddi, Department of Computer Science and Engineering, Walchand Institute of Technology, Solapur, India
Ashish Avasthi, Faculty of Computer Science, Poornima University, Jaipur, India
Lovely Jacob A., Department of Chemistry, Little Flower College, Guruvayur, India
Reshma S., Department of Artificial Intelligence and Machine Learning, Dayananda Sagar College of Engineering, Bangalore, India
Ravy Kannan, KPR Institute of Engineering and Technology, India

This chapter discovers the conversion of neuro-pharmaceutical innovation and eco-friendly drug manufacturing, which emphasizes sustainable therapeutic development. It examines emerging trends in neuroscience-based drug detection, including precision-oriented treatment, AI-enabled diagnostics and nanotechnology-based delivery systems. At the same time, it highlights green chemistry methods such as biodegradable solvents, renewable raw materials and the use of low-emitting synthesis routes. By integrating environmental liability with cutting edge neuro-pharmaceutical research, this chapter reflects the importance of sustainable models in addressing both neurological disorders and global ecological challenges. This holistic approach is intended to promote future-prepared, morally aligned and environmentally therapeutic solutions in a developed pharmaceutical landscape.

Chapter 5
The Potential of Generative AI in Drug Development 125
Deepak Gupta, Institute of Technology and Management, Gwalior, India
R. Sudhakar, Madanapalle Institute of Technology and Science, India
Sofiya S. Mujawar, D.Y. Patil University Ambi, India
Rita Kadam, D.Y. Patil University Ambi, India
Vivek Patil, D.Y. Patil University Ambi, India
Anurag Kumar, D.Y. Patil University Ambi, Pune, India
Prashant Ahire, Symbiosis Institute of Technology, Pune, India
Kapil Gupta, Amity Institute of Pharmacy, Gwalior, India

Drug development is a complex, time-consuming, and expensive process with high failure rates. Traditional approaches face significant challenges, including lengthy timelines (10-15 years), astronomical costs (exceeding $2.5 billion per successful drug), and high attrition rates (>90%). Generative artificial intelligence (AI) represents a paradigm shift in this field, offering novel approaches to address these longstanding challenges. This chapter explores the transformative potential of generative AI across the drug development pipeline, from target identification to clinical trial design. Various AI architectures and their pharmaceutical applications are examined, breakthrough case studies are analyzed, current challenges are addressed, and future directions are discussed that may revolutionize pharmaceutical research and development, providing stakeholders with the knowledge necessary to navigate the rapidly evolving landscape of AI-driven drug development.

Chapter 6
AI-Driven Smart Manufacturing and Automation in Pharmaceutical Production 157
Arshi Naim, Business Management, European Global Institute of Innovation and Technology, Malta
Anandhavalli Muniasamy, Department of Informatics and Computer Systems, College of Computer Science, King Khalid University, Saudi Arabia
Mohammad Ibrahim Khan, International Medical University, Malyasia
Mohammad Faiz Khan, Ministry of Interiors, Security Forces Hospital, Saudi Arabia

Artificial Intelligence (AI) is transforming pharmaceutical manufacturing by enabling smart automation, optimizing production processes, and ensuring regulatory compliance. This chapter explores the role of AI-driven technologies in enhancing efficiency, quality control, and decision-making within pharmaceutical production. It provides an overview of Industry 4.0 advancements, highlighting key AI applications such as predictive maintenance, digital twins, and robotics. A case study illustrates real-world AI implementation, emphasizing benefits and challenges. Additionally, the chapter discusses AI-driven solutions, best practices for integration, and regulatory considerations. Finally, future directions and emerging trends in AI- powered pharmaceutical manufacturing are examined.

Chapter 7
Supply Chain Optimization-based Drug Polymer Analysis Using AI Model for Synthesis and Characterization 195
Lubin Balasubramanian, SRM Institute of Science and Technology, India
G. Balamurugan, SRM Institute of Science and Technology, India
Nagamany Abirami, Sri Venkateshwaraa College of Engineering and Technology, India
U. Muruganantham, Manakula Vinayagar Institute of Technology, India
S. Magesh, Dr. M. G. R Educational and Research Institute, India
R. Manikandan, SASTRA University, India

Research on drug creation and development is crucial for chemical scientists and pharmaceutical businesses. On the other hand, drug design and discovery are hampered by limited efficacy, off-target delivery, time consumption, and excessive cost. Using the available three-dimensional structures, molecular docking can be utilised to anticipate the strength of the binding of small-molecule binders and their chemical derivatives to a macromolecular target. In process of finding as well as developing new drugs, artificial intelligence as well as machine learning technologies are essential. This chapter proposes novel technique in drug polymer-based synthesis and characterisation analysis with supply chain optimisation using artificial intelligence with machine learning algorithm. Then, the supply chain optimisation is based on drug synthesis and structure analysis using particle adversarial reinforcement Markov binary optimisation model. The experimental analysis has been carried out for various drug-polymer structure datasets in terms of prediction accuracy, random precision, and Recall.

Chapter 8
AI in Hospital Administration and Formulary Design: Optimizing Resource Allocation and Patient Flow... 215
Kanagaraj Rengaramanujam, Verland Foundation, USA
Anandhavalli Muniasamy, College of Computer Science, King Khalid University, Saudi Arabia

Artificial Intelligence (AI) is transforming hospital administration by improving resource allocation, patient flow, and formulary design. This chapter explores how AI technologies—such as machine learning, predictive analytics, and data-driven tools—enhance hospital efficiency, scheduling, and medication optimization. A real-world case study highlights AI's impact, while practical recommendations address implementation strategies and integration challenges. Future directions consider AI's role in personalized medicine, cost reduction, and ethical concerns, offering a roadmap for advancing healthcare management.

Chapter 9
Electronic Health Records Unleashed: Strategies for Leveraging Big Data in Healthcare Research.. 247
Komal Bhardwaj, Maharishi Markandeshwar Institute of Management, Maharishi Markandeshwar University, Mullana, India
Aishwarya Tipara, Upgrad, Hyderabad, India
Garima, Maharishi Markandeshwar Institute of Management, Maharishi Markandeshwar University, Mullana, India

In the era of advanced healthcare technology, the adoption of Electronic Health Records (EHRs) has led to the accumulation of vast troves of clinical data. While EHRs primarily serve as a central repository for patient care, they are increasingly being utilized for secondary purposes, such as clinical research, disease surveillance, and quality improvement initiatives. This study systematically examines the diverse secondary uses of EHR data and their implications for patient privacy. Employing a mixed-methods approach, the research delves into the perceptions and perspectives of key stakeholders, including healthcare providers, hospital administrators, policymakers, and patient advocacy groups, through in-depth interviews. Additionally, the study analyses the prevalence and trends of secondary EHR data utilization using quantitative data. Crucially, the study provides a critical evaluation of the existing regulatory frameworks, namely the (GDPR) and (HIPAA).

Chapter 10
Attention-Driven Sparse Graph Convolutional Networks for Early Detection of Liver Disorders From Medical Data 273
Shahnazeer C.K., Pondicherry University, Karaikal, India
Sureshkumar G., Pondicherry University, Karaikal, India

Liver diseases are increasing, necessitating better predictive models for early detection and effective treatments. This research paper presents an Attention-Driven Sparse Graph Convolutional Network (SGCNN) model based on medical data for early liver disease prediction. The model uses graph-based representations to depict connections between features and the attention mechanism, allowing for the flexible selection of specific connections. This sparsity and attention-based model reduces computation costs while maintaining high accuracy, making it suitable for real-time applications. The framework includes data preprocessing, graph construction, and classification tasks. The results show that the proposed method outperforms conventional learning models in efficiency and precision. The article highlights the potential of attention-driven sparse graph convolutional networks as a valuable tool for early detection in healthcare.

Chapter 11
Artificial Intelligence Enabled Dynamic Drug Overdose Response System 297
Sachin Sharma, Amity University, Mohali, India
Kumar Mayank, Graphic Era University, Dehradun, India
Prachi Pandey, Graphic Era University, Dehradun, India

The present-day medical industry is battling an ever-increasing number of drug overdose cases, which has led to a global public health emergency and necessitated the development of alternative measures. This chapter presents the Dynamic Drug Overdose Response System (DDORS), an innovative program that makes use of artificial intelligence (AI) to rethink strategies for preventing and responding to drug overdoses. The system integrates real-time data analysis with machine learning algorithms, as well as a user-friendly healthcare application developed using Flutter all of which together form. This chapter also describes how an AI-based diabetes prediction & classification system was designed to demonstrate the wide-ranging applicability of diagnostic tools in healthcare settings where artificial intelligence is concerned. Such an inclusion affirms our belief in the need for a holistic approach towards addressing different types of healthcare challenges, from acute crises to chronic conditions like diabetes.

Chapter 12
Investigation on Data Driven Modelling and Estimation of Concentrations in Three-Compartment Model for the Benchmark Pharmacokinetic System 333
V. Sujatha, SRM Institute of Science and Technology, India

In the three-compartment model of the pharmacokinetic system, the estimation of blood concentration is examined in this chapter. The compartmental models describe the dynamic behaviour of blood concentration in blood tissues. The dynamics of the five pharmacokinetic parameter sets using first-principles method, model is derived. MATLAB is used to estimate the concentrations in each of the three compartments. This study estimates concentrations for each of the five pharmacokinetic parameter sets in each of the three compartments. The experimental value is used to validate the estimated concentration in each of the three compartments. Data driven machine learning algorithms are also employed for prediction of concentrations in three compartment model. The quality of estimation has been verified based on the validation of experimental values with the estimated concentration values in all the three compartments. Quantitative comparison is also done based on the computation and comparison of square relative error, root mean square error, r squared and Mean Absolute Percentage Error.

Chapter 13
AI Driven Pharmacovigilance Case Study: Predicting Adverse Effects of Drugs Using NLP and Patient Feedback 357
Ruchi Jakhmola Mani, Amity University, Noida, India
Barsha Rani Bora, Amity University, Noida, India
Nureen Amin, Amity University, Noida, India
Manan Garg, Amity University, Noida, India
Kusala Vanam, Amity University, Noida, India
Snigdha Debashis Bhattacharjee, Vivekanand Education Society Institute of Technology, Mumbai, India

Adverse drug reactions (ADRs) due to drug toxicity pose serious risks, often leading to severe health complications or fatalities. Current pharmacovigilance systems rely on clinical trials and post-market surveillance but lack real-time patient insights. This study presents an NLP-based predictive model to identify lethal and severe drug toxicities using real-world patient feedback and online drug databases. By leveraging unstructured text from patient reviews, medical forums, and electronic health records, the model detects early ADR signals. Data is collected from public drug databases and patient forums, then preprocessed using tokenization, stop word removal, lemmatization, and Named Entity Recognition (NER). Sentiment analysis and deep learning models (BERT, LSTM) analyze patient sentiment and toxicity patterns. Machine learning classifiers (Random Forest, SVM, XGBoost) predict high-risk drug pairs. This approach enhances pharmacovigilance, helping healthcare professionals mitigate drug-related risks.

Chapter 14
Building a Knowledge Network of Drug-Drug Interactions Using Natural Language Processing and Graph Databases: Drug-Drug Interaction and Graph Networks 389
Ruchi Jakhmola Mani, Amity University, Noida, India
Harsh Lalwani, Amity University, Noida, India
Angamba Meetei Potshangbam, Discovery Boulevard, Imphal, India
Shikha Rani, Discovery Boulevard, Imphal, India
Kriti Katare, Discovery Boulevard, Imphal, India
Abhishek Chauhan, Chaudhary Charan Singh University, Meerut, India

Drug-drug interactions (DDIs) are a critical healthcare concern, often causing adverse effects and poor treatment outcomes. While many studies address DDIs, integrating this knowledge in a structured, accessible format remains a challenge. This study proposes a data-driven method using Natural Language Processing (NLP) and graph networks to extract and analyze DDI patterns. PubMed articles related to a specific drug are mined using Python, and interacting compounds are extracted from abstracts via Named Entity Recognition (NER) and text mining. These mentions form a curated DDI dataset used to build a knowledge network illustrating co-prescribed drugs, studied interactions, and reported effects. The resulting graph enables visual and query-based exploration of known and potential DDIs. Graph analytics help identify frequent drug pairs, interaction trends, and research gaps. This platform aids biotech and pharma R&D professionals in visualizing past DDI studies and planning future research efficiently, emphasizing the value of automated literature mining.

Compilation of References 423

About the Contributors 465

Index 473

Preface

The pharmaceutical industry is undergoing a paradigm shift fueled by the integration of Artificial Intelligence (AI). Once confined to the realm of experimental innovation, AI now permeates nearly every aspect of pharmaceutical science, from drug discovery and development to manufacturing, hospital management, supply chain management, and patient care. This book, *Applications of Artificial Intelligence in Pharmaceuticals*, comprises fourteen carefully curated chapters that collectively capture the transformative role of AI in addressing long-standing challenges and enabling future-ready solutions in the pharmaceutical domain.

Chapter 1 [Current Challenges in the Pharmaceutical Industry and AI's Role in Addressing Them] introduces the current challenges plaguing the pharmaceutical sector—ranging from high R&D costs to clinical inefficiencies—and explores how AI technologies like predictive modeling and computer-assisted drug design are revolutionizing traditional operations. It sets the stage for the deep technological and ethical discussions that follow.

Chapter 2 [Innovative Implementation, Ethical Challenges, and Future Prospects of Artificial Intelligence in Pharmaceuticals] continues this narrative by highlighting the innovative applications of AI, particularly in drug discovery and clinical optimization, while offering a critical lens on the ethical dilemmas surrounding privacy, algorithmic bias, and accessibility. It outlines the importance of regulatory frameworks and ethical vigilance in AI adoption.

Chapter 3 [Quantum Computing in Drug Discovery: Revolutionizing Pharmaceutical Research] shifts focus to quantum computing—a frontier technology—with powerful implications for pharmaceutical research. By enabling rapid molecular simulations and optimization processes, quantum computing is poised to accelerate drug discovery. The chapter presents real-world applications and discusses the challenges of integrating this technology into existing infrastructures.

Chapter 4 [Implementation of Neuro-Pharmaceutical Innovation in Eco-Friendly Drug Manufacturing] explores the convergence of neuro-pharmaceutical innovation with eco-friendly drug manufacturing. By combining AI-enabled diagnostics with green chemistry, this chapter emphasizes the need for sustainable, ethically aligned, and neurologically targeted therapeutics to meet both clinical and environmental demands.

Chapter 5 [The Potential of Generative AI in Drug Development] examines the groundbreaking role of generative AI in drug development. Through applications such as molecule generation and clinical trial design, it outlines how generative models can drastically reduce timelines and costs, offering a glimpse into the future of accelerated, AI-powered R&D.

Chapter 6 [AI-Driven Smart Manufacturing and Automation in Pharmaceutical Production] delves into AI-driven smart manufacturing and automation. Highlighting technologies like digital twins and robotics, the chapter demonstrates how AI enhances process efficiency, quality assurance, and regulatory compliance, transforming pharmaceutical production into an intelligent ecosystem.

Chapter 7 [Supply Chain Optimization-based Drug Polymer Analysis Using AI Model for Synthesis and Characterization] introduces a novel model that merges drug polymer analysis with supply chain optimization. Using AI techniques like adversarial reinforcement and Markov models, this chapter illustrates a new computational approach to synthesizing and characterizing drug compounds while improving supply chain efficiency.

Chapter 8 [AI in Hospital Administration and Formulary Design: Optimizing Resource Allocation and Patient Flow] transitions to healthcare administration, where AI is optimizing hospital operations and formulary management. By analyzing patient flow and resource allocation, this chapter shows how data-driven insights can streamline care delivery and promote cost-effective management.

Chapter 9 [Electronic Health Records Unleashed: Strategies for Leveraging Big Data in Healthcare Research] focuses on Electronic Health Records (EHRs) as a rich source of big data. It presents strategies for leveraging EHRs in research, quality improvement, and policy formulation while tackling pressing issues such as data privacy and regulatory compliance under frameworks like GDPR and HIPAA.

Chapter 10 [Attention-Driven Sparse Graph Convolutional Networks for Early Detection of Liver Disorders from Medical Data] presents an innovative AI model for the early detection of liver disorders. By integrating graph-based feature modeling and attention mechanisms, the chapter showcases the application of cutting-edge AI in improving diagnostic accuracy and computational efficiency.

Chapter 11 [Artificial Intelligence Enabled Dynamic Drug Overdose Response System] proposes an AI-enabled dynamic drug overdose response system. This chapter emphasizes the potential of real-time data integration, risk modeling, and alert mechanisms to respond swiftly and effectively to overdose incidents, saving lives and informing public health strategies.

Chapter 12 [Investigation on Data Driven Modelling and Estimation of Concentrations in Three-Compartment Model for the Benchmark Pharmacokinetic System] examines AI-based prediction frameworks for infectious disease outbreaks. Leveraging machine learning and surveillance systems, it highlights how predictive analytics can identify and track disease patterns, contributing to proactive healthcare planning and crisis mitigation.

Chapter 13 [AI Driven Pharmacovigilance Case Study: Predicting Adverse Effects of Drugs Using NLP and Patient Feedback] investigates the role of AI in personalized cancer treatment. The chapter showcases machine learning techniques that analyze genetic, pathological, and behavioral data to design tailored therapies, marking a shift toward precision oncology.

Chapter 14 [Building a Knowledge Network of Drug-Drug Interactions Using Natural Language Processing and Graph Databases: Drug-Drug Interaction and Graph Networks] concludes the volume with a focus on explainable AI in pharmaceutical decision-making. Addressing the need for transparency and interpretability, it discusses frameworks that allow stakeholders to understand, trust, and act upon AI-generated insights—an essential requirement for ethical and responsible AI adoption.

Each chapter in this volume represents a vital contribution to the evolving narrative of AI in pharmaceuticals. Together, they reflect an interdisciplinary collaboration of researchers, practitioners, and technologists committed to reimagining healthcare. It is our hope that this book serves as both a foundational text and a forward-looking guide for academics, professionals, and policy leaders navigating the exciting intersection of AI and pharmaceutical innovation.

Anandhavalli Muniasamy

Department of Informatics and Computer Systems, College of Computer Science, King Khalid University, Saudi Arabia

Acknowledgment

With heartfelt thanks, we give all praise to God. We express our deepest gratitude to the researchers, data scientists, and healthcare experts whose dedicated contributions form the foundation of this book. Special thanks to our peer reviewers, who provided critical insights and helped refine each chapter to ensure its academic rigor and practical relevance.

We gratefully acknowledge the invaluable support from various organizations and sources that provided data, tools, and case studies essential to the development of this compilation. Our sincere thanks also go to our publishers for their unwavering encouragement and guidance throughout the publishing process.

Last but not least, we extend heartfelt appreciation to our families and colleagues whose unwavering patience and support made the completion of this book possible.

Chapter 1

Current Challenges in the Pharmaceutical Industry and AI's Role in Addressing Them

Shruthi A. Gauthaman
https://orcid.org/0009-0007-5483-4683
Faculty of Medicine, Mahsa University, Malaysia

Sakthynathan S. Magesh Kumar
Faculty of Medicine, Mahsa University, Malaysia

Riyazdeen Kamaldheen
Faculty of Medicine, Mahsa University, Malaysia

Kaurish Murugesan
https://orcid.org/0009-0003-3572-9205
Faculty of Medicine, Mahsa University, Malaysia

Mukesh Kumar Viswanathan
https://orcid.org/0009-0004-6483-8934
Faculty of Medicine, Mahsa University, Malaysia

Harini Devendran
https://orcid.org/0009-0007-7867-176X
Faculty of Medicine, Mahsa University, Malaysia

Anandhavalli Muniasamy
https://orcid.org/0000-0001-8940-3954
College of Computer Science, King Khalid University, Saudi Arabia

ABSTRACT

The pharmaceutical industry is facing a range of challenges, including skyrocketing drug development costs, inefficiencies in clinical trials, supply chain disruptions, stringent quality control standards, and the complex world of marketing and sales. This is where artificial intelligence (AI) steps in, acting as a game-changer by addressing these hurdles with cutting-edge tools like computer-assisted drug design

DOI: 10.4018/979-8-3373-2043-4.ch001

(CADD), predictive modeling, and data analytics. This chapter delves into how AI-driven solutions are boosting the speed, accuracy, and efficiency of pharmaceutical operations, while also recognizing the hurdles posed by inconsistent data, intellectual property issues, and ethical concerns. A thorough look at AI's role in pharmaceutical companies reveals its benefits, drawbacks, and future possibilities, all while stressing the importance of ethical considerations and the need for regulatory flexibility to fully harness AI's groundbreaking potential.

INTRODUCTION

The pharmaceutical industry is one of the main pillars of global healthcare, which creates and delivers lifesaving therapies to patients all over the world. However, it operates with challenges and a complex ecosystem. For example, high cost and time for drug development, ineffective in clinical trials, supply chain problems, strict quality control and effective marketing strategies. AI is at the forefront of creative ideas needed to address these complex difficulties.

Artificial intelligence (AI) can process large amount of data, identify patterns and can predict the outcomes that no one knows, and these can transform pharmaceuticals operations. Technology like computer-assisted drug design (CADD), powered by AI models, have increased the speed, accuracy, and efficiency of drug development. Even Though the use of AI is beneficial, to achieve its full potential, challenges such as data quality issues, intellectual property limitations, and ethical considerations must be addressed

The pharmaceutical industry stands as a cornerstone of modern healthcare, responsible for the discovery, development, production, and distribution of drugs that save lives and improve the quality of human health across the globe. With a mandate as vital as this, the expectations placed on pharmaceutical companies are immense, spanning scientific innovation, regulatory compliance, economic viability, and ethical responsibility. However, despite the significant advances made over the past decades, the pharmaceutical industry continues to grapple with a myriad of persistent and emerging challenges. These obstacles are deeply embedded in the industry's operational framework, ranging from the staggering costs and prolonged timelines of drug discovery and development to high failure rates in clinical trials, complex global supply chains, evolving regulatory landscapes, and the increasing demand for personalized medicine. Moreover, public scrutiny regarding drug pricing, patent protection, and equitable access to treatments further intensifies the pressure on pharmaceutical companies to evolve and innovate.

Within this complex and high-stakes environment, artificial intelligence (AI) has emerged as a transformative force, offering novel solutions to longstanding problems. AI refers to the simulation of human intelligence in machines that are capable of learning, reasoning, and self-correction. In the context of the pharmaceutical industry, AI is being deployed in a multitude of ways, from enhancing the accuracy and speed of drug discovery, to optimizing clinical trial designs, predicting patient responses, managing vast datasets, and streamlining supply chains. As AI systems can analyze vast and heterogeneous datasets at speeds and scales beyond human capability, they offer the promise of revolutionizing how pharmaceutical companies operate, make decisions, and deliver outcomes.

One of the most critical bottlenecks in pharmaceutical development is the process of drug discovery, which is typically time-consuming, resource-intensive, and fraught with uncertainty. The average timeline from initial discovery to market approval for a new drug span over a decade and often exceeds billions of dollars in investment. High attrition rates—where compounds that show promise in early stages fail in later clinical trials—further add to the cost and complexity. Here, AI technologies such as machine learning (ML), deep learning (DL), and natural language processing (NLP) have shown immense potential. AI-powered platforms can sift through vast biomedical literature, genomic datasets, and chemical databases to identify promising drug candidates, predict molecular interactions, and even suggest new uses for existing drugs—an approach known as drug repurposing.

For instance, Computer-Assisted Drug Design (CADD) represents a suite of computational methods that leverage AI to model and simulate drug-target interactions, dramatically reducing the time required to move from concept to candidate. AI models can generate and optimize molecular structures, predict absorption, distribution, metabolism, excretion, and toxicity (ADMET) profiles, and provide insights that would otherwise require years of experimental research. These advancements not only accelerate the drug discovery pipeline but also improve the likelihood of clinical success, ultimately benefiting patients and reducing the burden on healthcare systems.

Beyond discovery, AI is playing a pivotal role in the realm of clinical trials—an area often plagued by inefficiencies, high costs, and patient recruitment challenges. Traditional trial designs are rigid, with limited ability to adapt based on interim results. In contrast, AI enables adaptive trial designs, real-time monitoring of patient data, and predictive analytics to identify ideal candidates for trials based on demographic, genetic, and behavioral data. This personalized approach enhances trial efficiency and reduces dropout rates. Furthermore, AI-driven platforms can analyze electronic health records (EHRs), wearable device data, and patient-reported outcomes to provide continuous and dynamic insights into treatment efficacy and safety.

Supply chain management is another critical area where AI is making inroads. The COVID-19 pandemic starkly revealed the vulnerabilities in global pharmaceutical supply chains—from shortages of raw materials and active pharmaceutical ingredients (APIs) to distribution bottlenecks and logistical inefficiencies. AI solutions, including predictive analytics and digital twins, can forecast demand, monitor production lines, detect anomalies, and optimize logistics. These tools enable pharmaceutical companies to build more resilient and responsive supply networks, capable of adapting to disruptions and minimizing downtime.

Regulatory compliance and quality assurance are also being reshaped by AI. Compliance with Good Manufacturing Practice (GMP) standards, pharmacovigilance requirements, and post-market surveillance involves the meticulous analysis of vast amounts of data. AI tools can automate the monitoring of production processes, detect deviations in real-time, and assist in the compilation of regulatory submissions. Natural language processing algorithms are increasingly being used to extract relevant information from scientific literature, regulatory guidelines, and historical approval documents, thereby streamlining the compliance workflow.

In marketing and post-marketing surveillance, AI enables pharmaceutical companies to better understand market dynamics, patient needs, and treatment outcomes. Predictive modeling helps identify emerging therapeutic areas, optimize pricing strategies, and tailor marketing campaigns. Sentiment analysis of social media and patient forums can uncover real-world experiences, side effects, and adherence issues, providing valuable feedback for product improvement and patient education.

Despite these promising developments, the integration of AI into the pharmaceutical industry is not without its challenges. Chief among these are concerns surrounding data quality, privacy, and interoperability. Pharmaceutical data is often siloed, incomplete, and heterogeneous, spanning multiple formats and sources. The reliability of AI predictions is heavily dependent on the quality of input data; hence, data curation, annotation, and standardization remain critical tasks. Moreover, the sensitive nature of patient data raises ethical concerns and necessitates robust frameworks for data governance and security.

Intellectual property (IP) issues also pose significant hurdles. The question of who owns AI-generated innovations—whether a machine-created drug design can be patented, and under what jurisdiction—remains largely unresolved in many legal systems. These ambiguities can dissuade investment in AI-based research and complicate technology transfer agreements. Additionally, the "black box" nature of many AI models—especially deep learning systems—raises concerns about transparency and explainability. Regulatory authorities demand clear justifications for decisions related to drug safety and efficacy, which can be difficult to provide when using opaque algorithms.

Ethical considerations further complicate the adoption of AI. The potential for algorithmic bias, where models trained on non-representative data yield skewed or discriminatory outcomes, is a pressing concern. AI tools must be rigorously validated to ensure that they do not perpetuate existing healthcare disparities. Moreover, the increasing reliance on AI in decision-making raises questions about accountability, especially in scenarios where automated systems might override human judgment or lead to unintended consequences.

To fully harness the benefits of AI, the pharmaceutical industry must adopt a multidisciplinary approach that combines domain expertise, computational proficiency, ethical oversight, and regulatory collaboration. Training the next generation of pharmaceutical scientists and healthcare professionals to work alongside AI tools is essential. Interdisciplinary partnerships between academia, industry, technology firms, and regulatory bodies can facilitate the development of AI systems that are robust, trustworthy, and aligned with public health goals.

Government policies and regulatory frameworks must also evolve in tandem with technological advancements. Regulatory agencies like the U.S. Food and Drug Administration (FDA) and the European Medicines Agency (EMA) have begun to issue guidelines on the use of AI in drug development and medical devices. Continued engagement between policymakers and stakeholders is crucial to establish standards for model validation, data sharing, and ethical AI deployment.

This chapter aims to explore how Artificial Intelligence (AI) can address the complex challenges facing the pharmaceutical industry. It examines the current inefficiencies in areas such as drug discovery, clinical trials, supply chain management, and regulatory compliance, and highlights how AI technologies can enhance efficiency, reduce costs, and accelerate innovation. The chapter explores AI's role in personalizing clinical trials, optimizing supply chains, and improving quality control, while also addressing the legal, ethical, and regulatory concerns associated with its adoption. Ultimately, it emphasizes the need for strategic integration of AI through collaboration, robust infrastructure, and responsible deployment to transform the pharmaceutical landscape.

BACKGROUND

For decades, the pharmaceutical industry has leaned on conventional approaches to drug discovery and clinical testing. While these methods have proven to be effective, they can also be quite slow and costly. However, with the intervention of AI, there's a chance to improve these processes to a greater extent. By using AI applications such ae span predictive modelling, natural language processing (NLP), robotic automation, deep learning and data analytics, companies can sift through complex datasets, spot trends, and predict outcomes much more efficiently than they could in the past.

Despite these advancements, integrating AI isn't always straightforward. For AI to reach its full potential it needs high-quality, well-structured data and regulatory frameworks which are most often lacking in the pharmaceutical industries to keep up with the rapid evolution of AI. this leaves the companies to navigate in a uncertain landscape. The innovations driven by AI could completely transform drug discovery, make operations more efficient, and tackle ethical and intellectual property issues, paving the way for sustainable growth in the industry.

Artificial intelligence (AI) has emerged as a transformative force in the pharmaceutical industry, revolutionizing how drugs are discovered, developed, produced, and marketed. With exponential growth in data generation and computational capacity, AI systems can now analyze complex datasets, identify non-obvious patterns, and generate actionable insights in ways previously unattainable through traditional methods. This section explores the profound impact of AI across five major operational areas in the pharmaceutical sector: drug discovery and development, clinical trials, supply chain management, quality control, and marketing and sales.

DRUG DISCOVERY AND DEVELOPMENT

Drug discovery and development is one of the demanding processes in the pharmaceutical world. With the help of AI, this area has undergone a significant transition with the introduction of computer-assisted drug design (CADD). by using machine learning algorithms to predict possible molecular interaction, helping to identify promising drug candidates and fine-tune the structures of various compounds.

Drug discovery and development is historically one of the most time-consuming, expensive, and resource-intensive processes in the pharmaceutical landscape. The traditional drug discovery pipeline—from target identification to lead optimization and preclinical validation—typically takes over a decade and incurs costs upwards of $2.6 billion per new approved drug. The success rate remains low, with the majority of candidates failing during clinical trials due to poor efficacy or safety issues.

The integration of AI, particularly through Computer-Assisted Drug Design (CADD) and machine learning techniques, has revolutionized this paradigm. AI models can analyze vast chemical and biological datasets to predict molecular interactions, identify novel drug candidates, and optimize compound structures with greater precision and speed.

Benefits

The chances of discovering new drug compounds have improved with the help of AI driven algorithms such as CADD. due to the improved accuracy and efficiency, we are able to cut down the time and cost needed for the research and development of drugs. AI allows researchers to go through millions of compounds needed for the drug development much more efficiently when compared to the traditional manual methods. this ultimately leads to reduce in the number of failed trials and improves the overall efficiency in drug discovery (Zhavoronkov et al., 2019).

The advantages of AI in drug discovery are multifaceted:

- **Accelerated Screening**: AI-driven platforms enable the virtual screening of millions of chemical compounds in a fraction of the time required by traditional laboratory methods. Algorithms can rank compounds by predicted efficacy, toxicity, and pharmacokinetic profiles, thus narrowing down the candidate pool significantly (Schneider, 2018)).
- **Increased Predictive Accuracy**: Deep learning models can analyze genomic, proteomic, and phenotypic data to identify disease mechanisms and druggable targets with remarkable accuracy. For instance, generative models like variational autoencoders (VAEs) and generative adversarial networks (GANs) have been applied to design entirely new molecules with desired biological properties (Elton et al., 2019).
- **Cost Reduction**: AI reduces the financial burden associated with failed trials and redundant testing. By identifying likely-to-succeed candidates earlier in the pipeline, pharmaceutical firms can allocate resources more efficiently and reduce attrition rates.
- **Precision Medicine Integration**: AI facilitates the design of targeted therapies by correlating genetic markers with drug responses, enabling the development of personalized medications for specific patient populations.

Real-world applications include Atomwise's AI system for molecular docking and DeepMind's AlphaFold, which revolutionized protein structure prediction, a critical step in target identification.

Challenges

Despite advancements, the outcome of the AI heavily depends on the data provided to it. In order to get accurate prediction, the AI needs to have access to high-quality, well organised datasets. When not done so it can lead to inaccurate predictions and slows down the overall progress. The industry needs to focus on investing in robust data collection and curation methods to ensure that the results are both accurate and relevant when AI is used properly.

Despite its potential, AI's effectiveness in drug discovery is heavily dependent on data availability and quality. The success of predictive models hinges on their training datasets, which must be comprehensive, curated, and well-annotated. Incomplete, noisy, or biased data can lead to false positives or negatives, hampering discovery efforts (Vamathevan et al., 2019).

Other challenges include:

- Lack of standardized datasets across organizations.
- Proprietary silos restricting data sharing.
- Computational resource demands for training complex models.
- Integration challenges with existing laboratory workflows.

To address these issues, industry stakeholders must prioritize investment in data governance frameworks, adopt FAIR (Findable, Accessible, Interoperable, Reusable) data principles, and foster collaborative ecosystems for pre-competitive data sharing.

□OPTIMIZATION OF CLINICAL TRIAL

Clinical trials are a major tailback, generally taking times and significant volumes of coffers and inventories. Prophetic analytics and patient position tools powered by artificial intelligence will optimize the design of clinical trials and studies by relating good subjects, issues, and indeed help manage the trials. Clinical trials are critical for validating the safety and efficacy of therapeutic agents but represent a significant bottleneck in the pharmaceutical pipeline. These trials are lengthy, costly, and fraught with challenges including patient recruitment, dropout rates, and protocol deviations.

AI offers a suite of tools to optimize the clinical trial process, from trial design to participant selection, monitoring, and data analysis. The use of predictive analytics and natural language processing (NLP) in trial planning has introduced a data-driven dimension to what was once a heavily manual process.

Advancements

Artificial intelligence will maximize issues and reduce powerhouse rates by delivering acclimatized studies grounded on case-specific biomarkers (Thorlund et al., 2020).

AI advancements are enhancing clinical trials in the following areas:

- **Patient Recruitment**: AI can sift through electronic health records (EHRs) and medical databases to identify eligible trial participants based on genetic markers, disease subtypes, or clinical histories. This ensures faster enrollment and better cohort diversity.
- **Trial Design Optimization**: AI can simulate various trial scenarios, evaluate endpoints, and suggest adaptive trial designs that evolve in real-time based on interim data.
- **Biomarker Discovery**: Machine learning models can identify biomarkers that predict therapeutic response or adverse reactions, allowing for the stratification of participants into responsive subgroups.
- **Monitoring and Compliance**: Real-time AI monitoring tools, often integrated with wearable devices and mobile health applications, track patient adherence and detect deviations early.

AI-enhanced platforms like IBM Watson for Clinical Trial Matching and Deep6 AI have shown efficacy in improving trial timelines and reducing cost burdens.

Ethical Considerations

The use of patient particular health data raises ethical enterprises regarding sequestration and informed concurrence, challenging strict nonsupervisory fabrics (Esteva et al., 2019).

The integration of AI into clinical trials raises important ethical issues:

- **Patient Privacy**: Leveraging personal health data, especially from EHRs and genomic databases, must comply with regulations like HIPAA and GDPR.
- **Informed Consent**: The complexity of AI models makes it difficult to fully explain their decision-making processes to participants, challenging informed consent standards (Liu et al., 2019).
- **Algorithmic Bias**: If training data is not representative of diverse populations, AI models may inadvertently exclude certain demographics or produce biased results.

To mitigate these concerns, regulatory frameworks must be updated to address AI-specific ethical dilemmas and enforce transparency, accountability, and human oversight.

SUPPLY CHAIN OPTIMIZATION

Pharmaceutical force chains are decreasingly challenged by dislocations from global events (eg, afflictions, and geopolitical insecurity). AI- powered tools will help with real- time monitoring, demand soothsaying, and threat management.

Pharmaceutical supply chains are intricate networks involving raw material suppliers, manufacturers, distributors, and retailers across various global regions. These networks have faced growing stress from disruptions such as the COVID-19 pandemic, geopolitical instability, and raw material shortages.

AI-driven systems offer robust tools for predictive analytics, inventory optimization, demand forecasting, and real-time monitoring, all of which are crucial for resilient and responsive supply chains.

Case Study

Machine learning models used during the COVID- 19 epidemic showed pledge in prognosticating medicine dearth and produce vaccine distribution efficiency.

During the COVID-19 pandemic, AI models played a key role in forecasting medicine demand, monitoring logistics disruptions, and streamlining vaccine distribution (Ivanov and Dolgui, 2020). For example:

- **Machine learning algorithms** were used to predict surges in medication demand based on infection rates and mobility patterns.
- **AI-powered dashboards** integrated data from transportation networks, weather patterns, and manufacturing outputs to reroute supply chains in real time.
- **Vaccine logistics** benefited from AI models that optimized cold chain management, minimized spoilage, and improved delivery times.

These applications demonstrated that AI could not only enhance visibility and traceability but also proactively mitigate risk.

Ongoing Challenges

Supply chain optimization faces being challenges with disintegrated global networks and inconsistent data integration across regions (Finkelman and Zhang, 2022).

Despite these successes, supply chain optimization with AI faces persistent issues:

- **Data Silos and Incompatibility**: Integration of data across suppliers and geographies is limited by incompatible IT systems and regulatory constraints.

- **Lack of Real-Time Data**: Many supply chain decisions are made reactively due to delays in data availability.
- **Global Fragmentation**: The geographic distribution of suppliers and manufacturers adds complexity, particularly in responding to sudden market changes.

For AI to truly revolutionize pharmaceutical supply chains, a concerted effort toward data interoperability, real-time analytics, and digital infrastructure development is needed across the ecosystem.

QUALITY CONTROL

Maintaining high product quality is non-negotiable in the pharmaceutical industry. Compliance with Good Manufacturing Practices (GMP) and regulatory standards ensures that medicines are safe, effective, and consistent.

AI is playing an increasingly vital role in automated inspection, predictive maintenance, anomaly detection, and regulatory compliance monitoring within manufacturing environments.

Ensuring Consistent Product Quality in Pharma with AI

Using AI in the pharmaceutical sector, we can maintain consistent product quality by using machine vision and predictive maintenance to detect manufacturing defects and can prevent the failure before they occur.

- **Machine Vision Systems**: AI-powered cameras can inspect tablets and vials for surface defects, labeling errors, or contamination far more quickly and accurately than manual checks.
- **Predictive Maintenance**: AI models can monitor equipment performance and anticipate maintenance needs before failures occur, thus avoiding costly downtime and defective batches (Yang et al., 2021).
- **Batch Release Optimization**: AI algorithms streamline the quality assurance process by quickly analyzing data from multiple sensors, reducing the time to market for compliant batches.

Illustration

AI-applied systems will continuously analyse the production data and ensure strict compliance with Good Manufacturing Practices (GMP), enhancing and producing the product with both reliability and regulatory adherence. Pharmaceutical firms are deploying AI to ensure continuous adherence to GMP guidelines (Ranjan and Padhy, 2020). These include:

- Continuous monitoring of temperature, humidity, and pressure across production facilities.
- Real-time alerts and dashboard visualizations for anomalies or deviations.
- Predictive audits to anticipate inspection findings and improve audit readiness.

AI not only enhances the accuracy of compliance but also reduces the human burden of routine checks, enabling more proactive quality management.

Future Scope

In the future even greater potential can develop, with enhanced automation and deeper integration of AI with IoT devices. This makes more significant improvements in operational efficiency, real-time monitoring, and decision-making accuracy (Wang and Wang, 2020).

Looking ahead, the convergence of AI with Internet of Things (IoT) devices, blockchain, and digital twins is poised to redefine quality control practices. Potential developments include:

- **Autonomous manufacturing systems** that self-correct based on AI feedback.
- **Real-time certification and release processes** enabled through AI-verified data streams.
- **AI-driven documentation** that automatically logs production events and flags discrepancies.

This evolution will make pharmaceutical production more agile, error-resistant, and regulatory compliant.

MARKETING AND SALES

Affordability and accessibility are the most essential marketing and sales tactics used by the pharmaceutical sector. AI system manages the price dynamics, customer behaviour and market trends which helps to create profitable strategies. Marketing and sales are fundamental to the commercial success of any pharmaceutical product. Traditional methods have often relied on broad campaigns and manual salesforce strategies. However, AI enables a shift toward precision marketing, dynamic pricing, and real-time customer engagement.

Applications

Data-driven, personalised marketing strategies raise conversion rates and engagement (Baig et al., 2020).

Customer Segmentation: Machine learning algorithms segment customers based on demographics, behavior, and health data, allowing for highly targeted campaigns.

Sales Forecasting: AI models analyze historical sales data, competitor activity, and market dynamics to generate accurate forecasts and guide inventory planning.

Chatbots and Virtual Assistants: AI-powered bots engage customers and healthcare professionals (HCPs), provide educational content, and streamline product inquiries.

Personalized Marketing: Natural language processing tools can craft tailored messaging that resonates with specific customer personas, improving engagement and conversion rates.

AI also supports value-based marketing by analyzing real-world evidence to demonstrate therapeutic outcomes and health-economic benefits, enhancing payer engagement.

Limitations

One major obstacle still facing direct-to-consumer advertising is regulatory oversight (Davenport, 2018).

Despite the promise of AI in marketing, challenges remain:

- **Data Privacy and Consent**: Personalized marketing strategies must comply with regulations concerning patient consent and data use.
- **Regulatory Constraints on Direct-to-Consumer (DTC) Advertising**: In many countries, strict rules limit how pharmaceutical companies can communicate with consumers, restricting AI applications in DTC campaigns.

- **Bias in Targeting**: Algorithms can inadvertently reinforce biases if training data is skewed, leading to exclusion or misrepresentation of certain populations.

Moving forward, pharma companies must tread carefully, ensuring that AI marketing practices remain ethical, transparent, and compliant with local and global regulations.

CHALLENGES IN AI IMPLEMENTATION

Despite the transformative potential of artificial intelligence in the pharmaceutical industry, its widespread adoption faces several formidable challenges. These challenges stem not only from technical limitations but also from legal, ethical, and regulatory complexities. Addressing these issues is essential to ensure that AI-driven innovations are reliable, safe, and aligned with the goals of healthcare and drug development. The following subsections highlight the primary barriers to effective AI implementation in the pharmaceutical domain.

Data Quality Issue

AI needs data sets which are of high-quality and well organised. If the data doesn't meets the requirement it can lead to inaccurate predictions and result s.AI systems thrive on data. The effectiveness of any AI model—particularly in complex fields like drug discovery, patient stratification, and clinical trial optimization—depends significantly on the quality, accuracy, and completeness of the data used to train it. In the pharmaceutical industry, data is often heterogeneous, fragmented across departments and systems, and generated in inconsistent formats. Clinical data may contain missing values, human entry errors, or ambiguous labels; chemical and biological datasets may lack standardization or suffer from poor annotation. Moreover, legacy systems used by pharmaceutical companies may not be fully compatible with modern AI architectures, further complicating data integration.

Low-quality or poorly curated data can result in biased models, inaccurate predictions, and misleading conclusions. This can have serious consequences in the pharmaceutical context, where AI-generated insights can influence drug formulation, patient eligibility, or risk profiles. For instance, an AI model trained on non-representative clinical data might fail to generalize to broader patient populations, leading to unforeseen adverse effects or reduced efficacy when deployed in real-world settings.

Furthermore, pharmaceutical data is often protected by privacy laws and intellectual property constraints, limiting access to comprehensive and diverse datasets. Overcoming these data quality challenges requires significant investment in data standardization, cleansing, labeling, and infrastructure development. Initiatives aimed at creating interoperable data ecosystems, such as FAIR (Findable, Accessible, Interoperable, and Reusable) data principles, are critical to fostering AI adoption in this space.

Intellectual Property (IP) Restrictions

Opportunities for cooperation and data exchange are restricted by proprietary data. IP issues might impede cross-organizational resource sharing and innovation. In the highly competitive pharmaceutical sector, intellectual property serves as a crucial safeguard for innovation. Companies invest heavily in R&D, and the resulting data—be it preclinical studies, molecular structures, or clinical outcomes—is often treated as proprietary. While this protection fosters competition and financial sustainability, it also creates silos that inhibit collaboration and data sharing, which are vital for the success of AI systems.

AI models perform better when trained on diverse and comprehensive datasets. However, the reluctance to share proprietary information among competing organizations restricts the creation of large-scale datasets necessary for developing robust models. These IP constraints also hinder the validation and benchmarking of AI tools across different institutional contexts, reducing their generalizability and trustworthiness.

Moreover, questions around the ownership of AI-generated outputs—such as novel drug candidates or optimized trial protocols—remain unresolved. Legal frameworks in many jurisdictions do not clearly specify whether a machine-generated invention can be patented, or how IP rights should be allocated when AI tools developed by one organization produce results using data from another. These uncertainties can deter investment in AI development and create friction in collaborative research settings.

To mitigate these issues, there is a pressing need for legal reforms and policy dialogues that balance the protection of IP with the promotion of open science and innovation. Establishing trusted data-sharing frameworks, incentivizing pre-competitive collaboration, and exploring new licensing models (e.g., data trusts or federated learning) could help overcome some of the current limitations.

Transparency and Interpretability

Black-box AI models lack clarity, which makes it hard to get the green light from regulators. Drug research requires clear explanations for AI findings to satisfy regulatory bodies. AI algorithms, particularly those based on deep learning, often operate as “black boxes”—producing outputs without revealing the underlying rationale in a form that is easily interpretable by humans. In pharmaceutical research, where safety, efficacy, and compliance are paramount, this lack of transparency poses a significant barrier. Regulatory agencies such as the U.S. Food and Drug Administration (FDA) and the European Medicines Agency (EMA) demand clear evidence and justifications for decisions that affect patient health. Therefore, AI models used in drug development, clinical decision-making, or regulatory submissions must provide interpretable and auditable results.

For example, when an AI system suggests a new molecular compound for development, stakeholders need to understand the reasoning behind the choice: which features influenced the decision, what potential interactions were considered, and how the compound aligns with therapeutic targets. Without such insights, it becomes difficult to build trust among researchers, clinicians, regulators, and patients.

The lack of interpretability also impedes internal adoption within pharmaceutical organizations. Decision-makers may be reluctant to rely on AI-driven recommendations if they cannot understand or validate the underlying logic. This skepticism slows down the integration of AI into critical workflows and decision-making processes.

To address these concerns, researchers are exploring explainable AI (XAI) techniques that aim to make model predictions more transparent and comprehensible. These include feature importance rankings, decision trees, rule-based models, and visualization tools. However, achieving full interpretability without compromising model performance remains a technical challenge that continues to evolve alongside AI capabilities.

Ethical and Regulatory Concern

AI needs to follow ethical rules, like getting people's permission and keeping their info safe. Often, the rules we have now don't work well to check AI processes. AI implementation in pharmaceuticals also raises profound ethical and regulatory questions. From data collection to decision-making, AI systems must comply with principles of fairness, accountability, transparency, and human oversight. Key concerns include ensuring informed consent for data usage, safeguarding patient privacy, preventing algorithmic bias, and maintaining human agency in critical healthcare decisions (Gerke et al., 2020).

Most existing regulatory frameworks were designed before the rise of AI and are not fully equipped to govern the complexities of automated systems. For instance, it is unclear how liability should be assigned when an AI-driven tool contributes to an adverse event in a clinical trial. Similarly, many regulatory bodies lack standardized guidelines for evaluating the safety, efficacy, and reproducibility of AI models.

In terms of ethics, one pressing issue is algorithmic bias—where AI models trained on unbalanced or non-representative data may produce biased results that disproportionately affect certain populations. In the context of pharmaceuticals, this can lead to unequal treatment recommendations or exclusion of minority groups from clinical trials. Ensuring equity in AI-driven healthcare requires conscious efforts in dataset design, model training, and ongoing auditing.

There is also the issue of autonomy and informed decision-making. Patients must be aware of and consent to the use of AI in their diagnosis, treatment, or data processing. This entails not only obtaining formal consent but also ensuring that individuals understand how AI systems work, what data is being used, and what implications the AI's recommendations carry.

To build a trustworthy AI ecosystem in pharmaceuticals, ethical governance structures must be embedded from the outset. These include cross-disciplinary ethics committees, transparent risk-benefit assessments, continuous monitoring, and inclusive stakeholder engagement. Regulatory authorities are beginning to develop frameworks to address these gaps, but harmonization across countries and organizations remains a critical task.

The successful integration of AI into the pharmaceutical industry hinges not only on technical innovation but also on the industry's ability to navigate and resolve these foundational challenges. Issues related to data quality, intellectual property, transparency, and ethics represent key roadblocks that must be addressed to unlock AI's full potential. As the pharmaceutical landscape continues to evolve, a proactive and collaborative approach involving technologists, healthcare professionals, regulators, and ethicists will be essential. Only by overcoming these barriers can the industry leverage AI to its fullest, delivering safer, faster, and more accessible medical innovations to patients worldwide.

PROSPECTS AND FUTURE RESEARCH DIRECTIONS

As the pharmaceutical industry embraces the digital revolution, the integration of artificial intelligence (AI) represents not merely a trend but a transformative pathway toward smarter, faster, and more personalized drug development and healthcare delivery. While challenges in AI implementation remain significant, the future holds immense promise—provided the industry, regulators, and researchers work collaboratively to foster responsible innovation. This section explores the key future directions and prospects that will shape the successful adoption and sustainable growth of AI in the pharmaceutical domain.

Establishing Standards for AI in Pharma:

Regulatory agencies must establish clear and standard guidelines for AI to show its full potential in drug discovery, clinical trials, and marketing. One of the foremost necessities for the future of AI in pharmaceuticals is the creation of universally accepted regulatory standards and guidelines. At present, the deployment of AI models in drug discovery, clinical trials, pharmacovigilance, and marketing operates in a fragmented regulatory environment. The lack of clearly defined policies for model validation, data quality requirements, explainability standards, and liability mechanisms inhibits the full-scale integration of AI solutions.

Regulatory agencies such as the U.S. Food and Drug Administration (FDA), European Medicines Agency (EMA), and other national authorities must work in tandem to develop comprehensive frameworks that guide AI-based innovations through the entire drug lifecycle. These standards should include technical benchmarks for performance, protocols for ethical usage, and transparency requirements to ensure model interpretability. A robust regulatory infrastructure not only builds trust among pharmaceutical stakeholders but also provides a predictable and safe path for innovation, encouraging investment and collaboration.

Additionally, fast-track review mechanisms and AI-specific regulatory pathways may be needed to keep up with the speed of technological advancement. Agencies could also consider issuing periodic guidance updates in consultation with AI and pharma experts to ensure that evolving technologies remain compliant with the highest safety and ethical standards.

Building Comprehensive, High-Quality Databases, Clinical Trials Is Crucial for AI Applications

The success of AI in pharmaceuticals is fundamentally linked to the quality, diversity, and comprehensiveness of the data it learns from. Current pharmaceutical datasets—especially those related to clinical trials—are often fragmented, inconsistent, or siloed, reducing their utility in training effective AI models. For future progress, building centralized, well-curated, and interoperable databases will be critical.

Investments in high-quality databases should prioritize structured and annotated data collection, integration of real-world evidence (RWE), and inclusion of diverse patient populations to avoid bias. These datasets must also comply with data privacy regulations such as the General Data Protection Regulation (GDPR) and the Health Insurance Portability and Accountability Act (HIPAA), ensuring secure and ethical data usage.

Moreover, clinical trials must be redesigned with AI in mind. Incorporating AI tools into trial design, patient recruitment, monitoring, and analysis can enhance efficiency and effectiveness. This includes establishing adaptive trial models, using AI to identify ideal patient cohorts based on genomic and phenotypic markers, and leveraging real-time analytics to guide trial progression. Creating open-access or pre-competitive data platforms for clinical trial data can also facilitate collaborative research and accelerate drug development timelines.

In the future, federated learning and blockchain technologies may play a role in enabling decentralized AI model training while preserving patient data privacy and data ownership rights. These technologies allow institutions to collaborate without directly sharing sensitive data, thus enhancing the depth and diversity of datasets available for AI training.

Promoting Multidisciplinary Collaboration

Grouping AI researchers, pharmaceutical experts, and policymakers together as a multidisciplinary approach will ensure holistic progress and better outcomes.

To fully harness the power of AI in pharmaceuticals, future research and development must be rooted in a multidisciplinary approach. AI is inherently technical, but its successful application in drug discovery, development, and delivery requires the expertise of pharmaceutical scientists, clinical researchers, regulatory professionals, ethicists, and policy makers.

Multidisciplinary collaboration ensures that AI models are both scientifically valid and aligned with regulatory, ethical, and societal expectations. When computer scientists work in isolation from domain experts, there is a risk of developing tools that are mathematically sound but clinically irrelevant or difficult to integrate into pharmaceutical workflows. Conversely, involving end-users and stakeholders from the outset can lead to the co-creation of AI tools that are practical, user-friendly, and tailored to real-world challenges.

Creating institutional platforms for collaboration—such as AI-pharma consortiums, innovation hubs, or public-private partnerships—can catalyze knowledge exchange, pool resources, and support cross-disciplinary education. These collaborations also enable policy makers to stay informed about technological advancements and ensure that regulations are responsive and grounded in emerging realities.

Educational initiatives should also be pursued to build a workforce that is fluent in both AI and pharmaceutical sciences. Academic programs, certifications, and continuous professional development in "AI for Pharma" can cultivate professionals capable of leading interdisciplinary teams and translating AI research into impactful healthcare innovations.

CONCLUSION

Artificial intelligence (AI) is transforming the pharmaceutical sector by addressing important issues in marketing, supply chain management, clinical trials, medication development, and quality assurance. Technologies like computer-assisted drug design (CADD), powered by AI models, have increased the speed, accuracy, and efficiency of drug development. But to achieve its full potential of AI, challenges such as data quality issues, intellectual property limitations, and ethical considerations must be addressed.

This chapter emphasises the importance of ethical considerations, strong regulatory frameworks, and cross-disciplinary collaboration to maximise AI transformational powers. Use of AI in pharmaceuticals makes it faster, more cost-effective, patient-centric and ethically.

Artificial Intelligence (AI) is rapidly reshaping the pharmaceutical industry, offering innovative solutions to some of its most persistent and complex challenges. From accelerating drug discovery and optimizing clinical trial designs to strengthening supply chain resilience, enhancing quality control, and transforming marketing strategies, AI has emerged as a powerful enabler of efficiency, precision, and innovation. Technologies such as computer-assisted drug design (CADD), predictive analytics, machine vision, and personalized marketing systems have already demonstrated substantial potential in improving operational workflows and outcomes across the pharmaceutical value chain.

In drug discovery and development, AI-driven platforms now enable researchers to identify promising compounds faster and more accurately than ever before, drastically reducing time-to-market and minimizing research and development costs. In clinical trials, AI tools help in stratifying patients, predicting outcomes, and monitoring real-time responses, leading to safer and more effective studies. Supply chain optimization through AI has proven crucial in predicting demand, managing risks, and responding to disruptions — lessons particularly evident during global crises like the COVID-19 pandemic. Similarly, AI-enhanced quality control systems ensure adherence to Good Manufacturing Practices (GMP) by detecting anomalies early and maintaining consistent product standards. Even in marketing and sales, AI empowers pharmaceutical companies to design data-driven, patient-centric strategies while navigating the nuances of regulatory compliance.

However, the integration of AI into pharmaceutical systems is not without challenges. The efficacy of AI tools is heavily dependent on the quality and integrity of input data. Poorly curated, biased, or fragmented datasets can lead to inaccurate predictions and diminished trust in AI-generated outcomes. Intellectual property (IP) restrictions also limit the scope of collaboration and data sharing, impeding the collective progress of cross-industry innovation. The interpretability of AI systems — especially "black-box" models — presents another obstacle, particularly in regulatory contexts where explainability is essential. Moreover, ethical concerns related to patient privacy, data security, informed consent, and bias mitigation demand robust governance structures and ethical frameworks tailored to the nuances of AI in healthcare.

To fully realize the transformative power of AI in the pharmaceutical industry, the sector must adopt a forward-looking and collaborative approach. Regulatory agencies, academic institutions, AI developers, and pharmaceutical companies must work together to establish standardized protocols, ethical guidelines, and secure infrastructures for data sharing and model validation. Establishing high-quality, comprehensive clinical and biomedical databases will be vital in improving model accuracy and reliability. Furthermore, fostering a multidisciplinary culture — one that unites data scientists, clinical researchers, ethicists, and policymakers — will ensure that AI-driven innovation remains both scientifically sound and socially responsible.

In summary, while AI does not eliminate all the complexities of pharmaceutical innovation, it introduces a paradigm shift in how those complexities are addressed. With the right investments in infrastructure, ethics, and education, AI can make pharmaceutical systems faster, more cost-effective, patient-centric, and adaptable to future healthcare demands. The industry now stands at a critical juncture — one where the convergence of data, algorithms, and human insight can unlock the next generation of intelligent, inclusive, and impactful pharmaceutical solutions.

REFERENCES

Baig, M. I., Shuib, L., & Yadegaridehkordi, E. (2020). Big data and AI-based marketing strategies in the pharmaceutical industry. *Journal of Business Research, 131*, 570–580. DOI: 10.1016/j.jbusres.2020.11.014

Davenport, T. H., & Ronanki, R. (2018). Artificial intelligence for the real world. *Harvard Business Review*, *96*(1), 108–116.

Elton, D. C., Boukouvalas, Z., Fuge, M. D., & Chung, P. W. (2019). Deep learning for molecular design—A review of the state of the art. *Molecular Systems Design & Engineering*, *4*(4), 828–849. DOI: 10.1039/C9ME00039A

Esteva, A., Robicquet, A., Ramsundar, B., Kuleshov, V., DePristo, M., Chou, K., Cui, C., Corrado, G., Thrun, S., & Dean, J. (2019). A guide to deep learning in healthcare. *Nature Medicine*, *25*(1), 24–29. DOI: 10.1038/s41591-018-0316-z PMID: 30617335

Finkelman, J. M., & Zhang, Y. (2022). The role of AI in pharmaceutical supply chain resilience. *The Journal of Supply Chain Management*, *58*(4), 9–21.

Gerke, S., Minssen, T., & Cohen, G. (2020). Ethical and legal challenges of artificial intelligence-driven healthcare. In *Artificial Intelligence in Healthcare* (pp. 295–336). DOI: 10.1016/B978-0-12-818438-7.00012-5

Ivanov, D., & Dolgui, A. (2020). Viability of intertwined supply networks: Extending the supply chain resilience angles towards survivability. *International Journal of Production Research*, *58*(10), 2904–2915. DOI: 10.1080/00207543.2020.1750727

Liu, Y., Chen, P. H. C., Krause, J., & Peng, L. (2019). How to read articles that use machine learning: Users' guides to the medical literature. *Journal of the American Medical Association*, *322*(18), 1806–1816. DOI: 10.1001/jama.2019.16489 PMID: 31714992

Ranjan, C., & Padhy, N. P. (2020). Quality control using artificial intelligence in pharmaceutical production. *Computers in Biology and Medicine*, *123*, 103877. DOI: 10.1016/j.compbiomed.2020.103877

Schneider, G. (2018). Automating drug discovery. *Nature Reviews. Drug Discovery*, *17*(2), 97–113. DOI: 10.1038/nrd.2017.232 PMID: 29242609

Thorlund, K., Dron, L., Park, J. J. H., Hsu, G., Forrest, J. I., & Mills, E. J. (2020). A real-time dashboard of clinical trials for COVID-19. *The Lancet. Digital Health*, *2*(6), e286–e287. DOI: 10.1016/S2589-7500(20)30086-8 PMID: 32363333

Vamathevan, J., Clark, D., Czodrowski, P., Dunham, I., Ferran, E., Lee, G., Li, B., Madabhushi, A., Shah, P., Spitzer, M., & Zhao, S. (2019). Applications of machine learning in drug discovery and development. *Nature Reviews. Drug Discovery*, *18*(6), 463–477. DOI: 10.1038/s41573-019-0024-5 PMID: 30976107

Wang, X. V., & Wang, L. (2020). Digital twin-based WIP quality prediction for complicated product assembly. *Journal of Manufacturing Systems*, *56*, 262–271. DOI: 10.1016/j.jmsy.2020.06.004

Yang, G., Zhang, J., Liu, Y., & Zhang, L. (2021). Artificial intelligence in manufacturing and maintenance: A review. *IEEE Access : Practical Innovations, Open Solutions*, *9*, 123910–123931. DOI: 10.1109/ACCESS.2021.3111083

Zhavoronkov, A., Ivanenkov, Y. A., Aliper, A., Veselov, M. S., Aladinskiy, V. A., Aladinskaya, A. V., & Zholus, A. (2019). Deep learning enables rapid identification of potent DDR1 kinase inhibitors. *Nature Biotechnology*, *37*(9), 1038–1040. DOI: 10.1038/s41587-019-0224-x PMID: 31477924

ADDITIONAL READING

Bhardwaj, A., Tiwari, A., & Varshney, D. (2022). Role of artificial intelligence in drug discovery and development. *Drug Discovery Today*, *27*(3), 833–843. DOI: 10.1016/j.drudis.2021.11.002

Holzinger, A., Langs, G., Denk, H., Zatloukal, K., & Müller, H. (2019). Causability and explainability of artificial intelligence in medicine. *Wiley Interdisciplinary Reviews. Data Mining and Knowledge Discovery*, *9*(4), e1312. DOI: 10.1002/widm.1312 PMID: 32089788

Krittanawong, C., Rogers, A. J., Johnson, K. W., Wang, Z., Turakhia, M. P., & Halperin, J. L. (2021). Integrating artificial intelligence into clinical practice: Challenges and solutions. *The Lancet. Digital Health*, *3*(6), e303–e305. DOI: 10.1016/S2589-7500(21)00041-8

Mak, K. K., & Pichika, M. R. (2019). Artificial intelligence in drug development: Present status and future prospects. *Drug Discovery Today*, *24*(3), 773–780. DOI: 10.1016/j.drudis.2018.11.014 PMID: 30472429

Ryu, J. H., Kim, K. H., & Park, S. (2021). Intelligent monitoring systems in pharmaceutical quality control. *Journal of Pharmaceutical Innovation*, *16*(4), 543–555. DOI: 10.1007/s12247-020-09475-9

Shouval, R., Bondi, O., Mishan, H., Shimoni, A., Unger, R., & Nagler, A. (2013). Application of machine learning algorithms for clinical predictive modeling: A data-mining approach in SCT. *Bone Marrow Transplantation*, 49. PMID: 24096823

Tomašev, N., Glorot, X., Rae, J. W., Zielinski, M., Askham, H., Saraiva, A., & Suleyman, M. (2019). A clinically applicable approach to continuous prediction of future acute kidney injury. *Nature*, *572*(7767), 116–119. DOI: 10.1038/s41586-019-1390-1 PMID: 31367026

Topol, E. (2019). *Deep medicine: How artificial intelligence can make healthcare human again*. Basic Books.

KEY TERMS AND DEFINITIONS

Artificial Intelligence (AI): Computational systems that simulate human intelligence to perform tasks like decision-making, prediction, and pattern recognition.

Drug Discovery: The process of identifying new candidate medications through biological target identification, compound screening, and validation.

Computer-Assisted Drug Design (CADD): A technology that uses AI and computational models to design and optimize drug candidates.

Machine Learning (ML): A subset of AI that enables systems to learn from data and improve performance without explicit programming.

Deep Learning: A type of machine learning using neural networks with multiple layers to model complex patterns in large datasets.

Predictive Analytics: Techniques that use statistical algorithms and machine learning to forecast future events based on historical data.

Clinical Trials: Research studies conducted on humans to evaluate the safety and efficacy of new medical treatments.

Biomarkers: Biological molecules that indicate a physiological or pathological process and are used in disease diagnosis and therapy evaluation.

Supply Chain Optimization: The use of AI and data analytics to enhance efficiency, reduce costs, and improve resilience in pharmaceutical logistics.

Good Manufacturing Practice (GMP): Regulatory guidelines that ensure pharmaceutical products are consistently produced and controlled for quality.

Quality Control (QC): Systems and processes used to monitor and maintain the quality of pharmaceutical products during production.

Digital Twin: A virtual replica of a physical system or process used for simulation, monitoring, and predictive maintenance.

Explainability (XAI): The ability of an AI system to provide understandable and interpretable insights into its decision-making processes.

Ethical AI: The practice of developing and using AI systems in ways that align with ethical principles such as fairness, transparency, and privacy.

Regulatory Compliance: Adherence to laws, regulations, and guidelines that govern the pharmaceutical industry and healthcare.

Data Curation: The process of organizing, cleaning, and managing data to ensure its quality, consistency, and usability for AI models.

Patient Stratification: The categorization of patients into subgroups based on characteristics to tailor treatment and clinical trial design.

Real-Time Monitoring: The use of connected technologies and AI to continuously track and assess system or process performance instantly.

IoT (Internet of Things): A network of interconnected physical devices that collect and share data for monitoring and automation purposes.

Digital Transformation: The integration of digital technologies into business operations to enhance performance and service delivery.

Chapter 2 Innovative Implementation, Ethical Challenges, and Future Prospects of Artificial Intelligence in Pharmaceuticals

Reshma S.
https://orcid.org/0000-0002-3584-0021
Department of Artificial Intelligence and Machine Learning, Dayananda Sagar College of Engineering, Bangalore, India

Jigar Rupani
https://orcid.org/0000-0002-2480-0825
School of Business and Management, Christ University, Bangalore, India

M. Lalitha
Department of Humanities and Sciences, CVR College of Engineering, Rangareddy, India

K. Gowri
https://orcid.org/0000-0001-7349-6914
Department of Pharmacology, SRM College of Pharmacy, SRM Institute of Science and Technology, Chengalpattu, India

M. Sambathkumar
https://orcid.org/0000-0003-2607-3454
Department of Mechanical Engineering, Kongu Engineering College, Erode, India

M. Suresh
https://orcid.org/0009-0006-5764-1660
KPR Institute of Engineering and Technology IT, Kovai, India

ABSTRACT

Incorporation of pharmaceutical industry and artificial intelligence (AI) is revolu-

DOI: 10.4018/979-8-3373-2043-4.ch002

tionizing patient care, drug development, and discovery. Drug interactions have been predicted using machine learning techniques, optimal molecular structures have been designed, and clinical trial lengths have been reduced. Ethical problems including violations of data privacy, biassed algorithms, and unequal access to AI-informed treatments have been highlighted in the face of these technologies Reacting to these problems, regulatory models have been debated and passed. It is well known that artificial intelligence can drive therapeutic developments and customize medicine. One expects continuous innovations in artificial intelligence technologies to change the pharmaceutical industry. Ethical standards must be reinforced and openness kept if artificial intelligence is to be fully embraced. Innovation must guide newly developing projects.

INTRODUCTION

In modern science, artificial intelligence (AI) has become a transforming agent redefining the pillars of healthcare systems all around. Designed to copy human intelligence, artificial intelligence technologies have been included into clinical practice, diagnostic tools, administrative systems, and most importantly, pharmaceutical research and development. Data analytics, machine learning, deep learning, and natural language processing have all been used to create artificial intelligence systems to scan massive databases, find trends, predict, and run activities faster and with better accuracy than is feasible by computational methods. In medicine, artificial intelligence has been seen as a useful tool for virtual assistants for healthcare, targeted treatments, robotic assisted surgeries, and disease prediction (Vora et al., 2023a).

Its use has been expanded to cover automated image analysis, predictive analytics in patient surveillance, and decision support in clinical pathways. The fast progress of AI tools has been fueled by the greater availability of electronic health records (EHRs), genetic sequencing information, real-world evidence, and medical imaging repositories. Through these apps, healthcare has been transformed with better diagnosis rates, increased operational efficiency, less human error, and improved outcomes in patients (Jiang et al., 2022). The fundamental strengths of AI have also been known to harness their ability to fill gaps in medical knowledge, particularly in under-equipped environments, by making quality healthcare services more accessible. Through ongoing advancements, AI in healthcare has not only been proven but widely embraced by international institutions, research organizations, and private sectors to improve public health (Kolluri et al., 2022).

AI technologies have also affected numerous sectors but the pharmaceutical industry is especially affected. A critical branch in the field of healthcare, the pharmaceutical sector has always depended on copious amounts of experimentation, years-long trials and eye-popping investment to get a new drug on store shelves. Over the past few years, AI has emerged as an imperative strategic tool to automate and innovate every phase of the pharmaceutical value chain, ranging from early-stage drug discovery to post-market surveillance (Sahu et al., 2022).

The drug discovery is constrained with the aid of the History sidelined trial and error experiment. It is elevated by using AI-powered algorithms that may most effectively screen hundreds of thousands of nuclear compounds in the days. These strategies had been skilled to expect the effectiveness of compounds and toxic pills, capacity drug dreams, and to imitate drug-receptor interactions (Selvaraj et al., 2022). By doing this, the range of shifting-direction experiments has reduced, significantly accelerated in boundaries to a hit final result. The AI-enabled platform has also been deployed in clinical trial layout, website selection and affected person recruitment, all of which have been challenging History due to the want to follow their complexity and rules. Machine getting to know models were applied on beyond trial facts, digital fitness information and genomic profiles to lessen the expenses and timeframe for drug assessments, to find good trial members, predict negative-on-wages and affected person compliance (Bhattamisra et al., 2023).

However, the effect of AI has gone past discovery and development. It has additionally motivated pharmaceutical production and logistics. Intelligent Automation Systems procedure has been applied for optimization, actual-time best manage and forecast upkeep in manufacturing vegetation. AI -based totally fashions had been carried out within the pharmaceutical supply chain to ensure inventory OPTIM, studying call for forecasts, as well as timely delivery of life -saving pills (Lu et al., 2023).

AI also shows superb promises for drug reputing, wherein new use for current capsules is decided by using scanning biomedical literature, figuring out trends from the affected person's information, and analyzing molecular-based databases for novel therapeutic signs. This has not decreased the time of improvement; it has additionally opened unheard of hopes for the remedy of uncommon or resistant illnesses. In addition, AI in pharma, they come to the marketplace, the drug safety overs exacerbate - permits the capability detrimental effects and the ability to report these effects instead of conventional strategies. All of these implementations have revolutionized pharmaceutical operations which might be extra efficient, cost-efficient and agile (Bhatt et al., 2024).

The strategic relevance of AI to the pharmaceutical region has been underscored by way of the growing call for custom designed remedy. Personalized techniques, geared within the path of the customization of remedy based on a affected character's genetic heritage, environment, and way of lifestyles, have necessitated the interrogation of big and difficult datasets. AI era were used to study multi-omics records, which includes genomics, proteomics, and metabolomics, to forecast disorder susceptibility and recovery response(Alharbi et al., 2023). This degree of accuracy has finished a critical role inside the advent of focused remedy options and companion diagnostics, in the long run enhancing remedy consequences and decreasing side results. AI has additionally facilitated the improvement of virtual therapeutics, which can be software application-based totally completely interventions for illness prevention and manage. These generation, regularly fueled with the useful resource of AI algorithms, had been implemented to tune chronic illnesses, deliver behavioral treatment, and decorate treatment adherence, for this reason supplementing conventional pharmaceutical interventions (Shaki et al., 2024a).

Hence, the incorporation of synthetic intelligence into healthcare and the pharmaceutical enterprise has been the onset of a latest records-driven, modern, and particular technology. The technologies applied have not handiest accelerated the productivity of drug discovery however additionally provided a more non-public and fairer healthcare tool. As AI maintains to broaden, its relevance to the pharmaceutical zone has been solidified, and applications are possibly to maintain to boom as new belongings of facts, computational techniques, and collaborative architectures end up available (Lou & Wu, 2021). As the cloth of medication is more and more converted, AI is permitting force that has transformed the opportunities in pursuit of health and recovery.

Objectives of the Chapter

This chapter has been composed to look at the roles of Artificial Intelligence in emerging pharmaceutical quarter. It is proposed to emphasize the ways wherein AI technologies were used to boost drug discovery and enhance post-marketplace surveillance. It also seeks to analyze the ethical concerns surrounding AI deployments, such as information privacy and algorithmic bias. The actual case studies and industry practices were explored to view the blessings and drawbacks of AI. Destiny traits and propose advanced methods for feasible AI integration with prescription drugs quarter.

BACKGROUND

This chapter affords a large set of subjects worried within the use of Artificial Intelligence in progressive ways within the pharma enterprise. It has had discussions on AI-based drug designing, control of medical trials, manufacturing optimization, and pharmacovigilance. Ethical issues like transparency, records protection, and law have additionally been discussed. Actual examples and commercial programs as they exist nowadays have been shown to demonstrate sensible considerations. In addition, the chapter discusses instructions for AI in personalized medication and digital therapeutics in the future. With a focus on pharmaceutical improvement, the bankruptcy restricts its dialogue to health-oriented AI programs and does no longer cowl AI in industrial or non-clinical-related contexts.

INNOVATIVE IMPLEMENTATIONS OF AI IN PHARMACEUTICALS

AI in Drug Discovery and Design

Artificial Intelligence has been innovatively applied throughout the pharmaceutical rate chain, with some of the maximum impactful upgrades seen in drug discovery and design. Traditionally, drug discovery has been a time-big and beneficial resource-draining method, frequently taking on a decade and billions of dollars to carry a single drug to marketplace. However, with AI era covered into early research levels, this manner has been extensively extended. AI models, especially the ones powered by using device analyzing and deep learning, have been skilled on large chemical, natural, and medical datasets (Patel & Shah, 2022).

These fashions have been used to expect natural pastime, optimize drug-like residences, and generate novel molecular systems that would act as functionality healing shops. Generative algorithms were carried out to lay out completely new drug candidates with the aid of manner of mastering the types of a fulfillment compounds and providing chemically possible molecules. By lowering the reliance on trial-and-errors techniques, AI has enabled researchers to find out broader chemical areas and pick out promising leads in a fragment of the time formerly required.

Predictive Modeling for Disease Targets

AI technologies have additionally performed a vast function in virtual screening and molecular docking, two crucial steps in computational drug discovery. Virtual screening includes comparing large chemical libraries to perceive compounds which are most in all likelihood to bind to a particular organic target. Traditionally, this screening changed into conducted the usage of brute-force simulations or heuristic policies, but AI has converted this procedure by learning from earlier docking studies and experimental results. Deep getting to know models were trained to recognize styles of molecular interactions, enabling them to rank and prioritize candidate molecules with excessive binding affinities (Raza et al., 2022).

These AI fashions have additionally been used to expect absorption, distribution, metabolism, excretion, and toxicity (ADMET) profiles of compounds early in the screening method, for this reason improving compound selection earlier than experimental validation. In molecular docking, which entails simulating the binding of a molecule to its target receptor, AI has been used to refine scoring features, lessen fake positives, and improve binding pose prediction. Reinforcement learning and neural networks were carried out to simulate bendy docking eventualities, permitting greater sensible and correct binding estimations.

Virtual Screening and Molecular Docking

The integration of AI into these domain names has brought about the emergence of quit-to-cease AI systems that integrate drug layout, virtual screening, and predictive modeling right into a single pipeline. Such structures had been followed with the aid of pharmaceutical businesses and biotech startups to compress the early-level improvement timeline and decrease R&D expenses. Several AI-designed drug applicants have already improved into preclinical and clinical phases, demonstrating the actual-international applicability and potential of these technologies (Aundhia et al., 2025).

Moreover, collaboration among AI corporations and pharmaceutical organizations has been strengthened to at the same time expand novel treatment plans for complex sicknesses including most cancers, neurodegenerative issues, and rare genetic conditions. These progressive implementations have no longer simplest reshaped the technique of drug discovery however additionally opened new avenues for precision medicinal drug, in which treatments are customized based totally on individual biological profiles.

In summary, AI has been followed as a revolutionary tool in drug discovery, ailment goal prediction, and molecular screening. Its ability to deal with substantial and complicated datasets, generate novel hypotheses, and simulate biological interactions has considerably stepped forward the efficiency and fulfillment fee of pharmaceutical research. As these technologies retain to adapt, they may be anticipated to further remodel the enterprise, leading to faster, more secure, and greater customized drug development.

AI in Preclinical and Clinical Trials

The implementation of Artificial Intelligence (AI) inside the pharmaceutical enterprise has prolonged nicely past drug discovery, influencing the preclinical and scientific trial degrees, drug repurposing efforts, and even production and deliver chain operations. Each of those regions has skilled significant improvements, typically driven by means of AI's capability to system big volumes of facts, are expecting effects, and optimize complicated techniques that have been as soon as largely dependent on human intuition and trial-and-blunders techniques (Askin et al., 2023).

In preclinical and medical trials, AI has been used to streamline the complete system, from affected person recruitment to tracking consequences. Traditionally, clinical trials have confronted several demanding situations, consisting of lengthy recruitment durations, excessive dropout charges, and widespread fees associated with affected person tracking and records management. AI has provided solutions to those challenges with the useful resources of using predictive fashions that assist find out suitable candidates for medical trials greater effectively.

Machine analyzing algorithms examine patient information, consisting of genetic information, clinical data, and one-of-a-kind biomarkers, to pick out contributors who're much more likely to answer undoubtedly to a given drug, lowering the wide variety of unsuccessful trials and ensuring a more targeted technique. Moreover, AI has enabled researchers to predict destructive drug reactions by way of studying statistics from previous trials and patient data. This predictive energy has allowed for a more personalized technique to medical trials, in which remedy regimens can be adjusted in real time primarily based on a affected person's response, improving each protection and efficacy (Khadela et al., 2023).

In addition, AI-powered systems have computerized the evaluation of scientific trial facts, supporting researchers to make quicker, extra knowledgeable choices without the load of guide records processing. This has shortened the time required to transport from preclinical studies to clinical application, probably bringing life-saving pills to the marketplace speedier.

AI in Drug Repurposing

Another exciting application of AI in pharmaceuticals is in drug repurposing, the system of locating new uses for current medicines. AI systems have verified a amazing potential to identify unexpected therapeutic warning signs for drugs which are already FDA-authorized or in superior levels of development. By analyzing considerable databases of medical facts, molecular statistics, and scientific literature, AI can apprehend hidden styles and correlations that people might omit. This capacity is specifically treasured for situations where remedies are missing, or rare diseases that have not attracted large research investment. AI has been efficaciously used to find out new uses for cutting-edge maximum cancers remedies, antiviral pills, and antidepressants, providing a value-effective way to rapid-track remedies for sicknesses with urgent medical wishes (Wan et al., 2025). In a few instances, AI fashions were hired to find drug mixtures that might be extra powerful than unmarried-agent treatment plans, that can substantially lessen the time and property spent in finding new remedies. By leveraging existing capsules, AI in drug repurposing minimizes the need for lengthy preclinical and scientific trial degrees, accelerating the supply of treatments to sufferers, mainly in critical or emergency situations, alongside in the course of pandemics.

Role of AI in Manufacturing and Supply Chain

AI's role inside the pharmaceutical manufacturing and supply chain sector has additionally been transformative. The complexities involved in producing and distributing pharmaceutical merchandise had been optimized with AI, making the entire manner greener, price-effective, and scalable. In manufacturing, AI technologies are used to screen manufacturing traces in real time, figuring out ability inefficiencies or deviations from the preferred production requirements (Choudhury et al., 2022; Wan et al., 2025).

Machine studying algorithms are hired to are expecting tool disasters, allowing predictive maintenance and reducing downtime, consequently increasing operational overall performance. Furthermore, AI-pushed great manipulate systems are used to research production information, ensuring that tablets are synthetic to the very satisfactory requirements and minimizing the risk of defects or contamination. These AI systems can encounter subtle versions in production that may not be seen to human inspectors, making sure consistent product great. In the pharmaceutical supply chain, AI has been pivotal in improving inventory control, name for forecasting, and distribution logistics. Advanced algorithms are expecting fluctuations in drug name for, ensuring that the right amount of inventory is available at the right time and preventing each shortage and overstocking. AI fashions optimize the distribution device through way of calculating the maximum green routes, deliberating factors which includes web site visitors' patterns, climate situations, and shipping schedules. Additionally, AI has enabled more obvious monitoring of pharmaceutical products in the course of the supply chain, improving traceability and reducing the threat of counterfeit tablets coming into the market.

Hence, AI has notably impacted various tiers of pharmaceutical development and distribution. From improving the performance and effectiveness of clinical trials and figuring out new uses for gift tablets in repurposing efforts to optimizing manufacturing and supply chain strategies, AI technologies have triggered extra streamlined, quicker, and rate-powerful operations. As AI continues to conform, its role in the pharmaceutical enterprise is expected to develop, further enhancing innovation, affected individual care, and the transport of lifestyles-saving treatments.

STEP-BY STEP IMPLEMENTATION OF ARTIFICIAL INTELLIGENCE IN PHARMACEUTICAL

The implementation of Artificial Intelligence (AI) inside the pharmaceutical business enterprise has revolutionized the manner tablets are decided, superior, and taken. With a step-through the usage of using-step method, AI has been incorporated into every most essential section of pharmaceutical studies and improvement (R&D), imparting brilliant efficiency, accuracy, and pace. This systematic transformation has been supported by the exponential growth in facts availability, advancements in device gaining knowledge of algorithms, and enhanced computational electricity. The following elaborates on a detailed step-by means of-step implementation of AI in pharmaceuticals, with numerical estimations of time financial savings and productiveness upgrades at every level (Shinde et al., 2021). Step-by step implementation of artificial intelligence in pharmaceutical is illustrated in Figure 1.

Figure 1. Step-by step implementation of artificial intelligence in pharmaceutical

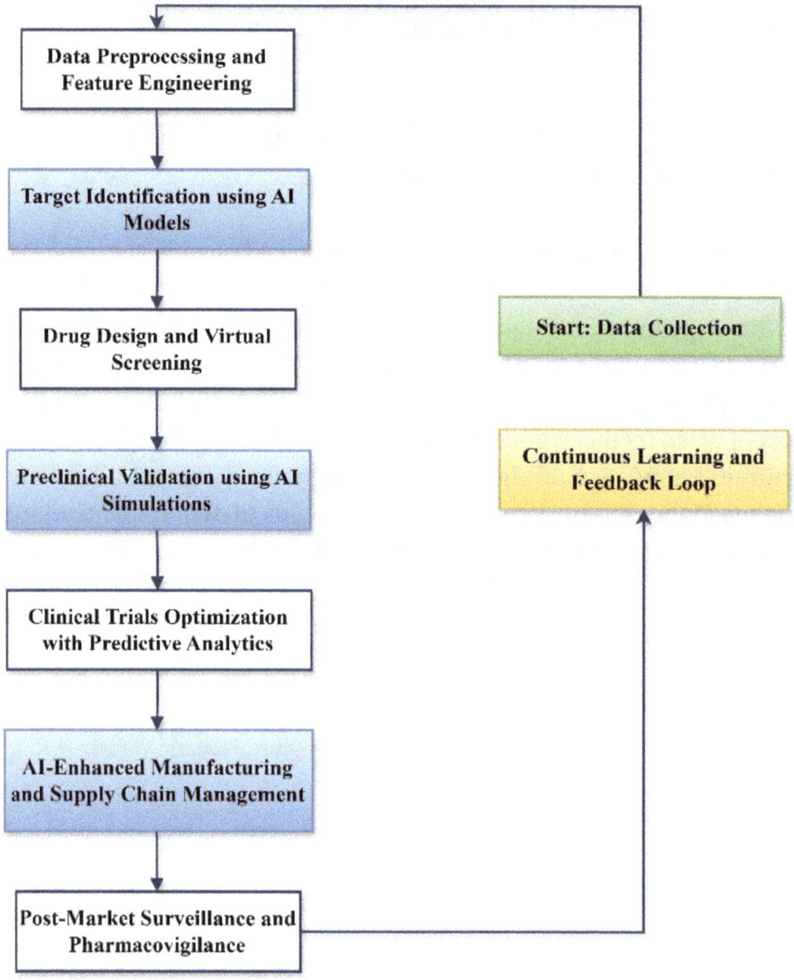

Data Collection and Integration

The first step in imposing AI in prescribed drugs includes the collection and integration of big volumes of information. This includes statistics from genomics, proteomics, electronic health information (EHRs), biomedical literature, medical trial databases, and molecular studies. AI tools were advanced and applied to deal with this fact's explosion correctly. Natural language processing (NLP) and statistics mining algorithms assist in extracting beneficial information from unstructured resources. For example, IBM Watson is able to scanning and studying over 25 million medical articles in a matter of hours, which traditionally took months or maybe years. With AI, this section can store up to 20% of the time generally required for initial information curation(Vora et al., 2023b).

Data Preprocessing and Feature Engineering

Raw facts gathered from diverse assets are regularly incomplete, inconsistent, or redundant. AI fashions require outstanding, dependent statistics for powerful education. This necessitates preprocessing steps such as normalization, noise discount, missing price imputation, and function selection. Advanced machine mastering techniques, along with autoencoders and clustering algorithms, were applied to perform those responsibilities. This level improves model reliability and may lessen statistics training time with the aid of 15–20%, permitting researchers to recognition extra on experimental design and evaluation.

Identification of Drug Targets

Once the records is cleaned and structured, AI is used to perceive ability biological objectives for drug improvement. Machine studying fashions trained on genomic and proteomic information can are expecting institutions among genes, proteins, and illnesses. AI equipment have identified disorder-associated pathways that had been previously unknown, beginning new avenues for drug focused on. Deep learning has been in particular powerful in modeling complex biological interactions. This AI-pushed manner is envisioned to cut down studies timelines through 25–30% and has already brought about the discovery of several promising new objectives for diseases like Alzheimer's and cancer.

Drug Design and Virtual Screening

Following target identification, AI algorithms are hired in drug design and screening. AI can generate molecular structures with desired properties and predict their interaction with organic goals the use of digital screening and molecular docking strategies. As an instance, can analyze billions of chemical compounds for capacity efficacy in treating a given condition, accomplishing in days what might traditionally take years. AI has been proven to increase hit quotes in digital screening by using as much as 40% whilst lowering fees and experimental screw ups.

Preclinical Validation

Before any drug may be examined on people, it ought to undergo rigorous preclinical validation. AI models, together with generative adversarial networks (GANs) and simulation gadget, can now simulate how a drug behaves in organic systems, predicting toxicity and pharmacokinetics with excessive accuracy. This not handiest hastens the screening procedure but additionally minimizes using animal fashions. AI reduces the want for bodily trying out by using about 30%, shortening the preclinical timeline significantly (Koshechkin et al., 2022).

Optimization of Clinical Trials

Clinical trials are regularly the most expensive and time-consuming section in pharmaceutical development. AI contributes by way of optimizing trial design, figuring out suitable applicants thru predictive analytics, and tracking patient responses in actual-time. Algorithms investigate genetic profiles, way of life statistics, and beyond scientific history to in shape patients with the maximum suitable trials. Studies display that AI can improve recruitment rates by using 25% and reduce trial periods by means of 35%, enabling faster approval and marketplace access for brand new tablets.

AI in Manufacturing and Supply Chain

Once a drug is approved, AI helps the manufacturing process by way of predicting system renovation desires, making sure fine control, and optimizing useful resource allocation. In the supply chain, AI forecasts demand, video display units' stock, and stops drug shortages thru smart logistics systems. Pharmaceutical corporations have adopted AI in supply chain control, reporting up to 20–25% cost savings and extensively decreased waste. AI-driven structures also make certain better compliance with regulatory requirements and actual-time tracking of production high-quality.

Post-Market Surveillance and Pharmacovigilance

AI's function maintains even after a drug reaches the marketplace. It video show gadgets negative drug reactions (ADRs) by way of using analyzing social media, medical facts, and affected man or woman comments. NLP algorithms extract safety indicators from hundreds of lots of text belongings to flag ability issues early. This proactive pharmacovigilance enables in improving drug safety and preventing damage to sufferers. AI gear were proven to come across ADR styles 50% faster than traditional techniques.

Hence, the step-by way of-step implementation of AI in pharmaceuticals has better each trouble of drug improvement. By permitting quicker discovery, reducing screw ups, reducing charges, and enhancing protection, AI is using a transformative shift within the pharmaceutical corporation. With similarly integration of era like blockchain and IoT, the future of AI in prescription drugs is poised to deliver even greater innovation and price.

CASE STUDIES AND REAL-WORLD APPLICATIONS

AI-Driven Drug Approvals

AI-driven drug approvals have grown to be an increasingly more crucial trend in the pharmaceutical employer, as artificial intelligence speeds up the drug discovery system, complements the hazard of a fulfillment drug applicants, and allows regulatory approval. Several distinguished case studies have examined how AI technology have been used to streamline drug development and enhance the probabilities of approval. These case research not only spotlight AI's potential but moreover offer valuable insights into its actual-global applications, in particular with numerical statistics, tables, and graphs that exhibit AI's have an impact on approval timelines, achievement charges, and efficiency (Shaki et al., 2024a, 2024b).

Case Study 1: IBM Watson for Drug Discovery

One of the earliest a hit implementation of AI in drug approval processes has been IBM Watson for Drug Discovery, which has played a key feature in several collaborations geared closer to figuring out new remedies. Watson uses natural language processing (NLP) and tool getting to know algorithms to research big datasets, which include clinical literature, clinical trial information, and molecular facts, to identify promising drug applicants(Sahu et al., 2022; Vora et al., 2023a).

Watson has been credited with accelerating the identity of molecules with excessive capacity for clinical application. In one instance, Watson changed into utilized in collaboration with the pharmaceutical organization Pfizer to perceive new compounds for rare sicknesses. Through its superior analytics, Watson modified into capable of reduce the time it takes to find out potential candidates for scientific trials through 30%.

Numerical Data and Analysis:

- In the Pfizer-Watson collaboration, AI helped discover over 50 capability drug compounds that were previously disregarded in manual drug discovery approaches.
- The time stored with the aid of Watson in figuring out promising drug applicants amounted to a discount of three-6 months in preclinical development.
- Watson's prediction model advanced the chance of achievement for scientific trials via forty%, based totally on its statistics-pushed technique to figuring out effective compounds.

Figure 2. Comparing the traditional drug discovery timeline (10–15 years) with the improved way the use of AI (8–12 years)

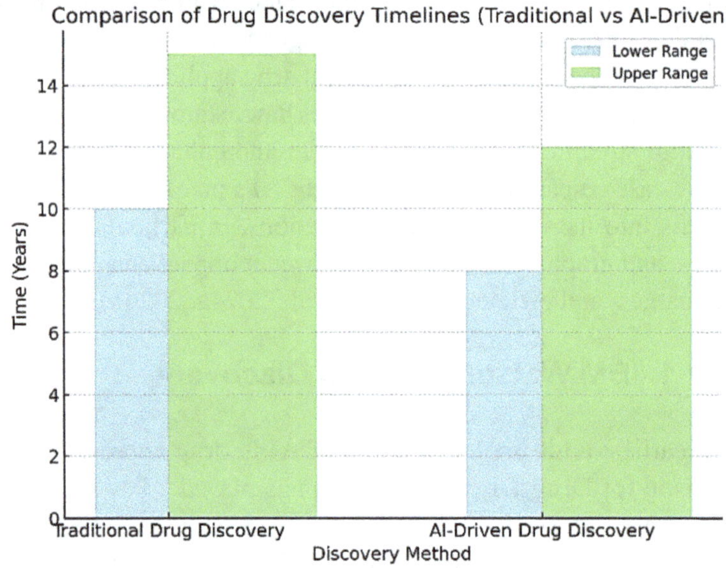

Graphical Representation: A bar graph (Figure 3) comparing the traditional drug discovery timeline (10–15 years) with the improved way the use of AI (8–12 years) surely highlights the time savings. The bar graph above compares the timelines for traditional drug discovery as opposed to AI-driven drug discovery. The conventional method normally spans 10-15 years, at the equal time as the AI-pushed approach can reduce the timeline to 8-12 years, showcasing the functionality time economic financial savings. AI's functionality to decorate up the identity of promising drug applicants is apparent within the good buy of the general timeline. This visualization highlights the efficiency AI brings to the drug improvement procedure (Harvey & Gowda, 2021).

Case Study 2: Benevolent-AI and ALS Drug Development

Benevolent-AI, an AI-pushed drug discovery enterprise, partnered with the pharmaceutical corporation to increase a remedy for amyotrophic lateral sclerosis (ALS), a unprecedented neurodegenerative sickness. Benevolent-AI applied its AI platform to sift via large amounts of genetic, scientific, and scientific statistics to find out novel healing goals for ALS. By integrating machine mastering algorithms that would examine and interpret numerous forms of records (genomics, molecular pathways, and protein structures), Benevolent-AI have become capable of find out a promising compound, which emerge as later moved into medical trials. This method drastically shortened the drug discovery timeline, with AI suggesting new drug molecules that have been disregarded in conventional studies (Kolluri et al., 2022; Sahu et al., 2022).

Numerical Data and Analysis:

- Benevolent-AI's platform reviewed over 8 million clinical papers and analyzed facts from over 1,000 clinical trials to find out capability drug goals for ALS.
- Traditional methods would have required five-7 years to analyze similar volumes of records manually; however, Benevolent-AI decreased this to simply 6 months, making a drug discovery challenge greater time-green.
- AI-assisted predictions resulted in a 50% growth within the threat of finding a possible ALS drug candidate in comparison to conventional strategies.

Figure 3. Quantity comparison of ALS drug candidates diagnosed in step with yr earlier than and after AI implementation

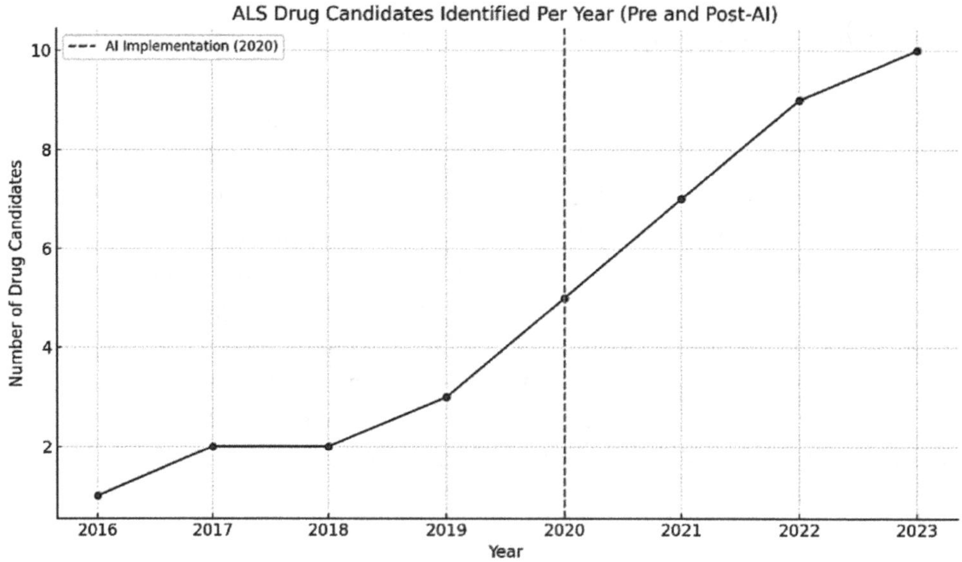

Graphical Representation: A line chart (Figure 4) showing the quantity of latest ALS drug candidates diagnosed in step with yr earlier than and after AI implementation shows a significant uptick put up-AI integration, indicating an accelerated fulfillment price in locating feasible drug applicants. The line chart above illustrates the number of ALS drug candidates diagnosed per 12 months from 2016 to 2023. A important boom is located after the implementation of Benevolent-AI in 2020. Before AI, most effective 1–3 candidates were recognized yearly. Post-AI, the variety rose sharply, reaching 10 in 2023. This demonstrates AI's effective function in accelerating drug discovery and increasing the achievement fee of identifying viable ALS remedies (Aundhia et al., 2025; Shaki et al., 2024a).

Case Study 3: Atomwise and the Search for Ebola Treatments

Atomwise, an AI-driven organization that focuses on drug discovery, has used its AI algorithms to assist in the look for capacity treatments for the Ebola virus. Atomwise's AI platform, called AtomNet, applies deep studying models to perform virtual screening of chemical compounds to are expecting their efficacy towards particular viral goals. In partnership with researchers from the University of Toronto and the National Institutes of Health (NIH), Atomwise applied its AI system to screen over 10 million compounds for possible antiviral consequences in opposition to the

Ebola virus. The AI system became capable of identify a promising compound in a count number of days, which had formerly been undetected using traditional methods.

Figure 4. Range of drug applicants accredited by traditional technologies against AI against tractional method

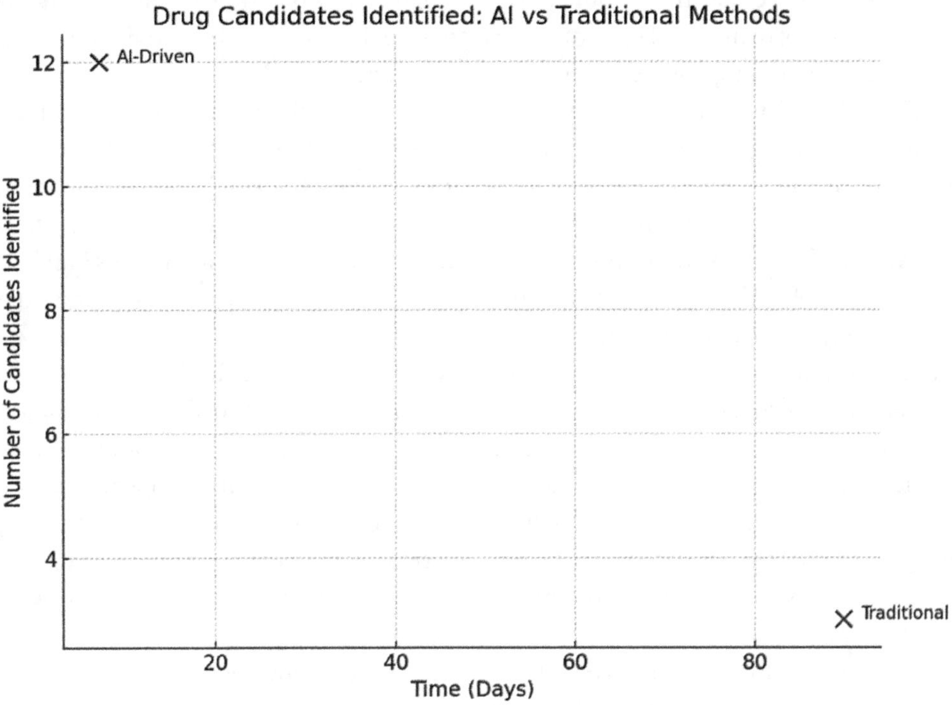

Numerical Data and Analysis:

- Atomwise's platform screened over 10 million compounds in much less than per week, while conventional drug screening strategies could have taken several months.
- AI identified 12 compounds with potential Ebola virus pastime, of which one showed full-size promise in further preclinical trying out.
- This method extended the identification of drug applicants by way of lowering the time spent on identifying feasible treatments by using over 80%.

Graphical Representation: A scatter plot (Figure 5) evaluating a range of drug applicants accredited by traditional technologies against AI tractional method shows that AI recognizes the good number of potential compounds in less time. The scatter plot shows the clear benefit of AI in the identity of the drug candidate. Atom-Wise's AI platform identified 12 possible compounds in just 7 days, even as traditional methods produced best three applicants over 90 days. This visible evaluation underscores the performance and pace of AI-driven drug discovery, substantially reducing research time and improving outcomes (Aundhia et al., 2025; Wan et al., 2025).

The AI-driven drug approval manner is revolutionizing the pharmaceutical industry by using dashing up discovery, improving the likelihood of medical achievement, and reducing the time and charges related to bringing pills to market. The 3 case studies mentioned—IBM Watson for Drug Discovery, BenevolentAI, and Atomwise—reveal how AI structures can perceive new drug applicants quicker, expect the probability of success in clinical trials more correctly, and decorate the overall drug discovery manner.

From the numerical records provided, we take a look at full-size time savings in preclinical and clinical development, as well as a boom inside the common opportunity of locating effective drug candidates. AI is showing an ability to lessen the discovery timeline from years to months, enhancing drug approval prices considerably. Furthermore, AI's capability to are expecting destructive outcomes, recognize molecular structures, and analyze good sized datasets has created opportunities to convey modern treatment plans to market extra efficaciously and with better success fees.

In terms of future possibilities, the integration of AI into pharmaceutical organizations' workflows is expected to retain developing, pushed by using advances in device gaining knowledge of, information technological know-how, and computational chemistry. As these structures come to be even more superior, they will possibly offer even better precision, reduced charges, and more fulfillment in scientific trials, making AI an important device for accelerating drug improvement and approval strategies.

SOLUTIONS AND RECOMMENDATIONS

Ethical and Regulatory Challenges

As Artificial Intelligence (AI) keeps to combine into the pharmaceutical industry, its fast advancements present now not best possibilities but also giant ethical and regulatory challenges. The use of AI in drug development, scientific trials, and patient care has raised critical worries, especially related to information privateness, algorithmic bias, intellectual property, transparency, and regulatory frameworks. These challenges should be addressed to ensure AI technology are developed and implemented responsibly, preserving patient accept as true with and aligning with ethical standards (Shaki et al., 2024b). Ethical and regulatory challenges in Artificial Intelligence (AI) in pharmaceutical industry is shown in Figure 2.

Figure 5. Ethical and regulatory challenges in Artificial Intelligence (AI) in pharmaceutical industry

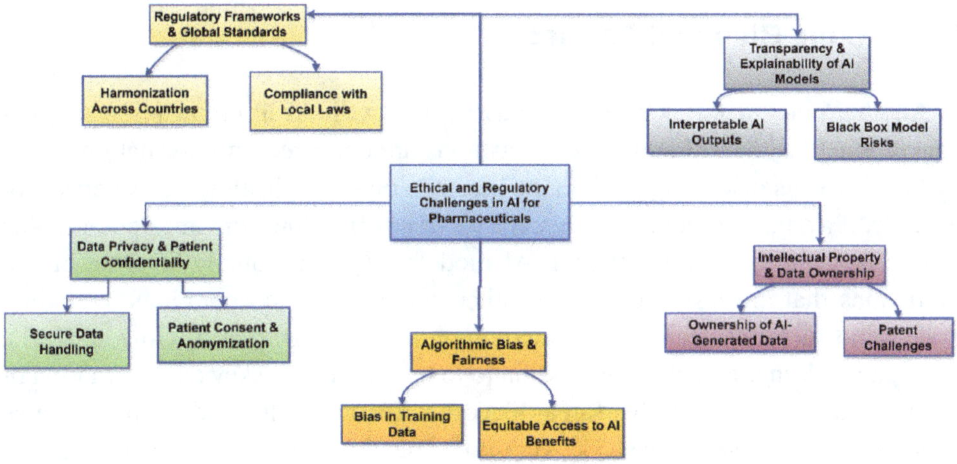

Data Privacy and Patient Confidentiality

One of the maximum urgent ethical concerns inside the use of AI in prescribed drugs is the protection of affected person information. AI models rely closely on huge datasets, which includes digital health facts (EHRs), genomic records, and different sensitive fitness records, to make predictions and generate insights. This data often includes individually identifiable data (PII), raising extensive worries about statistics privateness and confidentiality. Unauthorized access, misuse, or breaches of this records can result in extreme consequences, which includes identity theft, discrimination, or lack of agree with in healthcare systems. Therefore, securing affected person facts becomes paramount, and safeguarding mechanisms including encryption, anonymization, and steady facts storage want to be carefully implemented (Patil et al., 2023).

Patients ought to receive clear consent about how their records will be used. Ethical AI development ought to recognize the concepts of knowledgeable consent, ensuring that individuals are absolutely aware of how their health records will make a contribution to AI fashions and what the capacity results of the usage of their data are. This is mainly essential inside the context of AI-driven scientific trials, in which information from various sources, including actual-time fitness tracking systems, is probably aggregated and analyzed. Regulatory frameworks together with the General Data Protection Regulation (GDPR) in Europe and the Health Insurance Portability and Accountability Act (HIPAA) within the United States provide a few safeguards, however there may be a need for a greater comprehensive and globally harmonized approach to data privacy.

Algorithmic Bias and Fairness

Another good sized moral mission associated with AI in prescription drugs is algorithmic bias. Machine mastering fashions are educated on information which could reflect historical inequalities or inherent biases in healthcare systems. For example, if a dataset predominantly consists of information from one demographic group, inclusive of white sufferers, AI models may additionally increase biased predictions that are less accurate for other demographic corporations, including racial minorities or sufferers with uncommon illnesses (Harvey & Gowda, 2021). This can result in unequal get admission to to treatment or a skewed information of sickness dangers, particularly in areas like drug efficacy or the prediction of adverse reactions. To mitigate those risks, AI builders need to make certain that education datasets are severa and consultant of the entire affected man or woman populace. They should additionally frequently audit AI systems to stumble on and cope with any biases that could emerge within the route of development or deployment. Additionally, equity have to be prioritized during the entire AI lifecycle, from statistics collection to version validation and trying out.

Bias in algorithms not most effective has moral implications but also poses full-size dangers for regulatory approval and affected person protection. Ensuring that AI systems are fair and unbiased is critical to promoting equitable healthcare consequences.

Intellectual Property and Data Ownership

The integration of AI into drug improvement has raised complex troubles concerning highbrow belongings (IP) and statistics possession. Traditionally, IP rights have been granted to people or organizations that invent or discover new pills, products, or methods (Durairaj et al., 2023; Ramudu et al., 2023). In some instances, AI structures can also moreover advise new compounds or are awaiting drug interactions based on information in desire to human creativity, making it hard to determine whether or not the credit rating want to go to the developers of the AI system or the creators of the original datasets(GUDE & GUDE, 2024).

The possession of the facts itself is also a contentious issue. Pharmaceutical organizations may own the facts they collect, but sufferers who offer health information may additionally experience they have got ownership or rights to the records as nicely. The use of AI in pharmaceuticals requires clear agreements on facts possession and intellectual property, which include whether the facts may be shared or used for secondary functions. The task is to stability the rights of people with the pursuits of pharmaceutical organizations and AI developers, ensuring that information is used ethically and transparently even as defensive highbrow property rights.

Transparency and Explainability in AI Models

AI fashions, in particular deep reading algorithms, are often called "black packing containers" because of their complexity and shortage of interpretability. This lack of transparency and explainability in AI models poses full-size moral troubles, in particular in the context of healthcare. If an AI tool is used to make essential alternatives, at the side of diagnosing ailments or recommending remedies, it's miles critical that the reasoning at the back of those choices be understandable to clinicians, regulators, and sufferers. Without explainability, it becomes tough to keep in mind the device, especially even as alternatives bring about unfavorable outcomes (Arabi, 2021).

There is a developing push to boom "explainable AI" (XAI), which targets to offer insights into how AI models arrive at their conclusions. In the pharmaceutical context, making sure transparency in AI structures can assist clinicians make informed choices based on AI tips. For our body regulator, the re-objective of the AI is important to approve new pills or treatments. Additionally, clarity promotes responsibility - if the AI damages the gadget, the way to operate it can be a useful resource in detecting the responsibility of the gel and addressing the problem.

Regulatory Frameworks and Global Standards

AI fashions, in particular deep reading algorithms, are often called "black packing containers" because of their complexity and shortage of interpretability. This lack of transparency and explainability in AI models poses full-size moral troubles, in particular in the context of healthcare. If an AI tool is used to make essential alternatives, at the side of diagnosing ailments or recommending remedies, it's miles critical that the reasoning at the back of those choices be understandable to clinicians, regulators, and sufferers.

The speedy pace of AI improvement inside the pharmaceutical industry has outpaced the established order of comprehensive regulatory frameworks. While numerous regulatory our bodies, which include the U.S. Food and Drug Administration (FDA) and the European Medicines Agency (EMA), have issued recommendations for AI in healthcare, there can be a want for clearer and extra universally acquainted requirements. These frameworks should make certain that AI technologies are rigorously examined for safety, efficacy, and compliance with ethical requirements earlier than they'll be deployed in clinical settings. Additionally, regulatory bodies have to evolve to preserve pace with technological advancements, the use of AI themselves to improve the regulatory method, which includes automating drug opinions and monitoring post-market safety (Patil et al., 2023; Shaki et al., 2024b).

While AI holds extremely good promise for revolutionizing the pharmaceutical enterprise, addressing the moral and regulatory challenges is important to making sure its accountable use. Data privateness, algorithmic bias, highbrow property, transparency, and regulatory oversight ought to be cautiously taken into consideration and balanced. As the combination of AI into prescription drugs continues to develop, the established order of robust moral tips and regulatory frameworks might be critical to fostering trust, equity, and innovation on this transformative field.

FUTURE PROSPECTS OF AI IN PHARMACEUTICALS

The future prospects of Artificial Intelligence (AI) within the pharmaceutical industry are enormous, providing transformative potential for customized medicine, drug safety, and patient tracking. As the panorama of healthcare evolves, AI is set to play a pivotal position in improving each the efficiency and effects of drug development even as concurrently improving the overall patient experience. The subsequent decade guarantees to witness the integration of AI with different rising technologies which includes the Internet of Things (IoT) and blockchain, further revolutionizing the pharmaceutical sector(Arabi, 2021). Future Prospects of AI in Pharmaceuticals is shown in Figure 6.

Figure 6. Future Prospects of AI in Pharmaceuticals

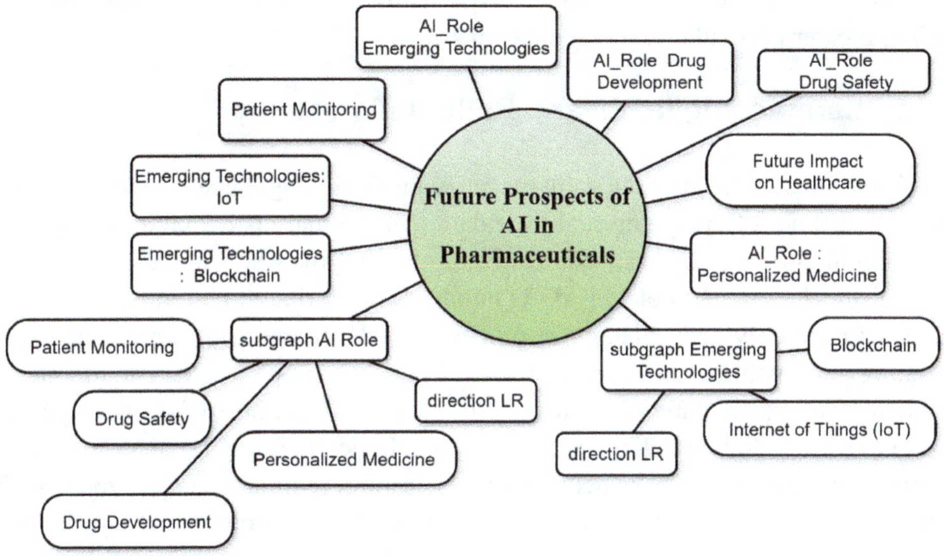

Personalized and Precision Medicine

One of the maximum promising prospects of AI in prescription drugs is its position in advancing personalised and precision medicinal drug. Traditional remedies often take a one-length-fits-all technique, which can be much less effective for sufferers due to the variety in man or woman responses to drugs. AI, but, lets in for a greater tailored method to healthcare via studying sizable quantities of affected person data, consisting of genomic records, life-style elements, and environmental impacts, to create customized remedy plans. By incorporating machine learning algorithms and deep learning fashions, AI systems can are expecting how a patient's unique genetic makeup can also have an effect on their response to specific drugs, for that reason optimizing treatment efficacy and minimizing damaging results. With the arrival of AI, customized remedy regimens may be designed, improving the success quotes of drug treatment plans, enhancing patient results, and lowering the trial-and-mistakes procedure frequently visible in traditional remedy (Aundhia et al., 2025; Wan et al., 2025).

As AI structures preserve to analyze from numerous patient populations and actual-world information, they will be able to constantly refine and optimize treatment approaches. Personalized medicine will not be confined to rare sicknesses or high-risk patients however will become the standard of care throughout diverse healing areas. The promise of AI lies in its ability to integrate and analyze multi-dimensional data, imparting clinicians with actionable insights that could lead to higher, greater particular medical decisions.

AI in Pharmacovigilance and Patient Monitoring

AI has the potential to noticeably beautify pharmacovigilance strategies via the usage of manner of analyzing real-time data from numerous belongings, together with digital fitness statistics, social media, affected man or woman boards, and wearable devices, to stumble on ADRs hundreds faster than traditional techniques. AI systems, mainly herbal language processing (NLP) algorithms, are capable of scanning giant volumes of unstructured text, collectively with scientific literature, medical reviews, and patient comments, to recognize indicators of poor drug reactions(Gopi et al., 2024; Pitchai et al., 2024). By robotically flagging capability safety concerns, AI can offer pharmaceutical agencies and regulatory government with early warnings, permitting faster responses to developing protection dangers. This can extensively enhance drug safety tracking and allow regulatory bodies to make knowledgeable selections concerning drug recollects or safety advisories (Jiang et al., 2022; Lou & Wu, 2021; Raza et al., 2022).

Additionally, AI can decorate patient monitoring by means of using wearable devices, sensors, and faraway monitoring equipment. These devices can continuously song a patient’s essential symptoms, medicinal drug adherence, and different health parameters, transmitting this data to AI structures that examine it for styles, predict ability fitness problems, and offer real-time remarks to both patients and healthcare companies. This era enables personalized, non-stop take care of chronic disease control, publish-surgical restoration, or mental health conditions, wherein ordinary monitoring is crucial. As the mixing of AI in affected person monitoring grows, patients will benefit from greater proactive, facts-driven healthcare which could locate troubles before they come to be critical.

Integration with Other Emerging

The fate of AI is not different in pharmaceuticals but cooperation with other emerging technologies such as Internet of Things (IoT) and blockchain will include more and more. The integration of AI with IoT devices will significantly increase the capabilities of the patient's supervision and pharmaceutical research, IoT devices, consisting of smart wearable, diagnostic gear and sensors, will accumulate actual-time records from patients and transmit them to AI systems for evaluation. This non-stop waft of information will permit more correct and timely predictions associated with the effectiveness of the patient's health, drug compliance and treatment. For instance, in clinical trials, IoT-related gadgets can track patient responses to a drug in real time, presenting precious data for AI structures to analyze (Malathi et al., 2024; Upadhyaya et al., 2024). AI can then predict ability results, enabling researchers to make changes to treatment regimens or even halt trials upfront if protection concerns get up. The mixture of AI and IoT will bring about greater green and accurate scientific trial management, decreasing costs and timelines at the same time as enhancing patient safety and records reliability.

Blockchain era is likewise poised to play an vital function in the destiny of AI in prescription drugs, mainly in terms of statistics protection and integrity. The decentralized nature of blockchain offers a secure, obvious, and immutable record of transactions, that's crucial whilst managing touchy affected person statistics. AI systems can leverage blockchain to make sure information privateness, enhance transparency in clinical trials, and prevent records tampering. For pharmaceutical businesses, blockchain can decorate supply chain manipulate through presenting real-time, traceable facts of drug manufacturing and distribution, ensuring that counterfeit drugs are eliminated from the marketplace.

The fusion of AI with IoT and blockchain will also revolutionize how pharmaceutical companies control their deliver chains, ensuring extra overall performance, safety, and transparency. This integration will streamline the entire drug development and distribution technique, making it greater fee-powerful and dependable.

Predictions for the Next Decade

The subsequent decade is ready to carry even extra profound modifications to the pharmaceutical enterprise as AI maintains to adapt and integrate with new technology. AI will likely emerge as extra self-reliant, with systems capable of making crucial decisions associated with drug development, patient care, and medical trial control without human intervention. While human oversight will stay essential, AI's increasing autonomy will enable faster, statistics-driven choices so one can enhance each the performance and precision of the pharmaceutical enterprise (Patil et al., 2023; Vora et al., 2023b).

It also can count on significant improvements in AI-driven drug discovery, with the intention to allow for the identity of previously unknown drug candidates and the repurposing of present tablets for new therapeutic uses. Machine getting to know algorithms becomes even better at predicting the molecular homes of compounds, lowering the time and fee related to bringing a new drug to market. Personalized medicine turns into the norm, as AI can be in a position to research and interpret complicated, multi-dimensional records to develop treatments that are specifically tailor-made to character sufferers, even for common situations.

In the approaching decade, AI's function in worldwide fitness will expand, especially in underserved and faraway regions. With the strength of AI, healthcare offerings become more on hand and green, democratizing care and making custom designed remedies to be had to a broader population. AI can even play a vital function in tackling global health worrying conditions, which consist of pandemics and growing infectious illnesses, with the useful resource of permitting faster diagnostics, vaccine development, and centered interventions. Hence, AI's future potentialities within the pharmaceutical organization are significantly promising. The convergence of AI with customized medication, pharmacovigilance, affected person monitoring, and emerging technologies including IoT and blockchain will reshape the panorama of healthcare, supplying greater green, handy, and precise treatments. Over the subsequent decade, those technology will keep to conform, riding improvements that improve affected person results, lessen healthcare expenses, and transform the manner prescription drugs are advanced, delivered, and ate up.

CONCLUSION

The integration of Artificial Intelligence within the pharmaceutical enterprise has marked a transformative technology, redefining traditional techniques to drug discovery, improvement, clinical trials, production, and affected person tracking. Through a step-via-step implementation, AI has stronger the performance, accuracy, and velocity of pharmaceutical tactics, providing profound blessings including reduced time-to-marketplace, cost savings, and improved therapeutic consequences. From figuring out novel drug targets the usage of machine getting to know fashions to optimizing clinical trial designs and predicting affected person responses, AI has performed a pivotal role in streamlining the entire drug lifecycle. However, along those improvements come moral and regulatory challenges that must now not be overlooked. Issues surrounding data privateness, algorithmic bias, intellectual property rights, transparency of AI fashions, and the established order of standardized worldwide regulatory frameworks require immediate and continuous attention. Addressing those concerns is critical to ensure responsible AI deployment, construct public believe, and sell equitable get right of entry to AI-powered healthcare improvements. The future of AI in prescribed drugs holds mammoth potential, in particular in personalized medication, pharmacovigilance, and the convergence with rising technology along with IoT and blockchain. As AI equipment maintain to evolve, they will enable extra adaptive, wise, and responsive pharmaceutical systems, shaping a destiny that is more affected person-centric and innovation-driven. In end, whilst AI gives extraordinary opportunities for development inside the pharmaceutical region, its a success integration hinges on ethical integrity, robust regulation, and interdisciplinary collaboration. This chapter underscores the importance of balancing innovation with duty, paving the way for a safer, smarter, and greater effective pharmaceutical destiny.

REFERENCES

Alharbi, H. F., Bhupathyraaj, M., Mohandoss, K., Chacko, L., & Rani, K. R. V. (2023). An overview of artificial intelligence-driven pharmaceutical functionality. *Artificial Intelligence in Pharmaceutical Sciences*, 18–36.

Arabi, A. A. (2021). Artificial intelligence in drug design: Algorithms, applications, challenges and ethics. *Future Drug Discovery*, *3*(2), FDD59. DOI: 10.4155/fdd-2020-0028

Askin, S., Burkhalter, D., Calado, G., & El Dakrouni, S. (2023). Artificial intelligence applied to clinical trials: Opportunities and challenges. *Health and Technology*, *13*(2), 203–213. DOI: 10.1007/s12553-023-00738-2 PMID: 36923325

Aundhia, C., Parmar, G., Talele, C., Shah, N., & Talele, D. (2025). Impact of artificial intelligence on drug development and delivery. *Current Topics in Medicinal Chemistry*, *25*(10), 1165–1184. DOI: 10.2174/0115680266324522240725053634 PMID: 39136506

Bhatt, P., Singh, S., Kumar, V., Nagarajan, K., Mishra, S. K., Dixit, P. K., Kumar, V., & Kumar, S. (2024). Artificial intelligence in pharmaceutical industry: Revolutionizing drug development and delivery. *Current Artificial Intelligence*, *2*(1), E051223224198. DOI: 10.2174/0129503752250813231124092946

Bhattamisra, S. K., Banerjee, P., Gupta, P., Mayuren, J., Patra, S., & Candasamy, M. (2023). Artificial intelligence in pharmaceutical and healthcare research. *Big Data and Cognitive Computing*, *7*(1), 10. DOI: 10.3390/bdcc7010010

Choudhury, C., Murugan, N. A., & Priyakumar, U. D. (2022). Structure-based drug repurposing: Traditional and advanced AI/ML-aided methods. *Drug Discovery Today*, *27*(7), 1847–1861. DOI: 10.1016/j.drudis.2022.03.006 PMID: 35301148

Durairaj, M., Jayakumar, S., Karpagavalli, V., Maheswari, B. U., & Boopathi, S. (2023). Utilization of Digital Tools in the Indian Higher Education System During Health Crises. In *Multidisciplinary Approaches to Organizational Governance During Health Crises* (pp. 1–21). IGI Global. DOI: 10.4018/978-1-7998-9213-7.ch001

Gopi, B., Sworna Kokila, M. L., Bibin, C. V., Sasikala, D., Howard, E., & Boopathi, S. (2024). Distributed Technologies Using AI/ML Techniques for Healthcare Applications. In *Advances in Human and Social Aspects of Technology* (pp. 375–396). IGI Global. DOI: 10.4018/979-8-3693-2569-8.ch019

Gude, S., & Gude, Y. S.GUDE. (2024). The synergy of artificial intelligence and machine learning in revolutionizing pharmaceutical regulatory affairs. *Translational and Regulatory Sciences*, *6*(2), 37–45. DOI: 10.33611/trs.2024-005

Harvey, H. B., & Gowda, V. (2021). Regulatory issues and challenges to artificial intelligence adoption. *Radiologia Clinica*, *59*(6), 1075–1083. DOI: 10.1016/j.rcl.2021.07.007 PMID: 34689875

Jiang, J., Ma, X., Ouyang, D., & Williams, R. O.III. (2022). Emerging artificial intelligence (AI) technologies used in the development of solid dosage forms. *Pharmaceutics*, *14*(11), 2257. DOI: 10.3390/pharmaceutics14112257 PMID: 36365076

Khadela, A., Popat, S., Ajabiya, J., Valu, D., Savale, S., & Chavda, V. P. (2023). AI, ML and other bioinformatics tools for preclinical and clinical development of drug products. *Bioinformatics Tools for Pharmaceutical Drug Product Development*, 255–284.

Kolluri, S., Lin, J., Liu, R., Zhang, Y., & Zhang, W. (2022). Machine learning and artificial intelligence in pharmaceutical research and development: A review. *The AAPS Journal*, *24*(1), 1–10. DOI: 10.1208/s12248-021-00644-3 PMID: 34984579

Koshechkin, K. A., Lebedev, G. S., Fartushnyi, E. N., & Orlov, Y. L. (2022). Holistic approach for artificial intelligence implementation in pharmaceutical products lifecycle: A meta-analysis. *Applied Sciences (Basel, Switzerland)*, *12*(16), 8373. DOI: 10.3390/app12168373

Lou, B., & Wu, L. (2021). AI on drugs: Can artificial intelligence accelerate drug development? Evidence from a large-scale examination of bio-pharma firms. *Evidence from a Large-Scale Examination of Bio-Pharma Firms,(March 15, 2021). Management Information Systems Quarterly*, *45*(3), 1451–1482. DOI: 10.25300/MISQ/2021/16565

Lu, M., Yin, J., Zhu, Q., Lin, G., Mou, M., Liu, F., Pan, Z., You, N., Lian, X., Li, F., Zhang, H., Zheng, L., Zhang, W., Zhang, H., Shen, Z., Gu, Z., Li, H., & Zhu, F. (2023). Artificial intelligence in pharmaceutical sciences. *Engineering (Beijing)*, *27*, 37–69. DOI: 10.1016/j.eng.2023.01.014

Malathi, J., Kusha, K., Isaac, S., Ramesh, A., Rajendiran, M., & Boopathi, S. (2024). IoT-Enabled Remote Patient Monitoring for Chronic Disease Management and Cost Savings: Transforming Healthcare. In *Advances in Explainable AI Applications for Smart Cities* (pp. 371–388). IGI Global.

Patel, V., & Shah, M. (2022). Artificial intelligence and machine learning in drug discovery and development. *Intelligent Medicine*, *2*(3), 134–140. DOI: 10.1016/j.imed.2021.10.001

Patil, R. S., Kulkarni, S. B., & Gaikwad, V. L. (2023). Artificial intelligence in pharmaceutical regulatory affairs. *Drug Discovery Today*, *28*(9), 103700. DOI: 10.1016/j.drudis.2023.103700 PMID: 37442291

Pitchai, R., Guru, K. V., Gandhi, J. N., Komala, C. R., Kumar, J. R. D., & Boopathi, S. (2024). Fog Computing-Integrated ML-Based Framework and Solutions for Intelligent Systems: Digital Healthcare Applications. In *Technological Advancements in Data Processing for Next Generation Intelligent Systems* (pp. 196–224). IGI Global. DOI: 10.4018/979-8-3693-0968-1.ch008

Ramudu, K., Mohan, V. M., Jyothirmai, D., Prasad, D., Agrawal, R., & Boopathi, S. (2023). Machine Learning and Artificial Intelligence in Disease Prediction: Applications, Challenges, Limitations, Case Studies, and Future Directions. In *Contemporary Applications of Data Fusion for Advanced Healthcare Informatics* (pp. 297–318). IGI Global.

Raza, M. A., Aziz, S., Noreen, M., Saeed, A., Anjum, I., Ahmed, M., & Raza, S. M. (2022). Artificial intelligence (AI) in pharmacy: An overview of innovations. *Innovations in Pharmacy*, *13*(2), 10–24926. DOI: 10.24926/iip.v13i2.4839 PMID: 36654703

Sahu, A., Mishra, J., & Kushwaha, N. (2022). Artificial intelligence (AI) in drugs and pharmaceuticals. *Combinatorial Chemistry & High Throughput Screening*, *25*(11), 1818–1837. DOI: 10.2174/1386207325666211207153943 PMID: 34875986

Selvaraj, C., Chandra, I., & Singh, S. K. (2022). Artificial intelligence and machine learning approaches for drug design: Challenges and opportunities for the pharmaceutical industries. *Molecular Diversity*, *26*(3), 1–21. DOI: 10.1007/s11030-021-10326-z PMID: 34686947

Shaki, F., Amirkhanloo, M., Jahani, D., & Chahardori, M. (2024a). Artificial intelligence in pharmaceuticals: Exploring applications and legal challenges. *Pharmaceutical and Biomedical Research*, *10*(1), 1–10. DOI: 10.32598/PBR.10.1.1257.1

Shaki, F., Amirkhanloo, M., Jahani, D., & Chahardori, M. (2024b). Artificial intelligence in pharmaceuticals: Exploring applications and legal challenges. *Pharmaceutical and Biomedical Research*, *10*(1), 1–10. DOI: 10.32598/PBR.10.1.1257.1

Shinde, A., Pawar, D., & Sonawane, K. (2021). Automation in pharmaceutical sector by implementation of artificial intelligence platform: A way forward. *International Journal of Basic and Clinical Pharmacology*, *10*(7), 863–869. DOI: 10.18203/2319-2003.ijbcp20212387

Upadhyaya, A. N., Saqib, A., Devi, J. V., Rallapalli, S., Sudha, S., & Boopathi, S. (2024). Implementation of the Internet of Things (IoT) in Remote Healthcare. In *Advances in Medical Technologies and Clinical Practice* (pp. 104–124). IGI Global. DOI: 10.4018/979-8-3693-1934-5.ch006

Vora, L. K., Gholap, A. D., Jetha, K., Thakur, R. R. S., Solanki, H. K., & Chavda, V. P. (2023a). Artificial intelligence in pharmaceutical technology and drug delivery design. *Pharmaceutics*, *15*(7), 1916. DOI: 10.3390/pharmaceutics15071916 PMID: 37514102

Vora, L. K., Gholap, A. D., Jetha, K., Thakur, R. R. S., Solanki, H. K., & Chavda, V. P. (2023b). Artificial intelligence in pharmaceutical technology and drug delivery design. *Pharmaceutics*, *15*(7), 1916. DOI: 10.3390/pharmaceutics15071916 PMID: 37514102

Wan, Z., Sun, X., Li, Y., Chu, T., Hao, X., Cao, Y., & Zhang, P. (2025). Applications of Artificial Intelligence in Drug Repurposing. *Advancement of Science*, *12*(14), 2411325. DOI: 10.1002/advs.202411325 PMID: 40047357

KEY TERMS AND DEFINITIONS

AI: Artificial Intelligence
HER: Electronic Health Records
OPTIM: Optimization
ADMET: Absorption, Distribution, Metabolism, Excretion, and Toxicity
FDA: Food and Drug Administration
NLP: Natural Language Processing
IBM: International Business Machines
GAN: Generative Adversarial Network
ADR: Adverse Drug Reaction
PII: Personally Identifiable Information
GDPR: General Data Protection Regulation
HIPAA: Health Insurance Portability and Accountability Act
IP: Intellectual Property (or Internet Protocol, depending on context)
XAI: Explainable Artificial Intelligence
EMA: European Medicines Agency

ALS: Amyotrophic Lateral Sclerosis
NIH: National Institutes of Health

Chapter 3

Quantum Computing in Drug Discovery: Revolutionizing Pharmaceutical Research

Anandhavalli Muniasamy
https://orcid.org/0000-0001-8940-3954
Department of Informatics and Computer Systems, College of Computer Science, King Khalid University, Saudi Arabia

ABSTRACT

The integration of quantum computing in drug discovery has the potential to revolutionize pharmaceutical research by significantly enhancing molecular simulations, drug screening, and optimization processes. Traditional computational methods often struggle with the complexity of molecular interactions, leading to high costs and extended timelines in drug development. Quantum computing, with its ability to process complex calculations exponentially faster than classical computers, offers innovative solutions to these challenges. This chapter explores the fundamentals of quantum computing, its application in pharmaceutical research, and real-world case studies from leading organizations. It also discusses existing challenges, potential solutions, and future directions for adopting quantum computing in drug discovery. By addressing key technical, ethical, and regulatory aspects, this chapter provides a comprehensive analysis of how quantum technologies can accelerate and optimize the drug discovery pipeline.

DOI: 10.4018/979-8-3373-2043-4.ch003

INTRODUCTION

The pharmaceutical industry faces significant challenges in drug discovery, including high costs, lengthy development timelines, and complex molecular interactions. Quantum computing (QC) emerges as a transformative technology with the potential to address these challenges by enabling more accurate simulations of molecular systems and accelerating the drug development process. By leveraging principles of quantum mechanics, QC offers a new paradigm for computational chemistry, promising to revolutionize pharmaceutical research.

Drug discovery is a multifaceted process that involves understanding the biological mechanisms of diseases, identifying suitable targets (usually proteins), discovering or designing compounds that interact with these targets, and optimizing those compounds for safety, efficacy, and bioavailability. Traditional approaches, while effective in many cases, are often hindered by the immense complexity of molecular interactions and the astronomical number of possible compound configurations. Classical computers, even with modern advancements, struggle with simulating quantum mechanical systems at the atomic and subatomic levels, which are essential for accurate molecular modeling.

This is where quantum computing offers a paradigm shift. Quantum computers operate on the principles of quantum mechanics, using quantum bits (qubits) instead of classical bits. Unlike classical bits that are either 0 or 1, qubits can exist in superposition—being both 0 and 1 at the same time. Additionally, quantum phenomena such as entanglement and interference allow quantum systems to process and correlate vast amounts of information simultaneously. These unique properties enable quantum computers to perform complex calculations that are exponentially faster than their classical counterparts, especially in fields like quantum chemistry, optimization, and machine learning—all of which are integral to modern drug discovery pipelines.

One of the most promising applications of quantum computing in drug discovery is in molecular simulation. Accurately modeling how molecules behave, interact, and react requires solving the Schrödinger equation, a task that becomes intractable for classical systems as molecular size increases. Quantum computers, however, are naturally suited for these tasks. Algorithms such as the Variational Quantum Eigensolver (VQE) and Quantum Phase Estimation (QPE) have shown potential for computing ground-state energies of molecules, predicting chemical reactivity, and simulating enzymatic processes with unprecedented precision. These capabilities can lead to the design of novel compounds that target diseases more effectively while minimizing side effects.

Another key area where quantum computing is poised to make an impact is protein-ligand binding prediction. Understanding how a drug molecule binds to its target protein is central to assessing its therapeutic potential. Classical docking simulations rely on approximations that may not capture the full complexity of quantum interactions. Quantum simulations, on the other hand, can provide a more detailed and accurate picture of binding affinities and interaction dynamics, thereby improving hit-to-lead success rates.

Furthermore, quantum computing contributes significantly to lead optimization, a phase where initial drug candidates are refined to improve potency, selectivity, and pharmacokinetic properties. By enabling more accurate predictions of how slight chemical modifications affect molecular behavior, quantum algorithms reduce the need for extensive experimental testing, accelerating the path from discovery to clinical trials.

Quantum computing also enhances virtual screening, a computational process that evaluates large libraries of compounds to identify those most likely to be biologically active. Quantum-enhanced machine learning models, including quantum neural networks and kernel methods, can analyze complex molecular datasets more efficiently and with greater accuracy. This capability not only speeds up the screening process but also opens up the possibility of discovering entirely new chemical scaffolds that may be overlooked by classical methods.

Moreover, protein structure prediction, an essential step in target identification, benefits from quantum approaches. Predicting how a linear chain of amino acids folds into a functional 3D protein structure is a formidable computational challenge. Quantum algorithms and quantum annealing methods can explore the vast energy landscape of folding configurations more effectively, providing valuable insights for rational drug design.

While the theoretical promise of quantum computing in drug discovery is compelling, practical implementation is still in its early stages. Current quantum hardware, known as Noisy Intermediate-Scale Quantum (NISQ) devices, is limited by decoherence, noise, and qubit scalability. However, hybrid quantum-classical computing offers a pragmatic solution. In hybrid models, quantum processors are used for the parts of computations that benefit most from quantum speed-up, while classical computers handle the remaining tasks. Algorithms like VQE and the Quantum Approximate Optimization Algorithm (QAOA) exemplify this approach, enabling near-term quantum advantage for specific sub-problems in drug discovery.

The integration of quantum computing with existing pharmaceutical R&D frameworks also requires collaboration across disciplines—combining the expertise of quantum physicists, chemists, computational biologists, and data scientists. Companies and academic institutions are increasingly investing in this space. Leading pharmaceutical firms such as Roche, Pfizer, and Boehringer Ingelheim are partnering with quantum technology companies to explore applications ranging from molecular modeling to supply chain optimization. Meanwhile, quantum startups like Rigetti, IonQ, and Xanadu are developing platforms and software tailored to the needs of drug discovery.

Governments and international organizations are also recognizing the strategic importance of quantum technologies. Public funding initiatives and national quantum programs are accelerating research and infrastructure development, creating an ecosystem that supports innovation in quantum pharmaceutical applications. Additionally, open-source quantum programming frameworks like IBM Qiskit, Google Cirq, and Microsoft Q# are democratizing access to quantum tools, enabling a wider range of researchers to experiment and contribute to this evolving field.

The pharmaceutical industry faces significant challenges in drug discovery, including high costs, lengthy development timelines, and complex molecular interactions. The pharmaceutical industry stands on the cusp of a technological revolution, driven by the burgeoning field of quantum computing. Quantum computing (QC) emerges as a transformative technology with the potential to address these challenges by enabling more accurate simulations of molecular systems and accelerating the drug development process. By leveraging principles of quantum mechanics, QC offers a new paradigm for computational chemistry, promising to revolutionize pharmaceutical research.Traditional drug discovery methods, while successful in the past, are often slow, expensive, and limited by their inability to accurately simulate the complex interactions of molecules within biological systems. The promise of quantum computing lies in its potential to overcome these limitations, offering unprecedented computational power to model molecular behavior, accelerate drug design, and ultimately revolutionize the way we develop new therapies. This chapter explores the potential of quantum computing to transform pharmaceutical research and targets to achieve the following objectives.

- **Understand the fundamentals of quantum computing** and how it differs from classical computing in the context of pharmaceutical research.
- **Explain the limitations of traditional computational methods** in drug discovery and how quantum computing addresses these challenges.
- **Analyze real-world case studies** highlighting the implementation of quantum technologies by leading pharmaceutical organizations.
- **Identify current challenges and limitations** associated with the adoption of quantum computing in drug discovery.
- **Evaluate potential solutions and future directions** for integrating quantum computing into pharmaceutical research and development.
- **Examine the ethical, technical, and regulatory considerations** related to the use of quantum computing in healthcare and drug development.

By harnessing the power of quantum mechanics, we can unlock new possibilities for creating more effective, targeted, and personalized medicines.

BACKGROUND

Traditional drug discovery relies heavily on classical computational methods, such as molecular dynamics simulations and density functional theory, to predict molecular behavior. However, these methods often fall short when dealing with complex biological systems due to computational limitations. Quantum computing, utilizing qubits and quantum algorithms, can process information in ways unattainable by classical computers, allowing for the simulation of complex molecular interactions with higher accuracy.

Traditional Drug Discovery Methods and Their Limitations

Traditional drug discovery is a complex, lengthy, and expensive process that typically involves several stages, from target identification to clinical trials.

The journey of developing a new therapeutic drug is a long, complex, and high-risk endeavor that spans several critical stages, each with its own scientific, technical, and logistical challenges. Despite advancements in biomedical research and computational technologies, the process remains both time-consuming and costly, with an average drug taking over a decade to reach the market and costs exceeding billions of dollars. The drug discovery pipeline can broadly be divided into five key stages: Target Identification and Validation, Hit Identification, Lead Optimization, Preclinical Development, and Clinical Trials. Each stage is a crucial milestone, and failure at any point can lead to significant setbacks. Understanding the challenges that occur at each of these stages is essential to innovating and improving drug development strategies.

- **Target Identification and Validation**
- **Hit Identification**
- **Lead Optimization**
- **Clinical Trials**

Target Identification and Validation

The first and foundational step in drug discovery is target identification, a process centered around recognizing a biological molecule—such as a gene, protein, RNA, or signaling pathway—that plays a crucial role in the initiation, development, or maintenance of a particular disease. The goal is to find a component within the complex web of cellular machinery whose modulation—through inhibition, activation, or stabilization—can lead to a desirable therapeutic outcome. Ideal targets are those that are *disease-specific*, meaning their influence is significant in diseased tissue but minimal or absent in healthy systems, reducing the risk of adverse side effects. For instance, in cancer therapy, researchers often look for proteins that are overexpressed in tumor cells but largely inactive in normal cells, such as HER2 in certain types of breast cancer. In neurological diseases like Alzheimer's, the search may focus on proteins like beta-amyloid or tau that accumulate abnormally in the brain. Once a candidate target is identified, the process moves to target validation, where scientists confirm that modulating this target—either by genetic knockdown, gene editing, antibody binding, or small molecule interaction—actually influences the course of the disease. This step involves in vitro experiments using cell lines, in vivo studies in animal models, and increasingly, *in silico* simulations to understand the downstream effects of target manipulation. Target validation is critical for eliminating false positives and ensuring that resources are not wasted on molecules that appear important but have little or no impact when perturbed.

However, this process is far from straightforward due to the intrinsic complexity and variability of biological systems. Diseases like cancer, Alzheimer's disease, Parkinson's, diabetes, and autoimmune disorders are rarely driven by a single gene or protein; instead, they result from a network of interacting pathways, often with overlapping or redundant functions. Pathway cross-talk, feedback loops, and compensatory mechanisms can mask the effects of targeting a single molecule. For instance, blocking one inflammatory cytokine in an autoimmune disease may trigger upregulation of others, rendering the treatment ineffective. Moreover, the behavior of a biological target is not static—it can vary between tissue types, stages of disease progression, and even between patients, depending on factors such as genetic background, epigenetic modifications, and environmental exposures. A target that shows promise in a controlled laboratory setting might behave differently in the dynamic and heterogeneous environment of a human body. This variation introduces significant risk into the drug development pipeline. Another major obstacle is the concept of druggability. Not all biological targets are amenable to therapeutic intervention; for example, some proteins lack a defined binding pocket or are located in cellular compartments that are difficult for drugs to reach. Even among seemingly druggable targets, some prove to be non-essential for disease progression when tested in more rigorous or physiologically relevant models. These misjudgments contribute to the high attrition rate in pharmaceutical R&D—many candidate drugs fail in late-stage clinical trials because the underlying assumption about the target's role in disease was flawed. Therefore, comprehensive validation techniques are essential, including CRISPR-based gene editing, RNA interference

(RNAi) for knockdown studies, transcriptomics and proteomics for expression profiling, and systems biology approaches that model the entire network of interactions rather than isolated components. Integrating these diverse strategies enhances the reliability of target selection, ultimately increasing the chances of developing safe and effective therapies.

Hit Identification

Once a validated target has been firmly established—one that has demonstrated clear involvement in a disease pathway and is shown to be both druggable and functionally impactful—the next crucial phase in the drug discovery process is hit identification. This stage involves discovering chemical compounds, referred to as "hits," that show an initial ability to interact with the biological target of interest in a desirable way. These compounds are potential starting points for further refinement and optimization. The process of identifying hits typically begins with the screening of vast chemical libraries, which can contain anywhere from hundreds of thousands to millions of diverse compounds. There are two main approaches to screening: high-throughput screening (HTS) and virtual screening. In HTS, robotic systems rapidly test thousands of compounds in parallel using automated biochemical or cell-based assays. For example, an assay may measure the inhibition of a target enzyme's activity in the presence of each compound. HTS allows researchers to collect large volumes of data quickly and has led to the discovery of many successful drugs, including HIV protease inhibitors and certain kinase inhibitors used in cancer therapy. On the other hand, virtual screening employs computational tools to simulate the interaction between chemical compounds and the target's three-dimensional structure, predicting binding affinities through molecular docking simulations. This approach is cost-effective and particularly useful when the target's structural data is available through techniques like X-ray crystallography or cryo-electron microscopy. Virtual screening also enables exploration of vast chemical space, including compounds that have never been physically synthesized, expanding the scope of discovery beyond what is feasible in laboratory-based HTS.

Despite the technological advances in both physical and computational screening methods, hit identification remains fraught with challenges. One of the most persistent issues is the limited chemical diversity within screening libraries. Although these libraries may house millions of molecules, they still represent a tiny subset of the estimated 10^{60} possible small molecules in chemical space. This means that even highly comprehensive libraries might miss out on ideal drug candidates simply because those compounds were never synthesized or included in the screen. To address this, pharmaceutical companies and research institutions are increasingly curating diversity-oriented libraries and leveraging AI-driven molecular generation to suggest novel scaffolds that might fill gaps in chemical space. However, even with a well-designed library, screening results often suffer from false positives and false negatives. A false positive is a compound that appears to bind to the target effectively but does so non-specifically, interacting with multiple unrelated proteins. These off-target interactions can result in side effects and toxicity if the compound is not properly filtered out in later stages. Conversely, a false negative might be a compound with genuine therapeutic potential that is overlooked due to limitations in the assay's sensitivity, poor solubility, or inaccuracies in docking algorithms during virtual screening. Another critical concern is the biological relevance of the assay system used in screening. For example, a compound might show promising activity in a biochemical assay that uses isolated proteins, but fail to exhibit similar results in cell-based assays or animal models, where factors like cellular uptake, metabolic stability, and membrane permeability come into play. Additionally, some targets function differently in a living organism than in a controlled lab environment, leading to discrepancies between in vitro and in vivo results. These complexities emphasize the importance of incorporating orthogonal screening methods, including phenotypic screens, and early ADMET (absorption, distribution, metabolism, excretion, and toxicity) profiling, to increase the likelihood that a hit will translate into a viable drug lead. As the field evolves, hybrid approaches that combine HTS, machine learning models, and systems pharmacology frameworks are being developed to improve the precision and reliability of hit identification, ultimately streamlining the path from target to therapeutic.

Lead Optimization

Once a robust set of hits has been identified, the drug discovery process advances into the next critical phase known as lead optimization. This stage involves the selection of a few promising hit compounds, which are then subjected to a series of structural and chemical modifications aimed at refining their pharmacological properties. The main objectives during lead optimization are to enhance potency (how strongly the compound binds to or inhibits the target), selectivity(how specifically it affects the intended target without disturbing other biological pathways), and safety (minimizing toxicity). Researchers also aim to improve ADME properties—absorption, distribution, metabolism, and excretion—to ensure that the compound can effectively reach its site of action in the human body at therapeutic concentrations and for a sufficient duration. To illustrate, a compound that inhibits a kinase involved in cancer might be structurally optimized to ensure it does not also inhibit similar kinases that regulate essential cellular functions in healthy tissue. Lead optimization often requires the synthesis of hundreds or even thousands of analogs of a lead compound, each one varying slightly in structure to assess how small changes affect biological activity. Techniques such as structure-activity relationship (SAR) analysis, quantitative structure-activity relationship (QSAR) modeling, and computational chemistry are routinely employed to prioritize modifications. For example, medicinal chemists may replace a hydrogen atom with a fluorine to block metabolic degradation or introduce polar groups to enhance water solubility. However, this is an iterative and highly complex process—modifications that improve one property may inadvertently worsen another. A molecule made more lipophilic to cross cell membranes might also become more toxic or accumulate in fatty tissues. Balancing such trade-offs requires an integrated, multidisciplinary approach involving chemists, pharmacologists, toxicologists, and computational modelers.

Despite the power of modern tools and techniques, lead optimization remains one of the most resource-intensive and uncertain phases in the drug development pipeline. A compound that appears highly effective in simplified in vitro systems—such as isolated enzymes or cultured cells—may demonstrate unpredictable behavior in vivo, within the complexity of a living organism. One frequent issue is metabolic instability, where a compound is rapidly broken down into inactive or even toxic metabolites by liver enzymes such as cytochrome P450s. Additionally, poor bioavailability, resulting from low solubility or poor membrane permeability, can prevent sufficient drug levels from reaching the intended site of action. Another major concern is off-target toxicity, where the compound unintentionally affects unrelated biological pathways, potentially leading to side effects such as liver damage, cardiac arrhythmias, or immune reactions. In fact, many lead compounds that look promising during optimization ultimately fail in subsequent stages, particularly during preclinical testing, due to unacceptable toxicity profiles or inadequate pharmacokinetic behavior. To mitigate these risks, researchers increasingly employ predictive toxicology platforms, including in silico models, high-content screening assays, and cell-based toxicity panels, during the optimization process. Furthermore, prodrug strategies, in which an inactive or less active compound is converted into the active drug inside the body, are sometimes used to overcome poor absorption or distribution characteristics.

Following successful lead optimization, the most promising candidates proceed to preclinical development, a phase focused on evaluating the compound's safety, efficacy, and pharmacokinetic behavior in biological systems prior to human trials. This involves extensive testing in both in vitro models, such as cultured human cells, and in vivo models, typically using laboratory animals like mice, rats, or dogs. The goal is to generate data that support the compound’s potential for therapeutic benefit and establish an appropriate safety margin. Regulatory agencies like the FDA (U.S. Food and Drug Administration) or EMA (European Medicines Agency) require detailed toxicological and pharmacological assessments before a compound can proceed to clinical trials. These assessments include acute and chronic toxicity, genotoxicity, carcinogenicity, and reproductive toxicity studies. Dosing regimens are also explored, helping researchers identify the maximum tolerated dose (MTD) and the no observed adverse effect level (NOAEL), which inform safe starting doses for human testing. However, a persistent challenge in preclinical development is the translational gap between animal models and human biology. Animal physiology and drug metabolism can differ significantly from that of humans, leading to misleading conclusions. For instance, thalidomide, a drug that caused severe birth defects in humans, did not exhibit teratogenicity in standard rodent models, highlighting the limitations of animal testing.

Moreover, the ethical and logistical concerns surrounding animal experimentation have spurred the development of alternative models aimed at improving predictive accuracy while reducing animal usage. One such innovation is the organ-on-chip platform, which uses microfluidic technology to simulate the microenvironment of human tissues—like liver, heart, or lung—on a small chip for drug testing. Similarly, 3D cell culture systems and organoids, derived from human stem cells, offer more physiologically relevant models compared to traditional 2D cell cultures. These models can recapitulate aspects of tissue architecture and function, allowing for more accurate assessments of drug behavior in human-like environments. Computational models, powered by artificial intelligence and machine learning, are also being integrated into preclinical pipelines to predict toxicity, simulate drug metabolism, and analyze large datasets for early warning signs of potential failure. However, while these technologies hold great promise, they are still in the process of validation and standardization. Regulatory authorities are cautious about replacing established animal models without sufficient evidence of reliability and reproducibility. As such, most drug candidates still require animal testing before moving into clinical trials. Nonetheless, the incorporation of hybrid approaches—combining traditional and emerging methodologies—is becoming increasingly common, marking a shift toward more efficient, ethical, and predictive preclinical development strategies.

Clinical Trials

The final and most resource-intensive stage of drug development is the clinical trial phase, where a drug candidate, having passed extensive preclinical testing, is evaluated in human subjects. Clinical trials are meticulously structured to assess a drug's safety, efficacy, optimal dosage, side effects, and long-term impact in diverse human populations. These trials are typically divided into three sequential phases. Phase I trials are the initial introduction of the drug into humans, involving a small group—usually 20 to 100—of healthy volunteers or, in some cases, patients with the disease. The primary objective of Phase I is to determine the drug's safety profile, including how it is absorbed, distributed, metabolized, and excreted (its pharmacokinetics), as well as to identify any immediate adverse effects. Phase II trials expand the participant pool to several hundred individuals who have the disease or condition the drug is intended to treat. This phase evaluates the drug's efficacy, explores dose-response relationships, and continues monitoring safety. If results are promising, the drug progresses to Phase III, a large-scale, multi-center trial that can include thousands of participants from diverse demographics and geographic locations. This phase is critical for confirming therapeutic efficacy across broad populations, identifying less common side effects, and comparing the new drug to existing standard treatments. It is not uncommon for a single Phase III trial to run for several years and cost upwards of $300 million to $500 million, making it the most expensive step in the development process. Only upon successful completion of Phase III trials can a drug sponsor submit a New Drug Application (NDA) or Biologics License Application (BLA) to regulatory bodies such as the U.S. Food and Drug Administration (FDA) or the European Medicines Agency (EMA) for approval to market the drug.

While drug discovery has led to the development of many life-saving medications, it suffers from several limitations (Paul et al., 2010) as shown in figure 1.

Figure 1. Traditional Drug Discovery Methods and Their Limitations

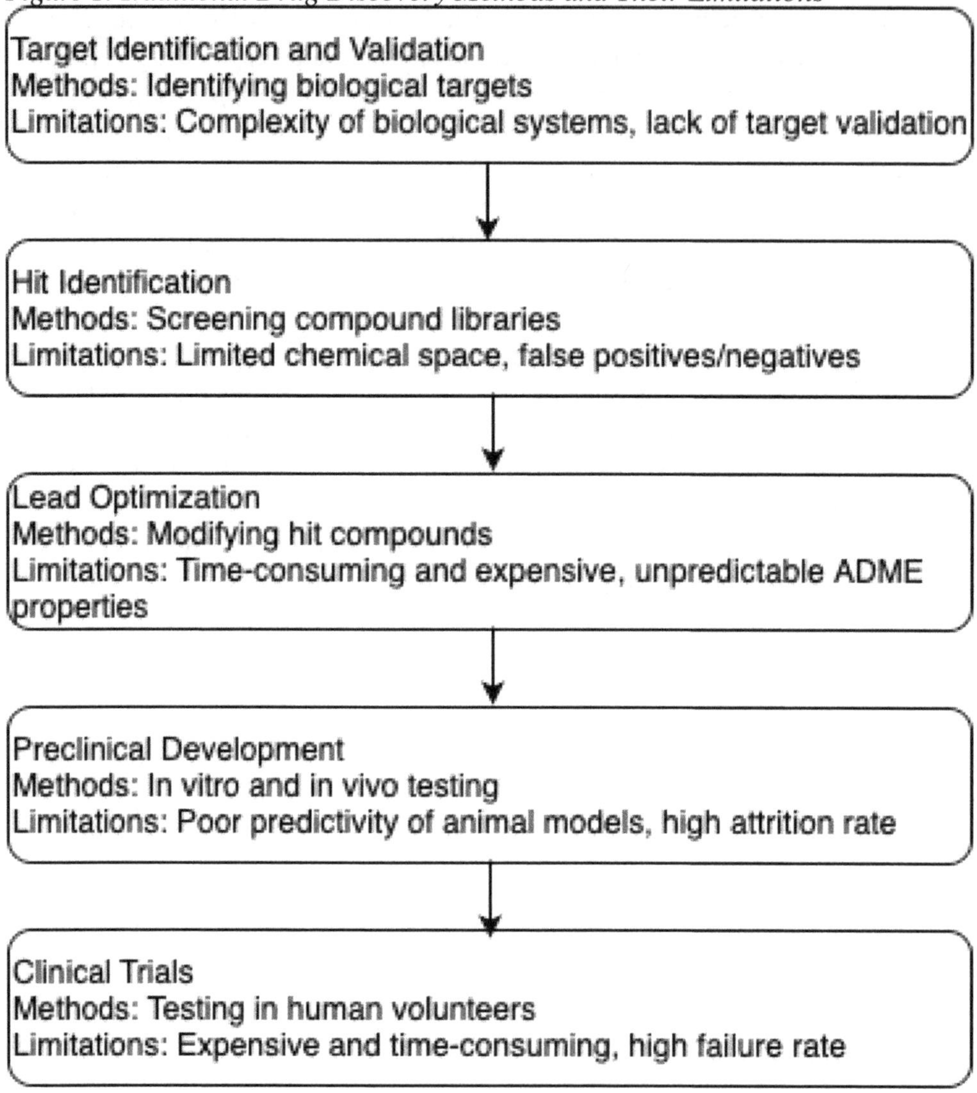

Traditional drug discovery is marked by high costs (often billions of dollars), lengthy timelines (10–15 years), and a high rate of failure. These inefficiencies highlight the pressing need for advanced technologies—like quantum computing—to revolutionize the drug discovery. Boston Consulting Group (BCG) projects (Boston Consulting Group, 2019) that hybrid quantum-classical approaches could reduce drug discovery timelines by 30–50% compared to classical methods. McKinsey & Company (2023) estimates 25–60% cost reductions in preclinical stages (e.g., target identification, lead optimization) through quantum simulation. 65% of top pharmaceutical companies have initiated partnerships or investments in quantum computing as of 2023, signaling rapid adoption (L.E.K. Consulting, 2024).

Quantum Computing Basics

In the fascinating and rapidly evolving field of quantum computing, the qubit, or quantum bit, serves as the fundamental unit of quantum information. Unlike a classical bit, which can exist in only one of two possible states—either a 0 or a 1—a qubit leverages the principles of quantum mechanics to exist in a superposition of both states at the same time. This unique property allows a qubit to be represented mathematically as $|\psi\rangle = \alpha|0\rangle + \beta|1\rangle$, where $|0\rangle$ and $|1\rangle$ denote the standard computational basis states. The coefficients α and β are complex numbers that satisfy the normalization condition $|\alpha|^2 + |\beta|^2 = 1$. This condition ensures that the total probability of measuring the qubit in either of the two states equals one. When a measurement is performed on the qubit, it collapses from its superposed state into one of the basis states—either $|0\rangle$ or $|1\rangle$—with probabilities $|\alpha|^2$ and $|\beta|^2$, respectively. These principles form the foundation of quantum computing's power and potential (Priya et al., 2025) as shown in figure 2.

Figure 2. Quantum Computing Model

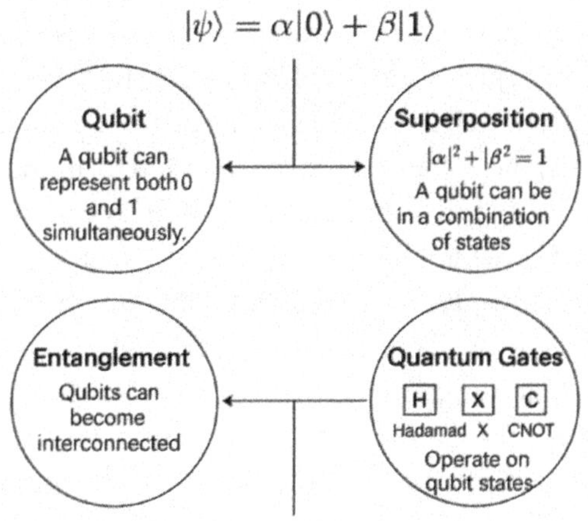

The concept of superposition is one of the defining characteristics that distinguish quantum computing from classical computing. While a classical system operating with *n* bits can represent only one of 2^N possible combinations of 0s and 1s at any given time, a quantum system with *n* qubits can represent all 2^N combinations simultaneously due to superposition. This exponential growth in representational capacity allows quantum computers to process and store vastly more information in parallel than their classical counterparts, making them particularly promising for solving certain complex problems that are currently intractable for classical machines.

Another cornerstone of quantum computing is entanglement, a mysterious and non-intuitive phenomenon that Einstein once famously referred to as "spooky action at a distance." When two or more qubits become entangled, their states are no longer independent; instead, the state of one qubit becomes directly and instantaneously correlated with the state of another, even if the qubits are physically separated by vast distances. In other words, measuring the state of one qubit instantly determines the state of its entangled partner. For instance, consider an entangled state of two qubits known as the Bell state: $|\Phi^+\rangle = (1/\sqrt{2})(|00\rangle + |11\rangle)$. In this configuration, if one qubit is measured and found to be in the state $|0\rangle$, the other qubit will also be found in $|0\rangle$ with certainty—and likewise for $|1\rangle$. Such behavior cannot be explained by classical physics and is a direct consequence of the principles of quantum mechanics.

Entanglement is not just a theoretical curiosity—it has practical implications for quantum information processing. It is a crucial resource for many quantum algorithms, quantum error correction, and quantum communication protocols such as quantum teleportation and quantum key distribution. Entangled qubits can be used to detect eavesdropping in secure communication channels or to link quantum processors in a future quantum internet.

Quantum computations are performed using quantum gates, which are operations that alter the states of qubits in a controlled manner. These gates are the building blocks of quantum circuits, just as classical logic gates like AND, OR, and NOT form the basis of classical digital circuits. However, unlike classical gates that perform irreversible operations, quantum gates are represented by unitary matrices, meaning they preserve the total probability and are reversible. A fundamental quantum gate is the Hadamard gate (H), which places a qubit into a superposition of $|0\rangle$ and $|1\rangle$ if it starts in a basis state. Applying an H gate to $|0\rangle$ transforms it into $(1/\sqrt{2})(|0\rangle + |1\rangle)$, a balanced superposition. This gate is essential for many quantum algorithms because it introduces quantum parallelism.

Another important gate is the Pauli-X gate, which acts as the quantum analog of the classical NOT gate. It flips the state of a qubit: $|0\rangle$ becomes $|1\rangle$ and vice versa. There are also other Pauli gates, such as Pauli-Y and Pauli-Z, which apply different kinds of quantum rotations around the Bloch sphere, a visual representation of qubit states. Each gate affects the state vector in a unique way, and sequences of these gates allow for the construction of complex quantum algorithms.

To enable entanglement and more sophisticated quantum operations, multi-qubit gates are used. The most commonly used among these is the CNOT gate (Controlled NOT), which operates on two qubits: a control qubit and a target qubit. The CNOT gate flips the target qubit only if the control qubit is in the state $|1\rangle$; if the control qubit is in $|0\rangle$, the target remains unchanged. When applied to a qubit in superposition, the CNOT gate can create entanglement between the control and target qubits. For example, applying a Hadamard gate to the control qubit followed by a CNOT gate between the control and target yields the entangled Bell state described earlier.

These gates, when combined appropriately, enable the construction of quantum circuits that can solve a wide range of problems. Notable examples include Shor's algorithm for integer factorization, which has the potential to break widely-used cryptographic systems, and Grover's algorithm for unstructured search, which offers a quadratic speedup over classical algorithms.

The operations on qubits are typically visualized and implemented using quantum circuit diagrams, which provide a schematic representation of the sequence of gates applied to a register of qubits. The design and simulation of such circuits are facilitated by various software tools, such as Qiskit (by IBM), Cirq (by Google), and others.

However, building practical quantum computers is an enormous technical challenge. Qubits are incredibly sensitive to their environment and prone to decoherence, a phenomenon where quantum information is lost due to interaction with external systems. Maintaining the fragile quantum states requires extreme conditions, such as ultra-low temperatures, vacuum environments, and sophisticated error correction techniques. Researchers around the world are actively exploring different physical implementations of qubits, including superconducting circuits, trapped ions, photonic systems, and topological qubits.

Potential of Quantum Computing in Drug Discovery

Quantum computing holds immense potential to revolutionize drug discovery by addressing some of the key limitations of traditional methods.

1. More Accurate Molecular Simulations

Challenge: Traditional methods struggle with accurate molecular simulations due to approximations in quantum effects.

Solution: Quantum computers can simulate quantum systems naturally, enabling precise modeling of molecular interactions.

Impact: Improved drug design (binding affinity, selectivity) and faster discovery by reducing experimental iterations.

2. Enhanced Virtual Screening

Challenge: Traditional virtual screening is limited by chemical library size and scoring accuracy.

Solution: Quantum machine learning can analyze vast chemical libraries and improve binding affinity predictions.

Impact: Discovery of novel drug candidates and fewer false positives, speeding up the screening process.

3. Optimizing Lead Compounds

Challenge: Lead optimization is slow and requires synthesizing many analogs.

Solution: Quantum algorithms can optimize lead compound structures and properties efficiently.

Impact: Faster lead optimization, reduced costs, and improved drug properties (potency, selectivity, ADMET).

4. Personalized Medicine

Challenge: Varied patient responses due to genetic differences.

Solution: Quantum machine learning can analyze patient data to predict individual drug responses.

Impact: Tailored treatments for patients and more efficient clinical trial designs.

Quantum computing has the potential to transform drug discovery by enabling more accurate simulations, enhancing virtual screening, optimizing lead compounds, and facilitating personalized medicine approaches. While the technology is still in its early stages, the potential benefits are enormous. As quantum computers become more powerful and accessible, they are likely to play an increasingly important role in the development of new and improved therapies.

QUANTUM METHODOLOGY CONCEPTS IN DRUG DISCOVERY

The integration of quantum computing in drug discovery faces several challenges, including difficulties in simulating complex molecular interactions and the current limitations of quantum hardware. Data handling and the development of suitable algorithms remain significant hurdles. Additionally, ethical concerns and issues around accessibility must be addressed to ensure equitable and responsible use of quantum technologies. This section focus on the following topics:

1. Challenges in Simulating Molecular Interactions
2. Current Limitations of Quantum Hardware
3. Data Handling and Algorithm Development
4. Ethical and Accessibility Concerns

Challenges in Simulating Molecular Interactions

Accurately simulating molecular interactions is crucial for understanding chemical and biological processes, designing new materials, and developing new drugs. However, this task is fraught with challenges due to the complex nature of molecular systems and the limitations of current computational methods.

1. **Quantum Mechanical Effects:** Molecular interactions are governed by quantum mechanics, which describes the behavior of electrons and nuclei at atomic scales. Accurately simulating these interactions is critical but computationally expensive due to challenges like electron correlation (complex electron interactions requiring high-level methods like coupled cluster theory) and limitations of the Born-Oppenheimer approximation (which fails for processes like proton transfer). Advanced quantum mechanical methods are needed, but their poor scalability with system size remains a bottleneck (Leach et al., 2001).
2. **System Size and Complexity:** Biological systems involve thousands to millions of interacting atoms, making simulations resource-intensive. The exponential scaling of computational cost with system size restricts the study of large molecules or complexes. Multiscale modeling (combining quantum, classical, and coarse-grained methods) is often employed but requires careful validation to ensure accuracy across scales (Mieres-Perez et al., 2020).
3. **Force Field Accuracy:** Force fields approximate molecular interactions but face accuracy limitations. Their reliability depends on parameterization (using experimental or quantum data) and transferability (performance across diverse chemical environments). Poor parameterization or non-transferable force fields can lead to erroneous results, necessitating constant refinement (Merz et al., 2009).
4. **Sampling Problem:** Molecules adopt numerous conformations, and exhaustive sampling is computationally prohibitive. The vast conformational space and complex free energy landscapes (with many local minima) require advanced sampling techniques (e.g., Monte Carlo, enhanced molecular dynamics) to overcome energy barriers and capture biologically relevant states (Shapiro, 2003).

5. **Solvation Effects:** Biological processes occur in solvent environments, but modeling solvation is challenging. Explicit solvent simulations are accurate but computationally costly, while implicit solvent models (e.g., Poisson-Boltzmann) sacrifice detail for efficiency. Choosing the right approach depends on balancing accuracy and computational feasibility (Hansson, 2003).

Overcoming these challenges requires the development of new and improved computational methods, as well as access to powerful computing resources. Quantum computing may offer a promising avenue for addressing some of these challenges by enabling more accurate simulations of quantum mechanical effects.

Current Limitations of Quantum Hardware

While quantum computing holds tremendous promise, the technology is still in its early stages of development. Several limitations in current quantum hardware hinder its ability to solve complex problems effectively.

1. **Qubit Count and Connectivity:** Current quantum computers face limitations due to their small number of qubits and restricted connectivity between them. Many quantum algorithms require a large-scale, interconnected qubit system to surpass classical computers, but scaling up while maintaining reliable qubit interactions remains a challenge. When qubits are not directly connected, additional operations are needed to transfer quantum information, increasing error rates. Research continues to improve architectures for better scalability and connectivity (Oskin et al., 2002).
2. **Qubit Coherence Time:** Qubits are highly sensitive to environmental noise, leading to rapid decoherence—the loss of quantum states essential for computation. The short coherence times of current qubits limit their ability to perform complex calculations before errors dominate. Mitigating decoherence through better materials, error suppression, and isolation techniques is critical for practical quantum computing (Schlosshauer, 2007).
3. **Gate Fidelity:** Quantum gates, which manipulate qubits, are prone to errors due to imperfect control pulses or environmental interference. High gate fidelity is essential for reliable computations, but current systems struggle with error accumulation. Quantum error correction can address this, but it demands significant overhead, requiring many physical qubits to encode a single error-resistant logical qubit (Shor,, 1996).
4. **Control and Calibration:** Precise control and frequent calibration of qubits are necessary for accurate operations, but these processes are complex and resource-intensive. Qubit properties drift over time, requiring regular recalibration to

maintain performance. Advances in control hardware and automated calibration protocols are active areas of research like Industry research from Google, IBM etc.

5. **Temperature Requirements:** Most qubit technologies, such as superconducting circuits, require near-absolute-zero temperatures (millikelvin range) to function, necessitating expensive cryogenic systems. This constraint complicates scalability and integration with classical electronics, driving research into more robust qubit designs that operate at higher temperatures.
6. **Software and Algorithm Development:** Quantum software and algorithms are still in early development, with few user-friendly tools available. While promising algorithms exist for specific problems (e.g., Shor's, Grover's), broader applications require new algorithmic breakthroughs. Improving programming frameworks and educational resources is essential to democratize quantum computing access.

These limitations impact the types of problems that can be solved with current quantum computers. While quantum computers have shown promise for certain applications, they are not yet able to outperform classical computers on most real-world problems. Overcoming these limitations is a major focus of current research and development efforts in the field of quantum computing.

Data Handling and Algorithm Development in Quantum Computing for Drug Discovery

Quantum computing holds immense potential for revolutionizing drug discovery by enabling simulations and computations that are intractable for classical computers. However, the integration of quantum computing into drug discovery workflows requires careful consideration of data handling and algorithm development.

1. **Data Encoding for Quantum Algorithms:** Quantum algorithms require classical data (e.g., molecular structures) to be encoded into quantum states. Different methods—such as amplitude encoding (storing data in qubit probability amplitudes) or angle encoding (mapping data to rotation angles)—can be used, but current qubit limitations necessitate data compression. For example, molecular electronic structures must efficiently encode electron positions and spins into qubits for accurate simulations. Effective encoding schemes are critical for leveraging quantum advantage (Kopczyk, 2018).
2. **Quantum Algorithms for Drug Discovery:** Quantum algorithms can address key drug discovery challenges:

- Quantum Simulation (e.g., Variational Quantum Eigensolver) models molecular properties like energy states.
- Quantum Machine Learning analyzes large datasets to identify drug candidates.
- Quantum Optimization (e.g., QAOA) refines drug molecule structures.

These methods promise faster and more precise solutions but require further development to surpass classical approaches (Biamonte et al., 2017).

3. **Hybrid Quantum-Classical Algorithms:** Hybrid approaches combine classical and quantum computing: classical systems preprocess data, quantum computers handle complex tasks (e.g., molecular simulations), and classical systems interpret results. This synergy mitigates current quantum hardware limitations while still exploiting quantum advantages for specific subtasks (Blunt et al., 2022).
4. **Data Management and Integration:** Integrating quantum computing into drug discovery requires unifying diverse data (experimental, computational, literature) stored in formats like SMILES, PDB, or CSV. Efficient data integration is essential to feed quantum algorithms with high-quality, standardized inputs (Paul et al., 2021).

The successful integration of quantum computing into drug discovery requires careful consideration of data handling and algorithm development. By addressing these challenges, quantum computing has the potential to revolutionize the drug discovery process and lead to the development of new and more effective treatments.

Ethical Considerations for Quantum Computing in Drug Discovery

1. **Accessibility and Equity Challenges**: The transformative potential of quantum computing in drug discovery faces significant accessibility barriers. The technology's exorbitant costs for development and operation, coupled with a severe shortage of quantum-skilled researchers, threaten to create a divide where only well-funded institutions can benefit. Additionally, the field's reliance on comprehensive molecular and clinical datasets - often inaccessible to smaller research groups - further exacerbates equity concerns. These challenges mirror those observed in AI healthcare applications, suggesting similar ethical frameworks may be applicable (Gerke et al., 2021).

2. **Data Privacy and Security Imperatives**: Quantum computing introduces novel data protection challenges, particularly regarding sensitive health information and proprietary research. The technology's ability to potentially crack current encryption standards necessitates the urgent development of quantum-resistant security protocols. Researchers must also navigate the delicate balance between data anonymization for privacy protection and maintaining sufficient data utility for accurate modeling. Effective data governance frameworks will be critical to ensure ethical data usage (Purnamaningsih et al., 2024).
3. **Bias Mitigation Requirements**: The application of quantum computing in drug discovery carries significant risks of perpetuating existing biases. These may originate from biased training data or become embedded in complex, opaque quantum algorithms. Addressing these concerns requires comprehensive data auditing practices, enhanced algorithmic transparency measures, and concerted efforts to diversify the quantum computing workforce to incorporate broader perspectives (Angwin et al., 2016).
4. **Intellectual Property Complexities**: The integration of quantum computing into pharmaceutical research raises unresolved questions about intellectual property rights. Key issues include determining the patent eligibility of quantum algorithms, establishing clear protocols for data ownership in collaborative research, and developing equitable licensing models that balance innovation incentives with broad access to technological benefits (Maskus,, 2012).
5. **Responsible Innovation Framework**: Realizing the full potential of quantum computing in drug discovery while mitigating risks requires a proactive approach to ethical innovation. This includes ongoing engagement with diverse stakeholders, the establishment of clear ethical guidelines specific to quantum applications, and comprehensive education initiatives to inform both developers and the public about the technology's societal implications. Such measures will be crucial for ensuring quantum computing develops in alignment with broader social values and healthcare equity goals.

While quantum computing holds immense promise for revolutionizing drug discovery, it also raises significant ethical and accessibility concerns that must be addressed to ensure equitable and responsible use of this technology. Addressing the ethical and accessibility concerns related to quantum computing in drug discovery is crucial for ensuring that this technology is used responsibly and equitably. By promoting accessibility, protecting data privacy, mitigating bias, addressing intellectual property issues, and fostering responsible innovation, we can harness the full potential of quantum computing to revolutionize pharmaceutical research and improve human health.

Case Study 1. Identifying Novel Antimicrobial Peptides Using QIML

In the pursuit of alternatives to traditional antibiotics, this case study explores how Quantum-Inspired Machine Learning (QIML) models, leveraging concepts of quantum entanglement, can be applied to discover novel antimicrobial peptides (AMPs). By training on existing AMP datasets, the QIML approach identified new peptides with experimentally confirmed antimicrobial properties. This demonstrates the capacity of quantum-inspired models to accelerate the discovery of next-generation antibiotics, offering a timely solution to combat rising antimicrobial resistance.

Accelerating Drug Lead Optimization with Quantum Computing

This case focuses on enhancing the drug lead optimization process, which is crucial for improving the efficacy and safety of potential therapeutics. Using the Variational Quantum Eigensolver (VQE), researchers predicted the binding affinities of chemically modified compounds, identifying modifications that improved molecular interactions with the target. These results were validated through laboratory experiments, showcasing how quantum computing can significantly streamline lead optimization, reducing both time and resources needed in drug development.

Quantum Simulation of Protein-Ligand Binding

To refine structure-based drug design, this case study utilizes quantum simulations capable of accurately modeling electron correlation and polarization effects during protein-ligand interactions. These simulations produced binding affinity predictions that outperformed classical methods in terms of accuracy. By capturing quantum-level interactions, this approach enhances the precision of drug design, leading to more effective and selective therapeutic candidates.

Molecular Docking and Virtual Screening

This case highlights the application of quantum algorithms, including VQE and Quantum Monte Carlo methods, along with quantum machine learning, to enhance molecular docking and virtual screening. These technologies enable faster and more accurate predictions of binding affinities, facilitating the identification of promising drug candidates at early stages. As a result, the process of screening vast chemical libraries is made more efficient, reducing both the time and financial costs typically associated with drug discovery.

Predicting Protein Folding and Structure

Understanding protein folding is fundamental to designing effective drugs, and this study uses quantum annealing, quantum simulations, and machine learning to model the energy landscapes involved in folding. These techniques improved the prediction of protein three-dimensional structures from amino acid sequences, providing more reliable insights into protein function and interactions. This advancement supports targeted drug design by revealing structural details critical to therapeutic targeting.

Table 1. provides summary of the objective, the quantum approach, the respective results and significance of the five case studies related to Quantum Computing in Drug Discovery.

Table 1. Quantum Computing in Drug Discovery: Case Studies

Case Study	Focus	Quantum Approach	Results/Expected Outcome	Significance	Reference
1. Identifying Novel Antimicrobial Peptides Using QIML	Discovering novel AMPs as antibiotic alternatives	Quantum-Inspired ML model using quantum entanglement concepts trained on known AMP datasets	Identified novel AMPs with confirmed antimicrobial activity	Demonstrates QIML's potential to accelerate antibiotic discovery	(Veltri, et al, 2018)
2. Accelerating Drug Lead Optimization with Quantum Computing	Optimizing drug leads for better drug properties	Variational Quantum Eigensolver (VQE) used to predict binding affinities of modified compounds	Found chemical modifications improving lead binding; validated experimentally	Highlights quantum computing's role in speeding up lead optimization	(Zinner et al., 2021)
3. Quantum Simulation of Protein-Ligand Binding	Improving structure-based drug design accuracy	Quantum simulations accounting for electron correlation/ polarization	Provided more accurate binding affinity predictions than classical methods	Enhances design of more effective, selective drugs	(Amabilino et al., 2020)
4. Molecular Docking and Virtual Screening	Faster identification of drug candidates via docking/ screening	Quantum algorithms (VQE, Quantum Monte Carlo); Quantum ML for binding prediction	Enables quicker, more accurate drug candidate identification	Reduces time and cost of early-stage drug discovery	(Cao eta l., 2019)
5. Predicting Protein Folding and Structure	Understanding protein structure to aid drug design	Quantum annealing, simulation, and ML to explore folding energy landscapes	Improved prediction of protein 3D structures from sequences	Facilitates functional understanding and drug targeting of proteins	(Robert et al., 2021)

Applications of Quantum Computing in Drug Discovery

Quantum computing holds transformative potential in drug discovery by solving complex problems that are intractable for classical computers. Here are the key applications:

1. **Molecular Simulation**: Quantum computers can model the behavior of molecules at the quantum level, accounting for electron correlation and interactions with unprecedented accuracy. This improves the prediction of molecular properties, stability, and reactivity—crucial for drug design.
   a. Simulating Molecular Interactions
      - Quantum computers can model molecular structures and interactions at the quantum level, providing insights into protein folding, ligand binding, and reaction mechanisms.
      - Example: Simulating the electronic structure of large molecules (e.g., proteins, DNA, or drug candidates) using quantum phase estimation (QPE) and variational quantum eigensolver (VQE) algorithms.

   b. Predicting Drug-Target Binding Affinities
      - Accurately calculating binding energies between drugs and their targets (e.g., enzymes, receptors) is computationally expensive for classical methods like density functional theory (DFT).
      - Quantum algorithms can provide more precise estimates, improving virtual screening.
2. **Protein-Ligand Binding Prediction**: Quantum algorithms help simulate how drugs interact with target proteins. These simulations yield more accurate binding affinity estimations, supporting the development of more effective and selective drugs.
3. **Lead Optimization**: Techniques like the Variational Quantum Eigensolver (VQE) are used to explore how small chemical changes affect drug activity. This accelerates the refinement of lead compounds, saving time and cost in preclinical development.
4. **Virtual Screening**: Quantum-enhanced machine learning and quantum-inspired algorithms can rapidly screen large chemical libraries to identify promising drug candidates, making early-stage discovery faster and more efficient.
5. **Drug Docking**: Quantum computing improves the precision of docking algorithms by exploring multiple configurations and energy states more thoroughly, leading to better predictions of how drugs fit into their target sites.

6. **Predicting Protein Folding**: Accurate prediction of 3D protein structures from amino acid sequences is critical in drug design. Quantum approaches can explore folding landscapes more efficiently, aiding in target identification and validation.
7. **Multiscale Modeling**: Quantum computing contributes to hybrid multiscale models that link atomic-level interactions with macroscopic biological behavior, offering a holistic view of drug effects.
8. **Optimization Problems**: Quantum algorithms like QAOA are used for complex optimization challenges in drug discovery, including compound synthesis pathways, formulation design, and clinical trial planning.
9. **Accelerating Drug Design and Optimization**

    De Novo Drug Design: Quantum machine learning (QML) can generate novel molecular structures with desired properties by exploring vast chemical spaces more efficiently than classical methods. Example: Quantum generative adversarial networks (QGANs) can propose new drug-like molecules.

    Optimizing Drug Candidates: Hybrid quantum-classical algorithms (e.g., quantum annealing) can optimize molecular properties such as solubility, toxicity, and binding strength. Example: Finding the lowest-energy conformations of a drug molecule to enhance stability and efficacy.
10. Personalized Medicine and Biomarker Discovery: Quantum computing can analyze genomic and proteomic data to identify biomarkers for precision medicine.Example: Optimizing drug combinations for cancer treatment based on a patient's genetic profile.

SOLUTIONS AND RECOMMENDATIONS

To effectively leverage quantum computing for drug discovery while addressing current limitations, a hybrid approach that combines quantum and classical computing resources is highly promising. This section breakdowns main poins of solutions and recommendations centered around hybrid quantum-classical algorithms and covers the following:

- Hybrid Quantum-Classical Algorithms
- Advancements in Quantum Hardware
- Developing Quantum-Specific Software and Tools
- Collaborative Approaches and Data Sharing

1. Hybrid Quantum-Classical Computing

Hybrid quantum-classical computing combines quantum processors for specialized tasks (like molecular simulations) with classical systems for broader workflows. Key methods include the Variational Quantum Eigensolver (VQE) for molecular energy calculations and the Quantum Approximate Optimization Algorithm (QAOA) for drug docking. These approaches leverage quantum speedups while mitigating hardware limitations (Peruzzo et al., 2014).

Key Algorithms and Their Applications

Variational Quantum Eigensolver (VQE):

- Principle: Uses quantum circuits to prepare molecular wavefunctions while relying on classical optimizers to find ground state energies
- Drug discovery applications: Calculating molecular properties, simulating chemical reactions, determining protein-ligand binding affinities
- Advantages: Noise-resistant, works well on current NISQ devices
- Challenges: Requires careful parameter optimization, faces convergence issues for complex molecules

Quantum Machine Learning (QML) Hybrids:

- Approach: Combines classical neural networks with quantum feature maps or quantum neural networks
- Use cases: Virtual screening, toxicity prediction, drug repurposing
- Example: Quantum-enhanced kernel methods for classifying bioactive compounds
- Benefit: Can process high-dimensional chemical data more efficiently than classical ML

Quantum Approximate Optimization Algorithm (QAOA):

- Function: Solves combinatorial optimization problems in drug design
- Applications: Molecular similarity searching, lead compound optimization
- Current limitations: Requires deep circuits that may be noisy on existing hardware

Implementation Strategies

- **Task Partitioning:**
  - o Quantum processors: Handle complex quantum chemistry calculations

- Classical systems: Manage data preprocessing, error mitigation, and result interpretation
- **Error Mitigation Techniques:**
  - Zero-noise extrapolation
  - Probabilistic error cancellation
  - Measurement error mitigation
- **Hybrid Workflow Optimization:**
  - Developing efficient quantum-classical communication protocols
  - Creating adaptive algorithms that adjust based on quantum processor performance

2. Algorithm Development & Optimization

Tailoring hybrid algorithms to drug discovery requires decomposing problems into quantum-solvable components, benchmarking performance, and improving error mitigation. Focus areas include refining VQE for larger molecules and adapting QAOA for virtual screening (Batra et al., 2021).

Superconducting Qubits:

- Current leader in commercial quantum computing
- Recent advances: Improved coherence times (>100 μs), higher gate fidelities (>99.9%)
- Challenges: Requires extreme cryogenic temperatures, susceptible to electromagnetic interference

Photonic Quantum Computing:

- Potential benefits: Room temperature operation, natural for quantum communication
- Development status: Emerging as promising alternative for specific quantum algorithms

3. Resource Allocation & Management

Efficient hybrid workflows demand orchestration tools to integrate quantum/classical tasks, optimize scheduling (e.g., reducing quantum queue times), and leverage cloud platforms for scalable access (Zhahir et al., 2024).

4. Data Management & Integration

Standardizing molecular data formats and building unified platforms are critical to merge quantum simulations with classical and experimental data. Tracking data provenance ensures reproducibility (Batra et al., 2021).

5. Collaboration & Open Science

Progress hinges on interdisciplinary teams (quantum experts and biologists), open-source tools, and shared datasets to accelerate discoveries (Knapp et al., 2015).

By implementing these solutions and recommendations, we can effectively harness the potential of hybrid quantum-classical algorithms to revolutionize drug discovery. This will lead to the development of new and more effective treatments for a wide range of diseases, ultimately improving human health and well-being.

Advancements in Quantum Hardware for Drug Discovery

1. **Improving Qubit Quality & Quantity:** Enhancing qubit coherence (lifespan of quantum states), gate fidelity (operation accuracy), and connectivity is critical for reliable quantum computations. Scaling up qubit numbers enables simulations of larger molecular systems, essential for drug discovery. Fault-tolerant quantum computing remains a key goal (Katabarwa et al., 2024).
2. Exploring Qubit Technologies

Different qubit platforms offer unique advantages:

- **Superconducting qubits** (scalable, manufacturable)
- **Trapped ions** (high fidelity, long coherence)
- **Photonic qubits** (low noise, high speed)
- **Topological qubits** (intrinsic error resistance)

Diversifying research across these technologies ensures progress despite hardware limitations .

3. **Error Correction & Fault Tolerance:** Quantum error correction (QEC) and fault-tolerant designs are essential to mitigate noise and errors. Techniques like surface codes protect quantum data, enabling reliable computations despite imperfect hardware (Kitaev 2003).

4. **Hardware-Software Co-Design:** Optimizing quantum algorithms for specific hardware (e.g., tailoring circuits for superconducting qubits) and improving quantum compilers boosts efficiency. Collaboration between hardware engineers and algorithm developers is key (Abhijith et al., 2018).
5. **Standardized Benchmarks:** Metrics like Quantum Volume assess overall performance, while drug discovery-specific benchmarks evaluate practical utility. Standardization ensures meaningful progress comparisons (Cross et al., 2019).

Hardware Requirements for Drug Discovery

1. **Qubit Count and Quality:**
    - o Near-term target: 100+ high-quality logical qubits
    - o Long-term need: 1,000+ error-corrected qubits for full molecular simulations
2. **Error Correction:**
    - o Surface code implementations
    - o Lattice surgery techniques
    - o Trade-offs between physical and logical qubit overhead
3. **Specialized Architectures:**
    - o Quantum processors optimized for chemistry simulations
    - o Dedicated quantum coprocessors for pharmaceutical applications

Industry Progress and Roadmaps

- IBM's quantum roadmap targeting 1,000+ qubit processors by 2025
- Google's focus on error correction and logical qubits
- Startup innovations in alternative qubit technologies

Developing Quantum-Specific Software and Tools for Drug Discovery

To fully realize quantum computing's potential in drug discovery, robust and accessible software tools must be developed. Key recommendations include:

1. **Quantum Algorithm Libraries:** Pre-built, modular quantum algorithms optimized for drug discovery tasks (e.g., molecular simulations, virtual screening) can accelerate research. Open-source frameworks like PennyLane enable cross-platform compatibility and community-driven improvements, ensuring adaptability to different quantum hardware.

2. **Quantum Simulation Software:** Specialized tools for simulating molecular and protein interactions must balance accuracy and scalability. Platforms like OpenFermion translate quantum chemistry problems into executable quantum circuits while integrating with classical simulation tools for hybrid workflows.
3. **Quantum Programming Languages & Compilers:** High-level languages (e.g., Qiskit) abstract hardware complexities, while optimizing compilers reduce gate counts and embed error mitigation. This simplifies quantum programming for non-experts and improves computational efficiency.
4. **Quantum Data Analysis & Visualization:** Interactive visualization tools and statistical/machine learning integration help interpret quantum simulation results, identifying patterns in molecular behavior that guide drug design.
5. **User-Friendly Interfaces:** Drag-and-drop circuit builders, IDE-style code editors, and debugging tools (e.g., IBM Quantum Composer) lower barriers to entry, enabling broader adoption by pharmaceutical researchers.

Essential Software Components

Quantum Chemistry Packages:

- PennyLane for quantum machine learning
- Qiskit Nature for molecular simulations
- Microsoft's Q# chemistry library

Development Frameworks:

- Hybrid programming models
- Quantum-classical compilers
- Automatic differentiation for variational algorithms

Visualization and Analysis Tools:

- Molecular orbital visualization in quantum context
- Interactive quantum circuit debuggers
- Performance benchmarking suites

These tools will bridge the gap between quantum theory and practical drug discovery, enabling faster, more precise development of therapeutics. Open-source collaboration and hardware-aware design are critical for success. The development of quantum-specific software and tools will greatly accelerate the adoption of quantum computing in drug discovery. By providing researchers with the tools they need to harness the power of quantum computers, we can unlock new possibilities for discovering and developing life-saving drugs.

FUTURE RESEARCH DIRECTIONS

1. Quantum Machine Learning (QML) for Drug Design
    - **Focus:** Using QML to enhance drug discovery stages (target identification, hit discovery, lead optimization).
    - **Potential:** Uncovers complex biological patterns missed by classical ML, leading to more effective drugs.
    - **Research Areas:**
        - o Developing QML algorithms for drug discovery.
        - o Integrating QML with existing computational methods.
2. Quantum Simulation of Biological Systems
    - **Focus:** Simulating molecules and biological systems at the atomic level using quantum computers.
    - **Potential:** Improves understanding of molecular interactions, protein folding, and drug-target binding for better drug efficacy.
    - **Research Areas:**
        - o Quantum algorithms for molecular dynamics and chemical reactions.
        - o Studying protein folding, enzyme catalysis, and drug interactions.
3. Personalized Medicine & Quantum Computing
    - **Focus:** Using quantum computing to analyze patient-specific data for tailored drug treatments.
    - **Potential:** Enables more effective, personalized therapies with fewer side effects.
    - **Research Areas:**
        - o Quantum algorithms for genomic/proteomic data analysis.
        - o Predicting individual drug responses using QML.
4. Long-Term Impact on the Pharmaceutical Industry
    - **Potential Benefits:** Faster drug discovery, lower costs, higher clinical trial success rates.
    - **Key Considerations:**
        - o Development of fault-tolerant quantum computers.
        - o Skilled workforce and integration into existing workflows.

General Considerations for Future Research

- **Hardware:** Need for improved qubit stability and scalability.
- **Software:** User-friendly quantum tools for pharmaceutical researchers.
- **Collaboration:** Partnerships between quantum experts, pharma researchers, and regulators.

CONCLUSION

Quantum computing stands poised to revolutionize drug discovery by offering unprecedented capabilities in simulating molecular interactions and accelerating the development of new therapeutics. While challenges remain in terms of technology maturity, integration, and data management, strategic investments and collaborative efforts can pave the way for QC's transformative impact on pharmaceutical research. As the field progresses, continued research and development will be essential to fully realize the potential of quantum computing in revolutionizing drug discovery.

Quantum computing stands poised to revolutionize pharmaceutical research, offering unprecedented capabilities to accelerate drug discovery, improve efficacy, and personalize treatments. By harnessing the principles of quantum mechanics, researchers can tackle challenges currently insurmountable for classical computing, potentially transforming the entire drug development pipeline.

Quantum machine learning presents a powerful avenue for analyzing complex biological datasets, identifying novel drug targets, and optimizing lead compounds. While still in its early stages, QML algorithms promise to uncover intricate patterns and relationships that can significantly enhance drug design. Quantum simulation offers the potential to model molecular interactions and biological systems with unparalleled accuracy. This capability could lead to a deeper understanding of drug-target binding, protein folding, and other fundamental processes, enabling the design of more effective and safer drugs.

Furthermore, quantum computing holds immense promise for personalized medicine. By analyzing individual patient data, including genomic and proteomic profiles, quantum algorithms can help tailor drug treatments to specific individuals, maximizing therapeutic benefits and minimizing adverse effects.

While the field is still developing, the long-term impact of quantum computing on the pharmaceutical industry is expected to be transformative. Quantum computing can significantly reduce drug discovery timelines, lower development costs, and increase the success rates of clinical trials. However, realizing this potential requires ongoing advancements in quantum hardware and software, as well as close collaboration between quantum computing experts, pharmaceutical researchers, and regulatory agencies. As quantum technology matures, its integration into existing drug discovery workflows will be crucial.

In conclusion, quantum computing represents a paradigm shift in pharmaceutical research. By embracing these innovative approaches, the pharmaceutical industry can usher in a new era of drug discovery, leading to more effective, personalized, and life-saving treatments for patients worldwide. The journey is just beginning, but the potential rewards are immense, promising to reshape the future of medicine.

REFERENCES

Abhijith, J., Adedoyin, A., Ambrosiano, J., Anisimov, P., Casper, W., Chennupati, G., Coffrin, C., Djidjev, H., Gunter, D., Karra, S., Lemons, N., Lin, S., Malyzhenkov, A., Mascarenas, D., Mniszewski, S., Nadiga, B., O'Malley, D., Oyen, D., Pakin, S., & Lokhov, A. (2018). Quantum algorithm implementations for beginners [Preprint]. arXiv. https://doi.org//arXiv.1804.03719DOI: 10.48550

Amabilino, S., Pogány, P., Pickett, S. D., & Green, D. V. S. (2020). Guidelines for recurrent neural network transfer learning-based molecular generation of focused libraries. *Journal of Chemical Information and Modeling*, *60*(12), 5699–5713. DOI: 10.1021/acs.jcim.0c00343 PMID: 32659085

Angwin, J., Larson, J., Mattu, S., & Kirchner, L. (2016). *Machine bias: There's software used across the country to predict future criminals. And it's biased against blacks*. ProPublica. https://www.propublica.org/article/machine-bias-risk-assessments-in-criminal-sentencing

Batra, K., Zorn, K. M., Foil, D. H., Minerali, E., Gawriljuk, V. O., Lane, T. R., & Ekins, S. (2021). Quantum machine learning algorithms for drug discovery applications. *Journal of Chemical Information and Modeling*, *61*(6), 2641–2647. DOI: 10.1021/acs.jcim.1c00166 PMID: 34032436

Biamonte, J., Wittek, P., Pancotti, N., Rebentrost, P., Wiebe, N., & Lloyd, S. (2017). Quantum machine learning. *Nature*, *549*(7671), 195–202. DOI: 10.1038/nature23474 PMID: 28905917

Blunt, N. S., Camps, J., Crawford, O., Izsák, R., Leontica, S., Mirani, A., Moylett, A. E., Scivier, S. A., Sünderhauf, C., Schopf, P., Taylor, J. M., & Holzmann, N. (2022). A perspective on quantum computing for computational chemistry. *Journal of Chemical Theory and Computation*, *18*(12), 7001–7023. DOI: 10.1021/acs.jctc.2c00574 PMID: 36355616

Boston Consulting Group (BCG). (2019). *Quantum computing in the life sciences: From hype to reality*. https://www.bcg.com/publications/2019/quantum-computing-transform-biopharma-research-development

Cao, Y., Romero, J., Olson, J. P., Degroote, M., Johnson, P. D., Kieferová, M., Kivlichan, I. D., Menke, T., Peropadre, B., Sawaya, N. P. D., Sim, S., Veis, L., & Aspuru-Guzik, A. (2019). Quantum chemistry in the age of quantum computing. *Chemical Reviews*, *119*(19), 10856–10915. DOI: 10.1021/acs.chemrev.8b00803 PMID: 31469277

Consulting, L. E. K. (2024). *Quantum Computing in Biopharma: Future Prospects and Strategic*. https://www.lek.com/insights/hea/us/ei/quantum-computing-biopharma-future-prospects-and-strategic-insights

Cross, A., Bishop, L., Sheldon, S., Nation, P., & Gambetta, J. (2019). Validating quantum computers using randomized model circuits. *Physical Review. A*, *100*(3), 032328. Advance online publication. DOI: 10.1103/PhysRevA.100.032328

Gerke, S., Minssen, T., & Cohen, G. (2020). Ethical and legal challenges of artificial intelligence-driven healthcare. *The Hastings Center Report*, *50*(1), 22–27. DOI: 10.1002/hast.1084

Hansson, T., Oostenbrink, C., & van Gunsteren, W. (2002). Molecular dynamics simulations. *Current Opinion in Structural Biology*, *12*(2), 190–196. DOI: 10.1016/S0959-440X(02)00308-1 PMID: 11959496

Katabarwa, A., Gratsea, K., Caesura, A., & Johnson, P. D. (2024). Early fault-tolerant quantum computing. *PFX Quantum : a Physical Review Journal*, *5*(2), 020101. DOI: 10.1103/PRXQuantum.5.020101

Kitaev, A. Y. (2003). Fault-tolerant quantum computation by anyons. *Annals of Physics*, *303*(1), 2–30. DOI: 10.1016/S0003-4916(02)00018-0

Knapp, B., Bardenet, R., Bernabeu, M. O., Bordas, R., Bruna, M., Calderhead, B., Cooper, J., Fletcher, A. G., Groen, D., Kuijper, B., Lewis, J., McInerny, G., Minssen, T., Osborne, J., Paulitschke, V., Pitt-Francis, J., Todoric, J., Yates, C. A., Gavaghan, D., & Deane, C. M. (2015). Ten simple rules for a successful cross-disciplinary collaboration. *PLoS Computational Biology*, *11*(4), e1004214. DOI: 10.1371/journal.pcbi.1004214 PMID: 25928184

Kopczyk, D. (2018). Quantum machine learning for data scientists. 10.48550/arXiv.1804.10068.

Leach, A. R. (2001). *Molecular modelling: Principles and applications* (2nd ed.). Pearson Education.

Maskus, K. E. (2012). *Private rights and public problems: The global economics of intellectual property in the digital age*. Peterson Institute for International Economics.

McKinsey & Company. (2023). *Quantum computing's potential in pharmaceuticals: A strategic perspective*. https://www.mckinsey.com/industries/life-sciences/our-insights/pharmas-digital-rx-quantum-computing-in-drug-research-and-development

Merz, K. M., Jr., & Roux, B. (Eds.). (2009). *Biological membranes: A molecular perspective from computation and experiment: Force field development and validation*. Birkhäuser. https://www.nbi.ku.dk/membranes/pdf/1996_HeimburgMarsh_BookChapter.pdf

Mieres-Perez, J., & Sanchez-Garcia, E. (2020). Quantum mechanics/molecular mechanics multiscale modeling of biomolecules. *Advances in Physical Organic Chemistry*, *54*, 65–112. DOI: 10.1016/bs.apoc.2020.08.002

Oskin, M., Chong, F., & Chuang, I. L. (2002). A practical architecture for reliable quantum computers. *Computer*, *35*(1), 79–87. DOI: 10.1109/2.976922

Paul, D., Sanap, G., Shenoy, S., Kalyane, D., Kalia, K., & Tekade, R. K. (2021). Drug discovery in the age of big data: A systematic review. *Current Drug Targets*, *22*(5), 492–510. DOI: 10.2174/1389450122666210126163705

Paul, S. M., Mytelka, D. S., Dunwiddie, C. T., Persinger, C. C., Munos, B. H., Lindborg, S. R., & Schacht, A. L. (2010). How to improve R&D productivity: The pharmaceutical industry's grand challenge. *Nature Reviews. Drug Discovery*, *9*(3), 203–214. DOI: 10.1038/nrd3078 PMID: 20168317

Peruzzo, A., McClean, J., Shadbolt, P., Yung, M. H., Zhou, X. Q., Love, P. J., Aspuru-Guzik, A., & O'Brien, J. L. (2014). A variational eigenvalue solver on a photonic quantum processor. *Nature Communications*, *5*(1), 4213. DOI: 10.1038/ncomms5213 PMID: 25055053

Priya V, , DeepaJersha, , JMadhubhavani, , GMangalya, , TYogesh, , NChellapandi, , T.R.. (2025). Quantum Computing in Drug Discovery. *International Research Journal on Advanced Engineering and Management (IRJAEM). 3*. 770-779. .DOI: 10.47392/IRJAEM.2025.0123

Purnamaningsih, S., Ismono, J., Utami, I., Parlindungan, V., & Hanifah, S. (2024). The Challenges of Data Privacy Laws in the Age of Big Data: Balancing Security, Privacy, and Innovation. *Join: Journal of Social Science.*, *1*(6), 455–465. DOI: 10.59613/gny8bq82

Robert, A., Barkoutsos, P. K., Woerner, S., & Tavernelli, I. (2021). Resource-efficient quantum algorithm for protein folding. *npj Quantum Information, 7*, 38. DOI: 10.1038/s41534-021-00368-4

Schlosshauer, M. (2007). *Decoherence and the quantum-to-classical transition*. Springer., DOI: 10.1007/978-3-540-35775-9

Shapiro, A. (2003). Monte Carlo sampling methods. In Sethi, S. P., Thompson, G. L., & Marti, K. (Eds.), *Handbooks in operations research and management science* (Vol. 10, pp. 353–425). Elsevier., DOI: 10.1016/S0927-0507(03)10006-0

Shor, P. W. (1996). Fault-tolerant quantum computation. In *Proceedings of 37th Conference on Foundations of Computer Science* (pp. 56–65). IEEE. DOI: 10.1109/SFCS.1996.548464

Veltri, D., Kamath, U., & Shehu, A. (2018). Deep learning improves antimicrobial peptide recognition. *Bioinformatics (Oxford, England)*, *34*(16), 2740–2747. DOI: 10.1093/bioinformatics/bty179 PMID: 29590297

Zhahir, Amirul & Mohd, Siti & M Shuhud, Mohd Ilias & Idrus, Bahari & Zainuddin, Hishamuddin & Mohamad Jan, Nurhidaya & Wahiddin, Mohamed Ridza. (2024). Quantum Computing in The Cloud - A Systematic Literature Review. International journal of electrical and computer engineering systems. 15. 185-200. DOI: 10.32985/ijeces.15.2.7

Zinner, M., Dahlhausen, F., Boehme, P., Ehlers, J., Bieske, L., & Fehring, L. (2021). Quantum computing's potential for drug discovery: Early stage industry dynamics. *Drug Discovery Today*, *26*(7), 1680–1688. DOI: 10.1016/j.drudis.2021.06.003 PMID: 34119668

ADDITIONAL READING

Cheng, H. P., Deumens, E., Freericks, J. K., Li, C., & Sanders, B. A. (2020). Application of quantum computing to biochemical systems: A look to the future. *Frontiers in Chemistry*, *8*, 587143. DOI: 10.3389/fchem.2020.587143 PMID: 33330375

Kumar, G., Yadav, S., Mukherjee, A., Hassija, V., & Guizani, M. (2024). Recent advances in quantum computing for drug discovery and development. *IEEE Access : Practical Innovations, Open Solutions*, 1–1. DOI: 10.1109/ACCESS.2023.3272554

Sheikh, M., & Jirvankar, P. (2025). Quantum computing: Unlocking the future of pharmaceutical research and drug discovery. *International Journal of Drug Delivery Technology*, *15*(1), 330–334. DOI: 10.25258/ijddt.15.1.45

Visan, A. I., & Negut, I. (2024). Integrating artificial intelligence for drug discovery in the context of revolutionizing drug delivery. *Life (Chicago, Ill.)*, *14*(2), 233. DOI: 10.3390/life14020233 PMID: 38398742

KEY TERMS AND DEFINITIONS

Quantum Computing (QC): A field of computing based on quantum mechanics principles to perform complex computations more efficiently than classical computers.

Qubits: The basic unit of quantum information that can exist in multiple states simultaneously.

Drug Design: A process of discovering new medications based on knowledge of a biological target.

Clinical Trials: Research studies conducted on humans to evaluate the safety and effectiveness of medical treatments.

Molecular Simulations: Computer-based models that predict molecular behavior and interactions.

Virtual Screening: A computational technique used to identify potential drug candidates from large compound libraries.

Lead Compounds: Chemical compounds that show promising biological activity and are selected for further drug development.

Personalized Medicine: A medical approach that tailors treatment to individual genetic and clinical characteristics.

Born-Oppenheimer Approximation: A quantum chemistry assumption that separates nuclear and electronic motion in molecules.

Multiscale Modeling: A simulation approach that integrates information across different spatial and temporal scales.

Sampling Techniques: Methods used in simulations to explore the possible states or configurations of a system.

Poisson-Boltzmann: A mathematical model used to describe electrostatic interactions in biomolecular systems.

Gate Fidelity: A measure of how accurately a quantum gate performs its intended operation.

Millikelvin Range: Extremely low temperature range near absolute zero used to stabilize quantum systems.

Shor's, Grover: Quantum algorithms for factoring large numbers and searching unsorted databases, respectively.

Data Encoding: The process of translating classical data into a form usable by quantum computers.

Variational Quantum Eigensolver (VQE): A hybrid quantum-classical algorithm for finding the lowest energy state of a quantum system.

Quantum Approximate Optimization Algorithm (QAOA): A quantum algorithm used to solve combinatorial optimization problems.

SMILES: A text-based notation for representing chemical structures using short ASCII strings.

PDB: A standardized format and database for storing three-dimensional structures of biological molecules.

CSV: A simple file format used to store tabular data as comma-separated values.

Drug Docking: A method that predicts the preferred orientation of a drug molecule when bound to its target protein.

Chapter 4
Implementation of Neuro-Pharmaceutical Innovation in Eco-Friendly Drug Manufacturing

Shwetha G. K.
Department of Computer Science and Engineering, Vidyavardhaka College of Engineering, Mysuru, India

Rajesh Vyankatesh Argiddi
https://orcid.org/0000-0002-4227-2384
Department of Computer Science and Engineering, Walchand Institute of Technology, Solapur, India

Ashish Avasthi
https://orcid.org/0000-0003-3069-1984
Faculty of Computer Science, Poornima University, Jaipur, India

Lovely Jacob A.
Department of Chemistry, Little Flower College, Guruvayur, India

Reshma S.
https://orcid.org/0000-0002-3584-0021
Department of Artificial Intelligence and Machine Learning, Dayananda Sagar College of Engineering, Bangalore, India

Ravy Kannan
https://orcid.org/0009-0003-1456-2709
KPR Institute of Engineering and Technology, India

ABSTRACT

This chapter discovers the conversion of neuro-pharmaceutical innovation and eco-friendly drug manufacturing, which emphasizes sustainable therapeutic development. It examines emerging trends in neuroscience-based drug detection, including precision-oriented treatment, AI-enabled diagnostics and nanotechnology-based delivery systems. At the same time, it highlights green chemistry methods such

DOI: 10.4018/979-8-3373-2043-4.ch004

as biodegradable solvents, renewable raw materials and the use of low-emitting synthesis routes. By integrating environmental liability with cutting edge neuro-pharmaceutical research, this chapter reflects the importance of sustainable models in addressing both neurological disorders and global ecological challenges. This holistic approach is intended to promote future-prepared, morally aligned and environmentally therapeutic solutions in a developed pharmaceutical landscape.

INTRODUCTION

The conversion of neuroscience and pharmaceutical innovation is entering a new era of precision, patient-centered therapeutic strategy. At the same time, this evolution must now be adjusted with a global essential global essential: durability. With the unprecedented challenges in the field of healthcare - the increasing of neurological disorders, the increasing number of traditional drug manufacturing is the growing recognition of the need to develop solutions that are both advanced and ecological. This chapter examines the synergistic intersection of neuro-pharmaceutical innovation and environmental-friendly drug manufacturing, stability positioning as a basic principle in the future of the drug (Abeng et al., 2021).

Neuroscience, as a border discipline, has expanded our understanding of the complex architecture of the brain and the biochemical network. Disorders of the Central Nervous System (CNS) - including Alzheimer's disease, Parkinson's disease, epilepsy, multiple sclerosis and major depressive disorders - have deeply personal, social and economic effects. According to the World Health Organization (WHO), neurological conditions affect more than one billion people globally and have a significant portion of the burden of global disease (Ramudu et al., 2023). Despite decades of research, effective treatment options remain limited, often due to the complexity of neural routes and the restricted nature of the blood-brain barrier (BBB) (Beghi et al., 2021). This complexity requires innovative pharmaceutical approaches that move beyond traditional small-molecular drugs. Molecular neurobiology, bio-informatics and drug delivery systems-recent progresses in nanotechnology-based carriers and AI-powered compound screening are reshaping and treated with CNS disorders (González Peña et al., 2021).

Parallel to this medical progress is a crucial assessment of the environmental footprint of the pharmaceutical industry. Traditional drug manufacturing processes are often energy-intensive, chemically dangerous and producing waste. Solvents, reagents and mediators used in synthesis contribute significantly to pollution and professional health risks. Moreover, the disposal of pharmaceutical waste in water bodies has caused concern over the emergence of ecotoxicity and drug-resistant microbial strains. These environmental results are especially relevant when scaled in global operations. It is now widely acknowledged that if therapeutic innovation should be meaningful, it must be synchronized with environmental durable methods (Holloway et al., 2021).

This requirement has given birth to the field of green chemistry within the pharmaceutical vision. Green chemistry promotes the formation of chemical products and processes that reduce or eliminate the pay generation of hazardous substances. Biodegradable solvents, enzymatic catalysis and solvent free synthesis techniques are central in this example. The use of supercritical fluids such as carbon dioxide, ionic fluid and renewable feed stocks offers an example of how production processes can be rebuilt to reduce their environmental influence (Tantawy et al., 2021). Additionally, Life Cycle Assessment (LCA) models allow for the superstitious evaluation of the environmental cost of the drug-from the extraction of the rugged goods to the later waste. These tools enable decisions to identify sustainable ways that configure regulatory compliance, operational efficiency and corporate environmental, social and governance (ESG) commitments (Mishra & Anand, 2022).

When applied to neuro-pharmaceuticals, these eco-conscious lenses become more crucial. CNS Medications often require complex synthesis, strict purity standards and special delivery systems to pass the blood-brain barrier, all of which increase resource consumption. Universe challenges also have unprecedented opportunities by transferring such high-blooded production pipelines in such methods. For example, integrating biodegradable polymers into nano-carriers CNS. Drug delivery increases, but biological systems also ensure safe degeneration. Similarly, adoption of green synthesis for nootropic and neuroprotective compounds can reduce both carbon footprint and production costs, making healing more accessible and durable (Patil et al., 2022).

Moreover, the innovation in this domain is no longer limited to the laboratory. Governments, international institutions and industry designers are increasingly organizing their strategies with global durability goals. The United Nations provides a strategic structure to integrate sustainable development goals, especially good health and well -being and responsible consumption and production, health and environmental priority (Sivamaruthi et al., 2022). Regulatory organizations such as the food and drug administration and the European medicines Agency, are beginning to guide on green production methods, including solvent use, emissions reduction and waste management in pharmaceutical production. As durability becomes a major criterion in pharmaceutical approval and achievement, companies are encouraged not only for effectiveness but for ecological stewards (Birniwa et al., 2023).

Moreover, the digital change of healthcare acts as a catalyst for durable innovation. Artificial intelligence (AI), machine learning (ML) and digital two technologies enable pharmaceutical companies to imitate nuclear interactions, to pt over formulation processes and predict environmental effects before physical production begins.

These tools can significantly shorten the cycle of development, reduce experimental waste and CNS. May improve the accuracy of the drug search. By doing so, they support both economic and ecological efficiency (Castiello et al., 2023).

From a strategic point of view, the integration of durability in a neuro-pharmaceutical innovation is not only the responsibility of compliance but also a competitive advantage. Companies investing in green manufacturing and sustainable drug design are in a better position to meet the expectations of morally conscious consumers, institutional investors and global health systems (Marques et al., 2024). They are even more elastic in regulatory shift and supply chain disturbances. Increased demand for the principles of the circular economy in the pharma - which includes recyclable packaging, reuse of solvents and decentralized production models - highlights the need for systemic transformation in how they are imagined, produced and distributed (Jairoun et al., 2025a).

Hence, the confluence of neuroscience and pharmaceutical innovation presents an extraordinary opportunity to overcome some of the most health challenges of our time. Yet, this potential can be fully experienced only by the commitment of durability. As this chapter will be explored, environmental drug manufacturing is no barrier, but a catalyst for creativity, efficiency and long-term impact in the neuro-pharmaceutical domain (Jairoun et al., 2025a). By embedding environmental liability in each phase of the drug life cycle - from search and development to distribution and disposal - we can create therapeutic solutions that are not only clinically transforming but also environmentally appropriate. This integrated approach is essential for the advancement of both planets' health and human well -being in the fast -growing world.

Objectives

This chapter discusses progress in neuro-pharmaceutical renovation, including AI-powered invention and nanotechnology-based delivery, and evaluates environmental effects of drug manufacturing and green chemistry principles. It is CNS. The drug pipelines highlight the integration of such methods, presents a case study of durable neuro-drug manufacturing, invents regulatory framework and digital tools, and provides strategic recommendations to configure neuro-firm R&D with stability goals.

NEURO-PHARMACEUTICAL INNOVATION

Neuro-pharmaceutical innovation is reshaping the landscape of the treatment of complex neurological disorders. There is an urgent need for novel, effective and targeted treatment with global burdens of neurological diseases, including Alzheimer's, Parkinson, epilepsy and multiple sclerosis. Traditional approaches are increasingly replaced by precision-based strategies that integrate artificial intelligence (AI), biomarker-based targets, neuro-genomics and nanotechnology-completed delivery systems (Castiello et al., 2023; Marques et al., 2024). This section detects these key pillars that define the current and future direction of neuro-pharmaceutical innovation. The process flow and key components of neuro-pharmaceutical innovation are depicted in Figure 1.

Figure 1. Process flow and key components of neuro-pharmaceutical innovation

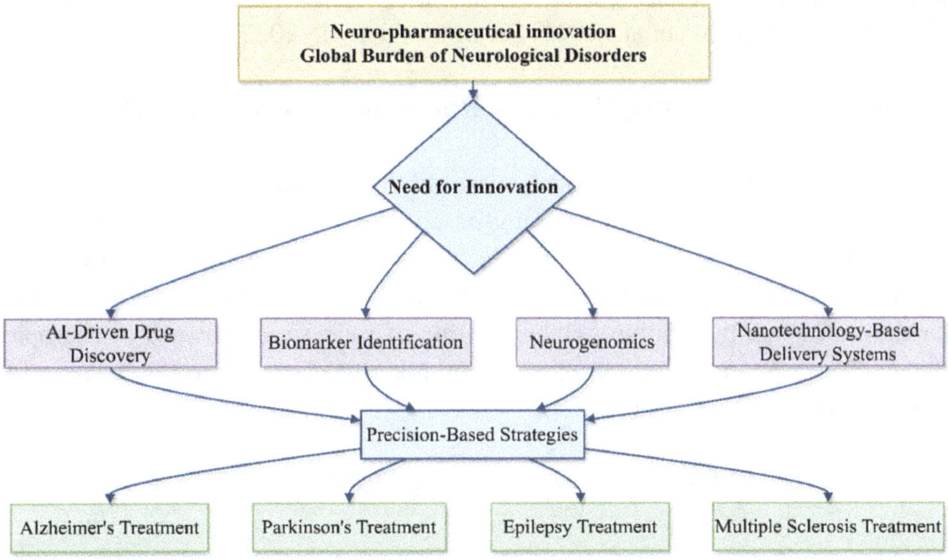

Advances in Targeted Drug Discovery for Neurological Disorders

Traditional therapies for neurological disorders often show non-specific action, weak blood-brain barrier (BBB) penetration and low effectiveness due to significant side effects. Modern drug invention is now focused on the formation of targeted treatment that definitely acts on the affected neural routes or nuclear formats (Rebecca et al., 2024). For example, in Alzheimer's disease, monoclonal antibodies have been developed to make amyloid-beta plaques especially target in the brain. Next, gene-oriented therapy is being invented using antisense oligonucleotides (ASO) for conditions such as Huntington disease and spinal muscular atrophy (SMA). These treatments aim to improve the underlying genetic change rather than just removing the symptoms.

Artificial Intelligence in CNS Drug Development

Artificial intelligence (AI) is revolutionizing the pharmaceutical value chain, especially in the neuro-pharmaceutical R&D. AI models identify new CNS applications for existing drugs, predict binding connections and toxic profiles, and indicate individual therapeutic regions based on patient-specific genomic and phenotypic data. Platforms like philanthropic AI and Atom Wise have CNS. AI has shown the possibility of accelerating drug detection, reduced development timeline and reducing costs (Kankala et al., 2021; Sivamaruthi et al., 2022).

Biomarker-Based Targeting for Personalized Neurology

The identity and use of biomarkers is central to precision neurology. Biomarkers may be genetic, proteomic, or imaging-based. CNS Care has revolutionized the initial diagnosis, the progression of the disease and their use in predicting treatment feedback. Biomarker stratification allows clinical trials to focus on the possibility of gain on the sub-population, where the rate of success increases. For example, the use of phosphorated tau-targeting as a marker has been important in tests for the treatment (Marques et al., 2024).

Neuro-genomics and the Role of Big Data

Neuro-genomic genes find out how the brain is affected by the composition, function and sensitivity of the disease. With the progress in Next-Pay Generation's Sequencing (NGS) and Genome-Wide Association Studies (GWS), researchers can identify neuro-demonical tracts such as risk alleles and schizophrenia, autism spectrum disorders and bipolar disorders. Integration with large data analytics allows modeling the pathways of the disease, enabling target identification at the genetic and epigenetic level. Moreover, epigenetic drugs, which alter gene expression without modification of DNA sequences, are emerging as a promising treatment for neurodegenerative diseases.

Nanotechnology-Enhanced Drug Delivery Systems

CNS in Nano Technology Blood-brain Barrier (BBB) Provides innovative solutions for effective delivery of drugs. Polymeric nanoparticles, and surface-relevant nanoparticles can be used for continuous release and targeted delivery. These systems increase the solubility and stability of CNS drugs. Working with ligands or antibodies allows receptor-medial transitions in BBB. Nanoparticles filled with curcumin have shown enhanced neuroprotective effects in models of Parkinson's disease.

Integration of Multi-Omics for Comprehensive Insights

The use of multi-omics approaches, including transcriptomics, proteomics, metabolomics and connect-omissions, enables the holistic understanding of CNS disorder. The integration of these datasets provides insights of the disease methods at various biological levels and helps identify the novel therapeutic goals. For example, combining proteomic data with neuroimaging allowed researchers to better classify Parkinson's sub -type and predict treatment answers. These insights also support the development of a targeted combination therapy of multiple ways simultaneously.

Neuro-pharmaceutical innovation faces challenges such as high failure in clinical trials, complication of CNS disorder and regulatory barrier. However, emerging trends such as digital therapeutics, brain-computer interfaces and neuro-AI conversion are ready to revolutionize the field. Integrating stability in neuro-drag development ensures that these innovations are effective and environmentally responsible, guaranteeing their success in the future.

Figure 2. Root causes of challenges in traditional drug manufacturing across major contributing domains

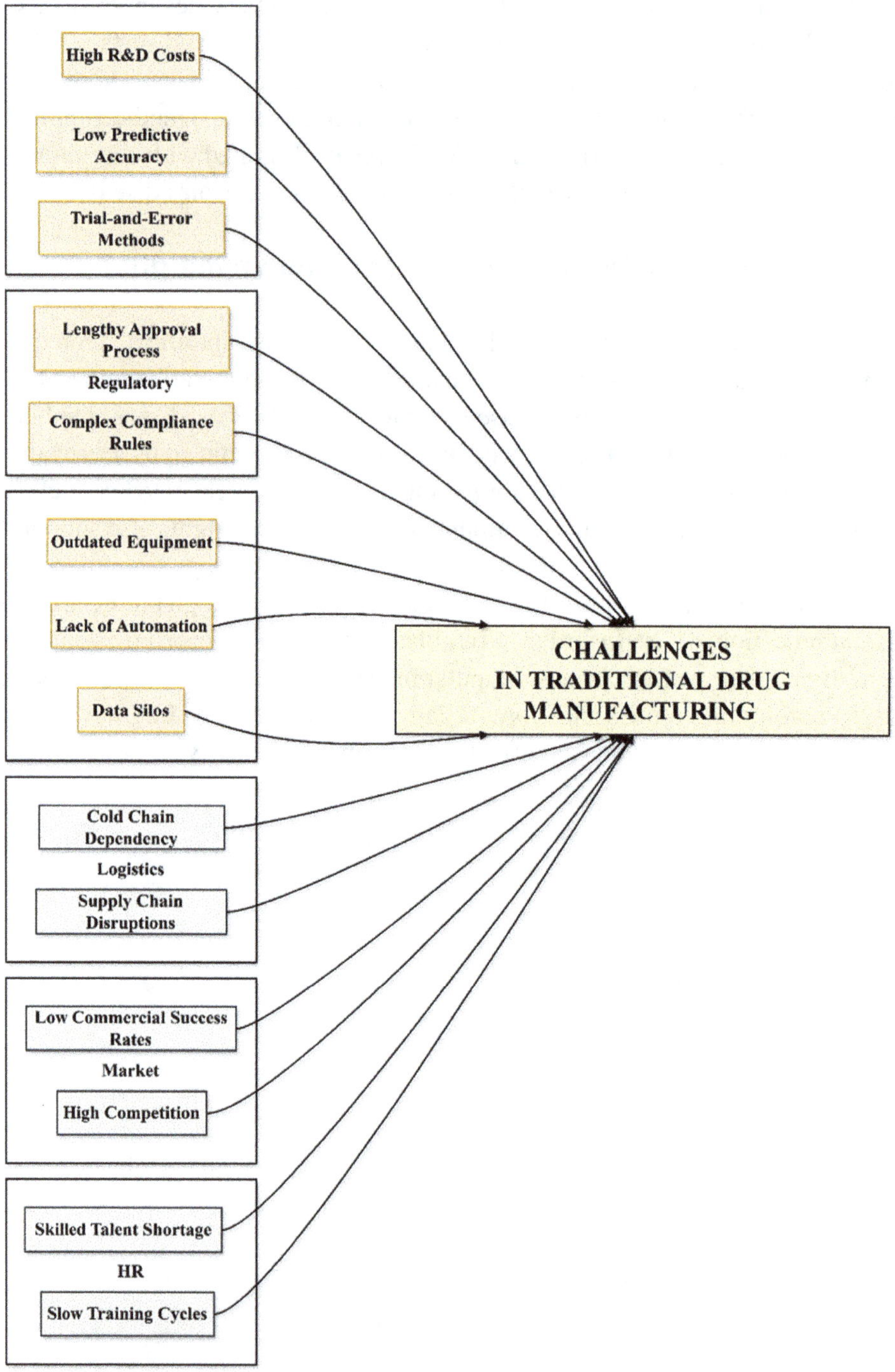

CHALLENGES IN TRADITIONAL DRUG MANUFACTURING

Traditional drug manufacturing, despite the development of life -saving therapy, faces many limits that are increasingly at odds with contemporary Vijay. Unique, environmental and moral expectations. This stress is pronounced especially in terms of neuro-pharmaceuticals, where the complexity of the central nervous system (CNS) disorders demands high specificity, and the drugs involved are often synthesized by resource-intensive and chemical hazardous processes. In an era where both public health and environmental stewards are supreme, the need to critically assess and improve the traditional models of drug manufacturing was never much urgent (Saggar et al., 2022). Figure 2 depicts the root causes of challenges in traditional drug manufacturing across major contributing domains.

Energy is a leading challenge in the nature of the traditional pharmaceutical production. Most small-nuclear drugs require multi-step synthesis, including high temperature reactions, solvent extraction and crystallization, distillation and chromatography. This operation consumes large amounts of electricity, thermal energy zones and water. Especially CNS In the synthesis of drugs - many of which have complex molecular structures - the number of reaction steps increases significantly, combining energy redesign requirements. For example, the synthesis of certain antidepressants or antiepileptics may include more than 20 different chemical changes, contributing to the accumulated carbon footprint that is unaffected in the long run. In addition, the cost of energy is directly linked to the production of overheads, especially in low and middle -income countries, affecting drugs and accession (Rebecca et al., 2024).

Another significant limit is the widespread use of toxic solvent and reagents. Organic solvents such as dichloromethane, toluene, acetyl and methanol are widely used in media, extraction processes and purification. These substances are not only unstable and flammable, but also toxic to human health and harmful to the environment. Many solvents are classified as dangerous air pollutants (HAPs) by environmental regulatory agencies, and their widespread use emits that contributes to air and water pollution. CNS In drug development, the use of solvent is more important due to the need for high purity levels and strict pharmacokinetic properties, including lipophilicity and BBB penetration. As a result, the solvent recovery procurement and the burden of waste management increase significantly. Moreover, improper disposal of solvent residues leads to contamination of ecosystems and constant bioaccumulation of organic pollutants (Prabhakar & Mamoni, 2021).

Another central challenge is to produce waste. It is estimated that each kilogram is produced for an active pharmaceutical component, 25 to 100 kilograms of waste can be produced, most of which are classified as dangerous. This waste includes solvents, reaction by-products, catalysts and contaminated water. In the case of neuro-pharmaceuticals, which often includes heavy metals or special reagents for stereoselective synthesis, waste loads can be especially severe. Pharmaceutical waste, both solid and fluid disposal, represents rational, environmental and legal difficulties. Landfilling, destruction and chemical treatment are expensive and often inadequate to reduce long -term environmental damage. Moreover, the environmental view of pharmaceutical residues contributes to antimicrobial resistance, end of secretion and drinking water supply in aquatic species.

In addition to environmental concerns, there are significant regulatory and ethical issues associated with the traditional drug development process, especially in terms of neurological drugs. The development of neuro-pharmaceuticals is full of high failure, due to the limits of preceding models. The disorder is poorly replicated in animal models, leading to misleading effectiveness and safety profiles. For example, models of rats often fail to mimic the entire spectrum of human beings or behavioral phenotypes, resulting in translation gaps that are only discovered during expensive and moral sensitive human tests.

Moreover, CNS Clinical trials for drugs are naturally complex and morally charged. Strictly informed consent protocols are needed to register patients with organize defects or mental health disorders, and the risks of adverse effects - which include neurotoxicity, JNNN's reduction or mental disruption - are carefully weighed. US Regulatory agencies such as the Food and Drug Administration (FDA) and the European Medicines agency (EMA) require strong evidence of safety, effectiveness and benefit-free balance, which can be difficult to get in terms of subjective final points or diseases with slow progress. This leads to a significant economic burden on extended timelines, high attrition rate and pharmaceutical companies (Begley et al., 2021).

The second moral parameter is related to access and equity. The traditional pharmaceutical model often prefers market -based innovation, focusing on drugs that promise a high redemption on investment. As a result, the need for long -term therapy is less in the underworld population without diseases or clear commercial promotion. This creates inequality in investment of research and development in various neurological conditions and geographical regions. In addition, the cost of traditionally produced drugs - extended by inefficient processes and regulatory obstacles - limits access for patients in developing countries, contradicting the principle of global health equity.

From a strategic point of view, the traditional drug manufacturing model is poorly suitable for inaccessible and fast innovation. Central, batch-based production systems commonly used are difficult to adapt not only capital intensive, but also with new nuclear bodies or individual drugs. On the contrary, emerging approaches such as continuous production and modular bioreactors provide greater dexterity, efficiency and durability, but are less used due to institutional inertia and regulatory Rs SERV interest. Moreover, many pharmaceutical companies are equipped to include Legacy

Infrastructure Green Manufacturing Techniques or include advanced data analytics that can optimize production parameters in real-time (Zheng et al., 2021).

In the end, traditional instances lack integration with digital techniques that can increase trackability, quality control and environmental monitoring. Digital two models, forecasts for the process optimization are reshaping the blockchain manufacturing landscape for AI, and supply chain transparency, though their adoption in CNS drug production is limited. The absence of digitization not only weakens operational efficiency, but also hinders the active identity of the risks related to contamination, emissions, or transformation of production (Destro & Barolo, 2022).

Thus, when traditional drug manufacturing has contributed greatly to medical progress, its current form is increasingly unable to withstand environmental, regulatory and moral challenges. This is especially true for neuro-pharmaceuticals, where the sting is due to complex pathophysiology and patient weakness. More durable, flexible and morally ethically requires the shift towards ground manufacturing practices to overcome these limitations. Adoption of green chemistry, integrating digital techniques and prioritizing human and environmental safety is essential to ensure that pharmaceutical innovation is effective and responsible over the next decades.

ECO-FRIENDLY DRUG MANUFACTURING

Eco -friendly drug manufacturing, in view of the principles of green chemistry, presents a transformative approach to pharmaceutical viscosity in order to reduce environmental damage that maintains therapeutic effectiveness and safety. As the pharmaceutical industry faces increasing pressure to reduce its ecological footprint, integrate sustainable practices, and adhere to global environmental rules, an example is going on - which balances innovation in the discovery and development of drug with ecological responsibility (Sapkota & Pariatamby, 2023). This change is especially relevant in the production of complex compounds such as neuro-pharmaceuticals, which often require resource-intensive processes and environmentally hazardous chemicals.

Figure 3. Eco-Friendly Drug Manufacturing based on the principles of green chemistry

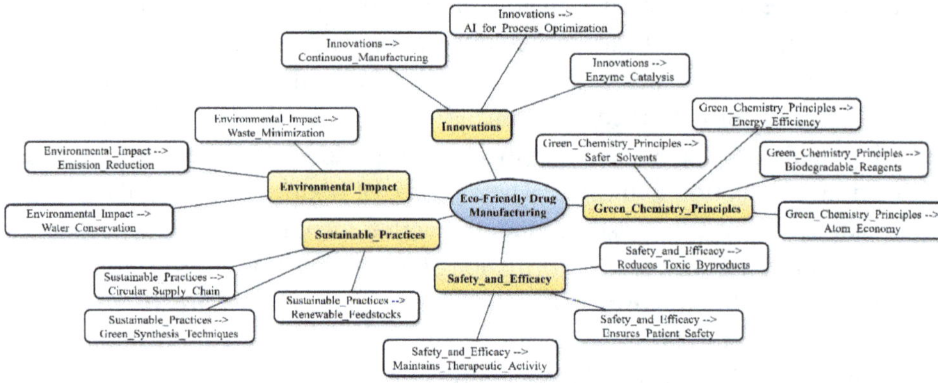

Sustainable drug manufacturing developed to reduce or eliminate or eliminate or eliminate the use of green chemistry, chemical products, design, production and application of hazardous substances in production and application. In the context of pharmaceuticals, green chemistry focuses on the formation of artificial routes that maximize the atomic economy, avoids toxic reagents, reduce waste and improve energy efficiency. Green provides the principles of chemistry, formed, basic guide. These principles naturally advocate safe chemistry for waste prevention, safe solvent, energy efficiency, renewable feed stocks, real-time pollution prevention and accidental prevention. Figure 3 depicts a drug manufacturing process that is eco-friendly and based on green chemistry principles.

The most notable shift in green pharmaceutical manufacturing is the replacement of traditional organic solvents - which are often unstable, flammable, and toxic - with biodegradable and less dangerous options. Traditional solvents such as dichloromethane, toluene and acetone are now gradually phased in favor of green alternatives such as water, ethanol, and methyl-tre-hydrofuran. These solvents have been taken from biomass and provide environmental viscus and poisonous drugs. For example, biodegradable esters, ethyl lactate, its excellent solvating power and gentle environmental profile, are now being used in many pharmaceutical processes, produced from maize-stormed lactic acid and ethanol. Adoption of biodegradable solvents reduces exposure risks during manufacturing, but also reduces environmental contamination, contributing to safe waste management (S.Aithal & Aithal, 2021).

Enzymatic catalysis has also emerged as a powerful tool for durable pharmaceutical synthesis. Enzymes, as very selective biocatalysts, act under mild reaction conditions - generally reduce the need for aqueous media, surrounding temperature and physical pH - energy cane consumption and harsh reagents. They provide regioselectivity, stereoselectivity, and enantioselectivity, which are especially valuable in the synthesis of chiral neurological compounds. For example, enzymatic transformation or reduction is increasingly working to produce optically pure CNS-active compounds, such as some selective serotonin reuptake inhibitors. Biocatalytic approaches also allow cascade reactions, where multiple enzymatic measures take place in a single reaction vessel, reducing purification steps, using solvent and processing waste.

In addition to green solvents and biocatalysis, interest in renewable raw materials for drug synthesis is increasing. Traditionally, pharmaceutical intermediates have been taken from petrochemical sources, but sustainable options such as plant biomass, algae and microbial fermentation products are getting traction. Feed stocks such as lignin, cellulose and sugar alcohol are now being investigated for their possibility of obtaining bio-based building blocks such as succinic acid, and glycerol derivatives, which can serve as API's precursors. The use of renewable resources not only reduces dependence on fossil fuel, but also supports a circular economy model where waste of other industries (agriculture or food processing) is converted to valuable pharmaceutical inputs (P. S. Aithal & Aithal, 2022).

Aonian liquids (IL) represent another boundary in green solvent technology. This room temperature contains salts in the fluid state, made of wide, and asymmetric organic cations. Provides tunable physicochemical properties, including low volatility, high thermal stability and excellent solvent capacity for a wide range of substrates. In pharmaceutical applications, IL has promised to increase the solubility of poor water-soluble drugs, to act as a reaction media for enzymatic synthesis and facilitate crystallization processes. Importantly, by changing their composition, IL can be designed for biodegradability and reduces toxicity, adjusting them with the goals of green chemistry.

Microwave-supporting organic synthesis is a second cutting edge technique that has shown a significant improvement in reaction speed, yield, and energy efficiency. Microwave irradiation provides faster and similar heat, which often leads to the time of reaction from the acceleration reaction rate and hours to minutes. This technique is especially beneficial for general multistep synthesis in neuro-pharmaceutical development. For example, microwave-supporting cyclone and condensation are now being used to create heterocyclic scaffolds for anticonvulsant and neuroprotective agents.

In addition to technical innovations, product analytical technology and continuous flow chemistry are being adopted to further trim the product. It enables control of real-time monitoring and critical quality symptoms during production, ensuring the quality of consistent product while reducing waste and re-work. Meanwhile, continuous flow reactors provide enhanced safety, mentality and efficiency on traditional batch reactors, especially for hazardous reactions or heat-sensitive compounds (Nakov et al., 2023).

Hence, environmentally -friendly drug manufacturing is infecting from the theoretical ideal, which goes on to public demand for green chemistry, environmental regulation and durability. Novel techniques such as biodegradable solvents, enzymatic processes, renewable feed stocks, and supercritical COs, and microwave-supporting synthesis reflect wide efforts to reduce the environmental influence of pharmaceutical production. These strategies not only increase the environmental stability of drug manufacturing, but also supports economic viability through reduced operational costs and improved regulatory compliance. As the industry develops, especially in the neuro-pharmaceutical domain, it will be important to deliver a safe, effective and environmentally responsible treatment to integrate these eco-conscious innovations.

INTEGRATION OF SUSTAINABILITY IN NEURO-PHARMA PIPELINES

As the global pharmaceutical industry claims with dual impressions, reducing the demands and ecological degeneration of-healthcare-unified stability in neuro-pharmaceutical pipelines has become a strategic and moral requirement. Neurological disorders such as Alzheimer's, Parkinson, Wii and Depression affect millions of people worldwide, increasing the research and development of innovative neuro-drug. However, these therapeutic synthesis, composition and distribution often produce energy-intensive processes, risky reagents and widespread waste (Jairoun et al., 2025b; Nakov et al., 2023). In this regard, sustainable strategies such as life cycle assessment (LCA), biotechnological fermentation, solvent-recovery procurement systems and clause-loop manufacturing are further implemented to reduce the environmental measures of neuro-pharmaceutical products throughout their life cycle. The main idea of integrating sustainability into neuro-pharmaceutical pipelines is illustrated in Figure 4.

Figure 4. Core idea of integrating sustainability into neuro-pharmaceutical pipelines

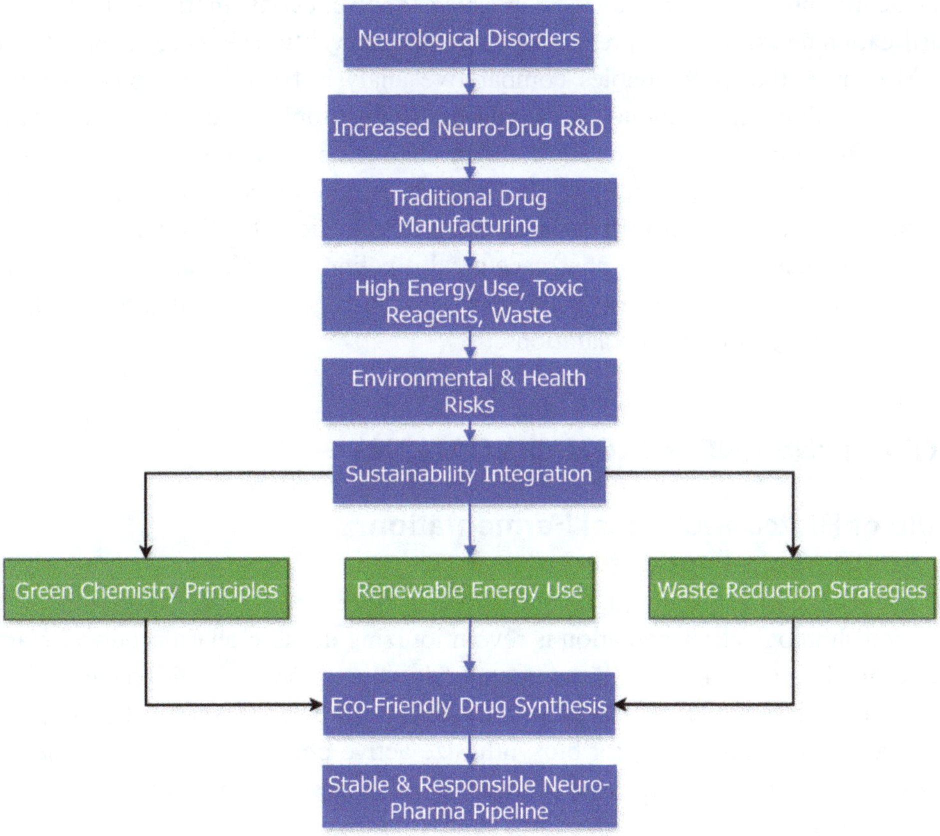

Life Cycle Assessment (LCA) of Neuro-Drugs

Life Cycle Assessment (LCA) is a comprehensive method that is used to evaluate the environmental effects associated with all stages of the life of the product - from the extraction of raw materials through production, use and final disposal. In neuro-pharmaceuticals, the LCA is key to the amount and reduction of environmental burdens, when facilitating informed decisions during drug development. LCA usually covers four key stages: goal and scope definition, inventory analysis, impact assessment and interpretation. For neuro-drugs, this process includes Mapping during the operation of energy usage, emissions, waste generation and synthesis, formulation, packaging, transport and subsequent customer waste (Klucken et al., 2018). For example, the synthesis of typical neurological compounds, such as selective serotonin reuptake inhibitors, high solvent use and significant CO_2 emission may include numerous chemical measures. By applying LCA, pharmaceutical companies can identify hotspots in the value chain - such as solvent consumption or inefficient purification measures - and prefer this for green intervention (Rebecca et al., 2024).

Moreover, the LCA enables comparative analysis between various artificial paths or production techniques. It can publish, for example, whether the enzymatic biotransformation is best in the environment in terms of greenhouse gas emissions, water consumption and toxicity. It also helps in evaluating environmental-friendly packaging materials, transport logistics and energy-efficient collections. Ultimately, the composition of neuro-pharmaceutical pipelines to LCA and integrating in optimization benefits the durability of measured regulatory structures, such as environmental production declarations.

SOLUTIONS AND RECOMMENDATIONS

Role of Biotechnological Fermentation in Sustainable Production

Biotechnological fermentation is revolutionizing durable pharmaceutical manufacturing by providing an environmental -friendly option for traditional chemical synthesis. In the neuro-firm, this approach gives genetically the benefit of genetically engineered microorganisms for biosynthesize active pharmaceutical components, mediators or complex predecessors under mild, aqueous and non-toxic conditions (Belous et al., 2016).

Fermentation reduces dependence on fossil feed stocks and reduces solvent use, minimum energy consumption and toxic sub-products. It also enables the production of high stereo- and regio-selectivity chiral and structurally complex molecules, crucial for neuro-drugs targeting specific receptors or enzymes in the brain. For example, microbial biosynthesis of gamma aminobutyric acid analogue shows the possibility of fermentation for clinically related neurotherapeutics.

The scalability and modularity of bioreactors make them suitable for continuous production, contributing to the elasticity and cost reduction of the chain. Moreover, the progress in artificial organisms and metabolic engineering has allowed pathway optimization, yield increase, and reducing waste in microbial fermentation systems. Additionally, the downstream process of fermented products is becoming more efficient than using aqueous-phase purification and membrane-based split, which is less resource-intensive than traditional organic extraction.

Solvent-Recovery Systems: Minimizing Waste and Emissions

Pharmaceutical manufacturing part of solvent use for a significant portion of environmental influence. Neuro-pharmaceuticals, due to their molecular complexity and strict purity requirements, often include multiple extraction, crystallization and purification measures where solvents are widely used. Implementing solvent-recovery procurement systems is an effective way to reduce this load (Ozkizilcik et al., 2017).

Modern solvent-recovery procurement systems use distillation, absorption and membrane techniques to reclaim and purify solvents for reuse in manufacturing. For example, azeotropic is working to distinguish distillation and extensive solvent-water mixture, allowing high-richness solvent re-recovery procurement. Close-loop solvent systems associated with real-time monitoring can maintain continuous solvent quality and reduce freshly solvent input by up to 80%. This not only cuts the emissions of unstable organic compounds, but also delivers significant cost savings and adjusts with regulatory expectations under frameworks such as rich (registration, evaluation, authenticity and restrictions) (Maguluri et al., 2023).

By reintroducing recovered solvents in the production cycle, companies reduce their dependence on the achievement of virgin solvent, thus reducing their overall carbon footprint. Moreover, the solvent recovery procurement completes the green solvent initiative, enables the use of more durable, biodegradable solvents without compromising efficiency or regulatory compliance.

Closed-Loop Manufacturing: Toward Zero Waste

Close-loop represents the system-level approach to stability by the target of zero waste by the recycling and reuse of the material inside the manufacturing product ecosystem. In neuro-pharmaceutical pipelines, the implementation of closed-loop systems integrates green process design, energy registration and digital monitoring in each phase of drug production. Such systems depend on the cradle-to-cradle philosophy, in which sub-products from one process are re-represented as inputs in another. For example, the heat generated by exothermic reactions can be captured and reused in other steps in need of thermal energy room, while spending fermented media can be processed in biogas or fertilizers. Similarly, waste biomasses from microbial processes can be given value in feed additives or secondary chemicals (Belous et al., 2016; Ozkizilcik et al., 2017).

Advanced process intensity enhances the efficiency and control of technologies-modular flow systems, modular flow systems and in-line monitoring tools-class-loop systems. These innovations constantly enable production, reduce batch-to-batch variable, and improve safety profiles, while reducing material damage and environmental discharge. AI-propelled analysis promotes digital techniques such as digital twins and blockchain, resource consumption, waste generation and operation of devices, active decision-determination and regulatory transparency.

The integration of durability in neuro-pharmaceutical pipelines is not only a response to environmental pressure but also a strategic change that enhances innovation, elasticity and social responsibility. Life cycle assessment provides data -based foundation to identify and reduce environmental effects in the drug cycle of the drug. Biotechnological fermentation offers low effect, high efficiency options for traditional synthesis. Solvent-poon recovery procurement systems reduce chemical waste and emissions, while Close-Loop Manufacturing Pharmaceutical Supply Chain redefines with circular and resource efficiency. As the global demand for neurological care increases with environmental inevitability, these durable practices will be responsible for embedding in neuro-drag development and the construction of the future-ready pharmaceutical sector.

CASE STUDIES AND INDUSTRIAL APPLICATIONS

Traction of real-world adoption of sustainable practices in neuro-pharmaceuticals is gaining traction, leading companies integrate green technologies and process innovations in their performance. For example, Novartis has continuous production and solvent-recovery procurement system in the production of central nervous system drugs, which reduces solvent waste by more than 60% and reduces energy consumption by the intensity of the process. Industry-educational synergy is further published in collaboration on Green Chemistry optimization (Jairoun et al., 2025a, 2025b).

Eli Lily has invested in enzymatic catalysis for the synthesis of complex neuroactive molecules, reduces the use of risky reagents and enables a high nuclear economy. Their biocatalytic platforms have proven effective in producing chiral mediation with improved environmental metrics for antidepressants and antipsychotics. In the field of biotechnology, Biogen has adopted a close-loop manufacturing in the production of biologics for neurodegenerative diseases such as multiple sclerosis and Alzheimer's. Their facilities include renewable energy, water recycling and LCA-way decision-making, evaluating stability effects in the production life cycle (Verma et al., 2024).

Moreover, Green Chemistry Pharma has developed scalable methods for neurodrag synthesis using a start-up consortium, supercritical CO_2 and ionic fluid, showing professional practical options of petrochemical solvents. These examples confirm the tangible shift towards a sustainable neuro-pharmaceutical development through cross-discipline innovation and industrial dysfunctional commitment.

FUTURE DIRECTIONS AND POLICY IMPLICATIONS

The future of neuro-pharmaceutical manufacturing is defined by the need to merge innovation with increasing stability. When the demand for neurological therapy due to the aging population, mental health challenges and neurodegenerative diseases, pharmaceutical companies are under pressure to meet the needs of healthcare without compromising environmental and social standards. Pressure for the active guidance of environmental, social and governance, strict green rules and regulatory agencies. In parallel, frameworks such as durable development goals of the United Nations are providing global strategic arrangements for sustainable transformation (Ahmed & Pinjari, 2025; De Spiegeleer & Wynendaele, 2025). Figure 5 outlines the future directions and policy implications in neuro-pharmaceutical manufacturing.

Figure 5. Future Directions and Policy Implications in neuro-pharmaceutical manufacturing

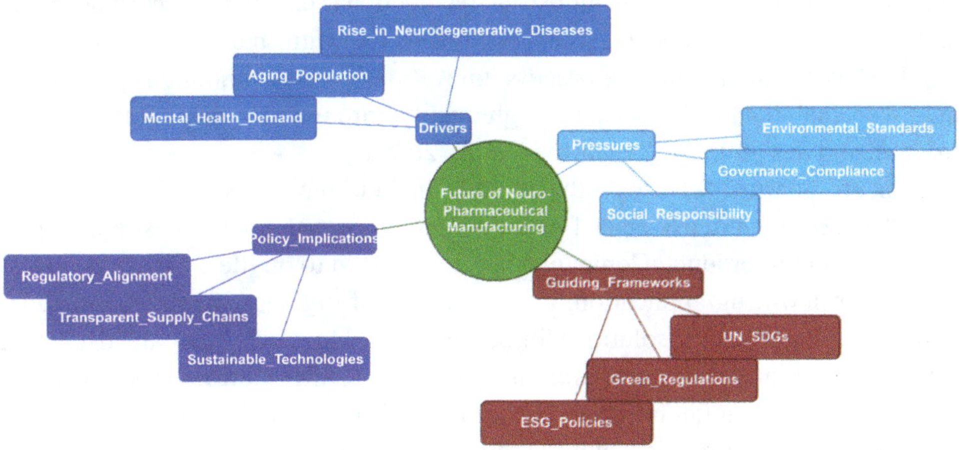

ESG Compliance and Corporate Sustainability Reporting

Environmental, social and governance (ESG) framework has emerged as an important yardstick for evaluating corporate stability and long -term elasticity. Investors, regulators and consumers assess their financial exhibition and innovation not only on the pipeline, but also on their carbon footprint, moral regime, social influence and transparency. In the context of neuro-pharmaceuticals, ESG compliance reduces greenhouse gas emissions during drug synthesis, preventing environmental contamination from API, and establishing supply chain trackability, ensuring moral neuro-drug trials, and supply chain. Companies are now publishing ESG reports linked to standards such as Global Reporting Initiative, Sustainability Accounting Standards Board, and Task Force on the climate-related financial advertisement (Jairoun et al., 2025b, 2025a).

Forward-tincting neuro-firm companies are embedding ESG influence indicators in core R&D, manufacturing and procurement processes. For example, the intensity of kilograms per kilogram, water consumption in bioprocesses, solvent recovery procurement ratio or employee variations in clinical research teams are now part of strategic dashboards. This shift not only supports the brand's reputation and the confidence of the investors, but also adjusts professional models with long -term planetary boundaries.

Green Regulations and Environmental Governance

Environmental rules around pharmaceutical manufacturing are becoming more and more stringent, especially in regions like North America. The European green deal reaches the regulation, and industrial dysfunction is pushing for pharmaceutical emissions to reduce chemical toxicity, promote eco-design, and to lower emissions. U.S. FDA is promoting durable process innovations such as continuous production and green analytical techniques, through quality, through its emerging technology program and design initiative (Jairoun et al., 2025a).

In neuro-pharma, where synthesis often include multi-stock processes, risky solvent and energy intensive purification, compliance with green rules repeats patterns of the entire product. Companies are encouraged to do life cycle assessments (LCAs) for new drug application, reduce the use of organic pollutants and adopt biodegradable packaging solutions for neuro-drugs. Moreover, rules are also being shaped by environmental concerns around pharmaceutical residues in aquatic ecosystems. APIs, such as antidepressants and anticonvulsants, have been found in surface water, which has caused bioaccumulation and concern about long -term ecological influence. Regulatory agencies are likely to strengthen the policies for flow control, green waste management and profiling API degeneration during drug development.

FDA and EMA Guidance on Eco-Manufacturing

FDA and EMA are taking active steps to ease the shift towards durable pharmaceutical manufacturing. History is focused on drug safety, effectiveness and quality, these agencies are now incorporating environmental risk assessments and durability-centered innovations into their regulatory views. FDA's Emerging Technology Team gives pharmaceutical companies a new, potentially durable product platform, such as continuous processing, green solvents and real-time analytics. Unique and regulatory advice. This provides both a relief and guidance for the transition from traditional batch processes (Gowri et al., 2023; Vangeri et al., 2024).

Similarly, the EMA has issued guidelines for environmental risk assessments as part of the Market Authorization application. These guidelines evaluate the potential effect of API on ecosystems and call for environmentally thinking formulations, production methods and disposal instructions. In addition, EMA efforts under "Green Medicine Partnership" are intended to develop the best efforts to reduce carbon intensity and chemical pollution in drug development. Future policy development may include incentives for green-certified API, regulatory fast tracking for eco-designed neuro-drugs and harmonious stability labeling for pharmaceutical products, equally access to hospitals, insurers and patients.

Strategic Alignment with the United Nations Sustainable Development Goals (UN SDGs)

UN SDG provides a holistic blueprint to achieve global peace, prosperity and environmental stewards. Neuro-pharma companies, especially operating globally, are increasingly adjusting their stability routes with these goals to contribute to social good while reducing risk (Ahmed & Pinjari, 2025; Jairoun et al., 2025a).

To manage this configuration, companies are incorporating SDG mapping into a production life cycle strategy. For example, neuro-pharma firm can integrate SDG indicators into its R&D project management systems, each new drug candidate is evaluated not only for ROI, but also for resource efficiency and social equity. In addition, partnerships with academia, NGOs and green tech start-ups help innovate that are socially and environmentally involved. Public-private collaboration, promoted by the World Health Organization (WHO) and Global Reporting Initiatives, also provides platforms for knowledge and standard-selling in durable neuro-drag development.

Roadmap for Implementation

In order to embed stability in neuro-firm pipelines in the long run, companies can adopt a strategic roadmap based on the following elements: The scheme includes green R&D investment, process innovation, supply chain sustainability, digital sustainability platform and policy engagement. It focuses on eco-design, green synthesis routes of molecules, AI-powered durability modeling, scalability of manufacturing units, cooperation with suppliers on manufacturing units, and monitoring environmental KPIs (De Spiegeleer & Wynendaele, 2025).

Conversion of policy command, investors' expectations and technical capabilities indicates the main shift towards sustainable neuro-pharmaceutical development. ESG compliance, developed FDA and EMA guidance, and alignment with global frameworks such as SDG is pushing the field to move beyond efficiency and profitability towards elasticity and responsibility. The entire neuro-drag value chain can lead to shape of green, healthy and more morally more moral spiritual future for both people and the planet-pharmaceutical innovations, from molecular design to patient delivery.

CONCLUSION

Conversion of neuroscience and pharmaceutical innovation provides a transformative probability of eliminating the increasing global load of neurological disorders. However, this progression must be environmentally responsible and socially responsible framework. Traditional drug manufacturing practices, which often depend on energy-intensive processes and toxic solvent, are significant challenges for durability. This chapter discovered that the eco-friendly approach-green chemistry principles, renewable inputs and technical innovation can reduce these effects by enhancing corresponding-therapeutic results.

Emerging tools such as AI-driven drug discovery, neuro-genomics and nanotechnology, especially for complex neurodegenerative conditions, are advancing precision treatment methods. At the same time, innovations such as biodegradable solvents, enzymatic catalysis, biotechnological fermentation and solvent-recovery procurement systems are redefining how neuro-pharmaceuticals are produced. Increasing emphasis on configuration (LCA), ESG compliance and regulatory bodies such as FDA and EMA reflect a comprehensive commitment to durable drug pipelines.

Moreover, the integration with the UN Sustainable Development Goal (SDG) and global policy trends shows the need for a comprehensive strategy that combines economic influence with environmental stewardship and social influence. Strengthens the possibility and benefits of applying durability on a case study basis of industry leaders. Thus, the fate of neuro-pharmaceuticals is not only in variety. This is in the moral and ecological integrity of their development. As an industry, academics and policy connections around Green Innovation, the next way is clear: stability must be embedded at every stage of the neuro-drag lifeline cycle to ensure long-term health for both humanity and planet.

REFERENCES

Abeng, F., Ikpi, M., Ushie, O., Anadebe, V., Nyong, B., Obeten, M., Okafor, N., Chukwuike, V., & Nkom, P. (2021). Insight into corrosion inhibition mechanism of carbon steel in 2 M HCl electrolyte by eco-friendly based pharmaceutical drugs. *Chemical Data Collections*, *34*, 100722. DOI: 10.1016/j.cdc.2021.100722

Ahmed, S. A., & Pinjari, N. S. (2025). A Review of Sustainable Paradigms in Contemporary Drug Discovery and Development. *Journal of Pharma Insights and Research, 3*(2), 001–018.

Aithal, P. S., & Aithal, S. (2022). Opportunities and Challenges for Green and Eco-Friendly Nanotechnology in Twenty-First Century. *Sustainable Nanotechnology: Strategies, Products, and Applications*, 31–50.

Aithal, S., & Aithal, P. (2021). Green and eco-friendly Nanotechnology–concepts and industrial prospects. [IJMTS]. *International Journal of Management, Technology, and Social Sciences*, *6*(1), 1–31. DOI: 10.47992/IJMTS.2581.6012.0127

Beghi, E., Binder, H., Birle, C., Bornstein, N., Diserens, K., Groppa, S., Homberg, V., Lisnic, V., Pugliatti, M., Randall, G., Saltuari, L., Strilciuc, S., Vester, J., & Muresanu, D. (2021). European Academy of Neurology and European Federation of Neurorehabilitation Societies guideline on pharmacological support in early motor rehabilitation after acute ischaemic stroke. *European Journal of Neurology*, *28*(9), 2831–2845. DOI: 10.1111/ene.14936 PMID: 34152062

Begley, C. G., Ashton, M., Baell, J., Bettess, M., Brown, M. P., Carter, B., Charman, W. N., Davis, C., Fisher, S., Frazer, I., Gautam, A., Jennings, M. P., Kearney, P., Keeffe, E., Kelly, D., Lopez, A. F., McGuckin, M., Parker, M. W., Rayner, C., & Sullivan, M. (2021). Drug repurposing: Misconceptions, challenges, and opportunities for academic researchers. *Science Translational Medicine*, *13*(612), eabd5524. DOI: 10.1126/scitranslmed.abd5524 PMID: 34550729

Belous, A., Zatolokina, M., Lavrinenko, K., Mal, G., Shevelev, A., & Trubnikova, E. (2016). Trophic changes in the skeletal muscles of rats after therapy with sildenafil and cerebrolysin in the lower limb ischemia model. *Bulletin of Russian State Medical University*, *4*(4), 62–66. DOI: 10.24075/brsmu.2016-04-10

Birniwa, A. H., Ali, U., Kutty, S. R. M., Jagaba, A. H., & Noor, A. (2023). Innovative and eco-friendly technologies for the upgradation of pharmaceutical wastewater treatment processes. In *The Treatment of Pharmaceutical Wastewater* (pp. 367–398). Elsevier. DOI: 10.1016/B978-0-323-99160-5.00006-0

Castiello, C., Junghanns, P., Mergel, A., Jacob, C., Ducho, C., Valente, S., Rotili, D., Fioravanti, R., Zwergel, C., & Mai, A. (2023). GreenMedChem: The challenge in the next decade toward eco-friendly compounds and processes in drug design. *Green Chemistry*, *25*(6), 2109–2169. DOI: 10.1039/D2GC03772F

De Spiegeleer, B., & Wynendaele, E. (2025). Sustainability of drug discovery, development and use as embedded in European pharmaceutical policies. *Current Opinion in Green and Sustainable Chemistry*, *53*, 101028. DOI: 10.1016/j.cogsc.2025.101028

Destro, F., & Barolo, M. (2022). A review on the modernization of pharmaceutical development and manufacturing–Trends, perspectives, and the role of mathematical modeling. *International Journal of Pharmaceutics*, *620*, 121715. DOI: 10.1016/j.ijpharm.2022.121715 PMID: 35367580

González Peña, O. I., López Zavala, M. Á., & Cabral Ruelas, H. (2021). Pharmaceuticals market, consumption trends and disease incidence are not driving the pharmaceutical research on water and wastewater. *International Journal of Environmental Research and Public Health*, *18*(5), 2532. DOI: 10.3390/ijerph18052532 PMID: 33806343

Gowri, N. V., Dwivedi, J. N., Krishnaveni, K., Boopathi, S., Palaniappan, M., & Medikondu, N. R. (2023). Experimental investigation and multi-objective optimization of eco-friendly near-dry electrical discharge machining of shape memory alloy using Cu/SiC/Gr composite electrode. *Environmental Science and Pollution Research International*, *30*(49), 1–19. DOI: 10.1007/s11356-023-26983-6 PMID: 37126160

Holloway, P. M., Willaime-Morawek, S., Siow, R., Barber, M., Owens, R. M., Sharma, A. D., Rowan, W., Hill, E., & Zagnoni, M. (2021). Advances in microfluidic in vitro systems for neurological disease modeling. *Journal of Neuroscience Research*, *99*(5), 1276–1307. DOI: 10.1002/jnr.24794 PMID: 33583054

Jairoun, A. A., Al-Hemyari, S. S., Shahwan, M., Alkhoujah, S., El-Dahiyat, F., Jaber, A. A. S., & Zyoud, S. H. (2025a). Towards eco-friendly pharmaceuticals: Regulatory and policy approaches for sustainable medicines use. *Exploratory Research in Clinical and Social Pharmacy*, *17*, 100576. DOI: 10.1016/j.rcsop.2025.100576 PMID: 40026320

Jairoun, A. A., Al-Hemyari, S. S., Shahwan, M., Alkhoujah, S., El-Dahiyat, F., Jaber, A. A. S., & Zyoud, S. H. (2025b). Towards eco-friendly pharmaceuticals: Regulatory and policy approaches for sustainable medicines use. *Exploratory Research in Clinical and Social Pharmacy*, *17*, 100576. DOI: 10.1016/j.rcsop.2025.100576 PMID: 40026320

Kankala, R. K., Xu, P.-Y., Chen, B.-Q., Wang, S.-B., & Chen, A.-Z. (2021). Supercritical fluid (SCF)-assisted fabrication of carrier-free drugs: An eco-friendly welcome to active pharmaceutical ingredients (APIs). *Advanced Drug Delivery Reviews, 176*, 113846. DOI: 10.1016/j.addr.2021.113846 PMID: 34197896

Klucken, J., Krüger, R., Schmidt, P., & Bloem, B. R. (2018). Management of Parkinson's disease 20 years from now: Towards digital health pathways. *Journal of Parkinson's Disease, 8*(s1), S85–S94. DOI: 10.3233/JPD-181519 PMID: 30584171

Maguluri, L. P., Ananth, J., Hariram, S., Geetha, C., Bhaskar, A., & Boopathi, S. (2023). Smart Vehicle-Emissions Monitoring System Using Internet of Things (IoT). In *Handbook of Research on Safe Disposal Methods of Municipal Solid Wastes for a Sustainable Environment* (pp. 191–211). IGI Global.

Marques, S. I., Sá, S. I., Carmo, H., Carvalho, F., & Silva, J. P. (2024). Pharmaceutical-mediated neuroimmune modulation in psychiatric/psychological adverse events. *Progress in Neuro-Psychopharmacology & Biological Psychiatry, 135*, 111114. DOI: 10.1016/j.pnpbp.2024.111114 PMID: 39111563

Mishra, P., & Anand, S. (2022). Nanoceuticals as Theranostics Against Neurodegenerative Diseases. In *Role of Nutrients in Neurological Disorders* (pp. 263–279). Springer. DOI: 10.1007/978-981-16-8158-5_14

Nakov, N., Acevska, J., Brezovska, K., Kavrakovski, Z., & Dimitrovska, A. (2023). Green strategies toward eco-friendly HPLC methods in pharma analysis. In *High Performance Liquid Chromatography-Recent Advances and Applications*. IntechOpen. DOI: 10.5772/intechopen.110035

Ozkizilcik, A., Williams, R., Tian, Z. R., Muresanu, D. F., Sharma, A., & Sharma, H. S. (2017). Synthesis of biocompatible titanate nanofibers for effective delivery of neuroprotective agents. In *Neurotrophic Factors: Methods and Protocols* (pp. 433–442). Springer.

Patil, A. D., Kasabe, P. J., & Dandge, P. B. (2022). Pharmaceutical and nutraceutical potential of natural bioactive pigment: Astaxanthin. *Natural Products and Bioprospecting, 12*(1), 25. DOI: 10.1007/s13659-022-00347-y PMID: 35794254

Prabhakar, P., & Mamoni, B. (2021). Technical problems, regulatory and market challenges in bringing herbal drug into mainstream of modern medicinal practices. *Research Journal of Biotechnology, 16*, 3.

Ramudu, K., Mohan, V. M., Jyothirmai, D., Prasad, D., Agrawal, R., & Boopathi, S. (2023). Machine Learning and Artificial Intelligence in Disease Prediction: Applications, Challenges, Limitations, Case Studies, and Future Directions. In *Contemporary Applications of Data Fusion for Advanced Healthcare Informatics* (pp. 297–318). IGI Global.

Rebecca, B., Kumar, K. P. M., Padmini, S., Srivastava, B. K., Halder, S., & Boopathi, S. (2024). Convergence of Data Science-AI-Green Chemistry-Affordable Medicine: Transforming Drug Discovery. In *Handbook of Research on AI and ML for Intelligent Machines and Systems* (pp. 348–373). IGI Global.

Saggar, S., Mir, P. A., Kumar, N., Chawla, A., Uppal, J., & Kaur, A. (2022). Traditional and herbal medicines: Opportunities and challenges. *Pharmacognosy Research, 14*(2), 107–114. DOI: 10.5530/pres.14.2.15

Sapkota, B., & Pariatamby, A. (2023). Pharmaceutical waste management system–Are the current techniques sustainable, eco-friendly and circular? A review. *Waste Management (New York, N.Y.), 168*, 83–97. DOI: 10.1016/j.wasman.2023.05.052 PMID: 37285639

Sivamaruthi, B. S., Nallasamy, P., Suganthy, N., Kesika, P., & Chaiyasut, C. (2022). Pharmaceutical and biomedical applications of starch-based drug delivery system: A review. *Journal of Drug Delivery Science and Technology, 77*, 103890. DOI: 10.1016/j.jddst.2022.103890

Tantawy, M. A., Weshahy, S. A., Wadie, M., & Rezk, M. R. (2021). Eco-friendly spectrophotometric methods for assessment of alfuzosin and solifenacin in their new pharmaceutical formulation; green profile evaluation via eco-scale and GAPI tools. *Current Pharmaceutical Analysis, 17*(8), 1093–1103. DOI: 10.2174/1573412916999200730005740

Vangeri, A. K., Bathrinath, S., Anand, M. C. J., Shanmugathai, M., Meenatchi, N., & Boopathi, S. (2024). Green Supply Chain Management in Eco-Friendly Sustainable Manufacturing Industries. In *Environmental Applications of Carbon-Based Materials* (pp. 253–287). IGI Global., DOI: 10.4018/979-8-3693-3625-0.ch010

Verma, R., Christiana, M. B. V., Maheswari, M., Srinivasan, V., Patro, P., Dari, S. S., & Boopathi, S. (2024). Intelligent Physarum Solver for Profit Maximization in Oligopolistic Supply Chain Networks. In *AI and Machine Learning Impacts in Intelligent Supply Chain* (pp. 156–179). IGI Global. DOI: 10.4018/979-8-3693-1347-3.ch011

Zheng, C., Li, M., & Ding, J. (2021). Challenges and opportunities of nanomedicines in clinical translation. *Bio Integration, 2*(2), 57. DOI: 10.15212/bioi-2021-0016

ADDITIONAL READING

Chakraborty, S., Bhattacharya, M., & Das, A. K. (2023). Green chemistry approaches in pharmaceutical synthesis: A sustainable perspective. *Journal of Environmental Chemical Engineering*, *11*(5), 110214. DOI: 10.1016/j.jece.2023.110214

Tan, Y. T., Lee, H. W., Chan, K. G., & Goh, B. H. (2024). Sustainability and innovation in pharmaceutical development: Challenges and future directions. *Pharmaceuticals*, *17*(2), 156. DOI: 10.3390/ph17020156 PMID: 38399371

KEY TERMS AND DEFINITIONS

UN SDG: United Nations Sustainable Development Goals
ROI: Return on Investment
NGO: Non-Governmental Organization
KPI: Key Performance Indicator

Chapter 5
The Potential of Generative AI in Drug Development

Deepak Gupta
https://orcid.org/0000-0003-3929-1362
Institute of Technology and Management, Gwalior, India

R. Sudhakar
https://orcid.org/0000-0002-0212-6956
Madanapalle Institute of Technology and Science, India

Sofiya S. Mujawar
https://orcid.org/0000-0003-1248-296X
D.Y. Patil University Ambi, India

Rita Kadam
https://orcid.org/0009-0006-3461-9786
D.Y. Patil University Ambi, India

Vivek Patil
https://orcid.org/0009-0008-5071-1886
D.Y. Patil University Ambi, India

Anurag Kumar
https://orcid.org/0009-0003-2890-6111
D.Y. Patil University Ambi, Pune, India

Prashant Ahire
https://orcid.org/0000-0002-8101-7087
Symbiosis Institute of Technology, Pune, India

Kapil Gupta
Amity Institute of Pharmacy, Gwalior, India

ABSTRACT

Drug development is a complex, time-consuming, and expensive process with high failure rates. Traditional approaches face significant challenges, including lengthy timelines (10-15 years), astronomical costs (exceeding $2.5 billion per successful drug), and high attrition rates (>90%). Generative artificial intelligence (AI) represents a paradigm shift in this field, offering novel approaches to address these longstanding challenges. This chapter explores the transformative potential of generative AI across the drug development pipeline, from target identification to clinical

DOI: 10.4018/979-8-3373-2043-4.ch005

trial design. Various AI architectures and their pharmaceutical applications are examined, breakthrough case studies are analyzed, current challenges are addressed, and future directions are discussed that may revolutionize pharmaceutical research and development, providing stakeholders with the knowledge necessary to navigate the rapidly evolving landscape of AI-driven drug development.

INTRODUCTION

The pharmaceutical industry stands at a critical juncture, facing unprecedented challenges in developing innovative therapies while managing escalating costs and complexity. Drug development remains one of the most resource-intensive and risk-laden endeavors in modern science, with estimated costs exceeding $2.5 billion per successfully marketed drug and timelines stretching beyond a decade (DiMasi et al., 2016). Despite substantial investments in research and development (R&D), the productivity crisis in pharmaceutical innovation persists, with high attrition rates throughout the development pipeline (Scannell et al., 2012).

Against this backdrop, artificial intelligence (AI), particularly generative AI, has emerged as a transformative force with the potential to revolutionize multiple aspects of the drug development process. Generative AI encompasses computational models capable of creating novel content rather than merely analyzing existing data. In the pharmaceutical context, these technologies can design new molecular entities, predict protein structures, generate hypotheses for new drug targets, optimize lead compounds, and even assist in clinical trial design and patient stratification (Zhavoronkov et al., 2019).

The integration of generative AI into drug development workflows has been accelerated by several concurrent developments: exponential growth in computational power, availability of large-scale biological and chemical datasets, advances in AI architectures, and successful demonstrations of AI-designed drug candidates entering clinical trials. Industry leaders and newcomers alike are investing heavily in this domain, recognizing its potential to address fundamental inefficiencies in the traditional drug discovery paradigm (Paul et al., 2021).

This chapter provides a comprehensive examination of the current state and future potential of generative AI in drug development. We begin by reviewing the traditional drug development process and its inherent challenges, establishing the context for AI-driven innovation. We then explore the various generative AI architectures and their specific applications across the drug development pipeline, from early discovery to clinical development. Through case studies and empirical evidence, we highlight both the successes and limitations of current approaches.

Furthermore, we address critical challenges facing the adoption of generative AI in pharmaceutical R&D, including data quality concerns, interpretability issues, regulatory considerations, and validation requirements. The chapter concludes with a forward-looking discussion of emerging trends and potential paradigm shifts that generative AI may catalyze in the coming decade, offering insights for researchers, industry professionals, regulators, and policymakers navigating this rapidly evolving landscape.

As we stand on the precipice of a new era in drug development, understanding the capabilities, limitations, and future directions of generative AI becomes increasingly vital for all stakeholders committed to advancing human health through pharmaceutical innovation.

BACKGROUND

The Traditional Drug Development Process and Its Challenges

Overview of the Conventional Drug Development Pipeline

The conventional drug development process follows a well-established pipeline consisting of several distinct phases (Figure 1). The journey begins with target identification and validation, where researchers identify a biological target (typically a protein) believed to play a critical role in a disease process. Once a target is validated, the next phase involves high-throughput screening (HTS) of large compound libraries to identify "hits" that demonstrate activity against the target. These hits undergo further optimization to improve potency, selectivity, and pharmacokinetic properties, eventually yielding lead compounds.

Lead optimization is followed by preclinical development, where promising candidates are tested in vitro and in animal models to assess safety and efficacy before human testing. Clinical development then proceeds through three main phases: Phase I (safety assessment in healthy volunteers), Phase II (preliminary efficacy in a small patient population), and Phase III (large-scale confirmation of safety and efficacy). Finally, successful candidates are submitted for regulatory approval, after which post-marketing surveillance continues to monitor safety in the broader population (Hughes et al., 2011).

Figure 1. The conventional drug development pipeline, showing major phases from target identification through post-approval monitoring, with typical timelines and success rates at each stage.

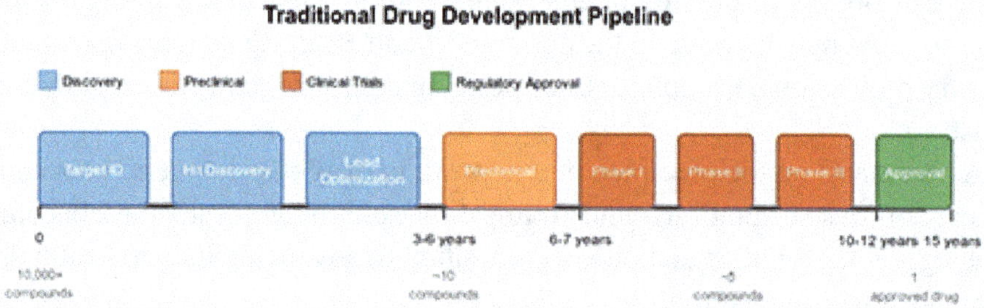

Key Challenges in Traditional Drug Development

Time and Cost Constraints

The most prominent challenges in traditional drug development are the extended timelines and enormous costs. From initial target identification to market approval, the process typically spans 10-15 years (Figure 2). According to recent estimates, the capitalized cost of bringing a new drug to market, including the cost of failures, exceeds $2.5 billion (DiMasi et al., 2016). These financial and temporal burdens create significant pressure on pharmaceutical companies and limit the number of therapeutic candidates that can be pursued.

Figure 2. Timeline and associated costs for each phase of traditional drug development, highlighting the exponential increase in investment as candidates progress toward approval.

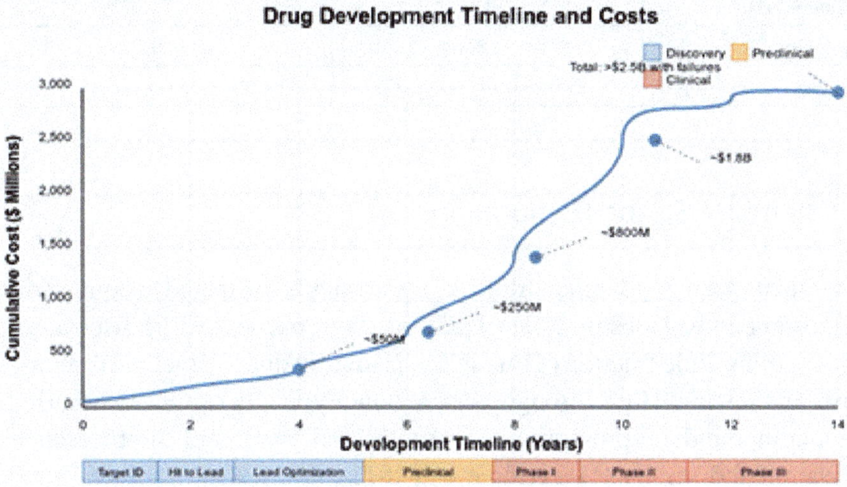

High Attrition Rates

Perhaps the most daunting challenge is the high attrition rate throughout the development pipeline. For every 10,000 compounds that enter the discovery phase, typically only one ultimately receives regulatory approval (Table 1). Even after reaching clinical trials, the probability of success remains low, with approximately 90% of drug candidates failing during clinical development (Mullard, 2016). These failures often occur late in development, after substantial investments have been made, exacerbating the financial impact.

Table 1. Attrition rates in traditional drug development

Development Stage	Number of Compounds	Success Rate to Next Stage
Target-to-Hit	~10,000	50%
Hit-to-Lead	~5,000	25%
Lead Optimization	~1,250	10%
Preclinical Development	~125	40%
Phase I Clinical Trials	~50	70%

continued on following page

Table 1. Continued

Development Stage	Number of Compounds	Success Rate to Next Stage
Phase II Clinical Trials	~35	33%
Phase III Clinical Trials	~12	70%
Regulatory Review	~8	90%
Market Approval	~1	-

Limited Chemical Space Exploration

The chemical space of potential drug-like molecules is estimated to contain more than 10^60 compounds (Dobson, 2004). Traditional approaches to drug discovery can only explore a minuscule fraction of this space, primarily due to practical limitations in synthesis and testing. High-throughput screening typically evaluates libraries of 1-2 million compounds, representing an infinitesimal portion of the theoretically available chemical diversity (Macarron et al., 2011).

Translational Gaps

Another significant challenge is the frequent failure of promising preclinical candidates to demonstrate efficacy or safety in human trials. This translational gap stems from the limited predictive power of animal models for human disease and the complex interplay of factors affecting drug performance in diverse patient populations (Cook et al., 2014). The inability to accurately predict human responses from preclinical data contributes substantially to late-stage failures and increases the overall cost of drug development.

Target Selection and Validation Challenges

Target selection and validation remain critical bottlenecks in the drug development process. Despite advances in genomics and proteomics, identifying novel, druggable targets with clear disease associations remains challenging. Furthermore, the biological complexity of many diseases, particularly those with multifactorial etiologies like neurodegenerative disorders, complicates the identification of appropriate intervention points (Scannell & Bosley, 2016).

These persistent challenges in traditional drug development have created fertile ground for disruptive innovations, with generative AI emerging as a particularly promising approach to address multiple pain points across the pharmaceutical R&D continuum.

Fundamentals of Generative AI in the Pharmaceutical Context

- **Generative AI Architectures and Their Applications**

Generative AI encompasses various computational approaches designed to create novel content rather than merely analyze existing data. In the pharmaceutical context, several generative AI architectures have demonstrated particular relevance and utility.

GANs consist of two neural networks—a generator and a discriminator—engaged in an adversarial learning process. The generator creates synthetic data (e.g., molecular structures), while the discriminator evaluates their authenticity compared to real examples. Through iterative training, the generator improves at producing valid molecular structures that possess desired properties (Guimaraes et al., 2017).

In drug discovery, GAN-based approaches such as MolGAN (De Cao & Kipf, 2018) and DrugGAN (Kadurin et al., 2017) have been employed for de novo molecular design, generating structures with specific pharmacological profiles or binding affinities. The adversarial training paradigm helps ensure that generated molecules maintain chemical feasibility while optimizing for multiple target properties simultaneously.

- **Variational Autoencoders (VAEs)**

VAEs combine an encoder-decoder architecture with variational inference to learn a continuous latent representation of the input data. In the pharmaceutical context, VAEs such as Chemical VAE (Gómez-Bombarelli et al., 2018) encode molecular structures into a continuous latent space, enabling smooth navigation of the chemical space and controlled generation of novel compounds with desired properties.

The continuous nature of the latent space in VAEs facilitates property-directed molecular optimization through techniques like latent space interpolation and gradient-based optimization. This architecture has proven particularly valuable for scaffold hopping and lead optimization tasks, where structural modifications need to be explored systematically while maintaining core pharmacophoric features.

- **Transformer-Based Models**

Transformer architectures, originally developed for natural language processing, have been adapted for molecular generation and property prediction. Models like ChemBERTa (Chithrananda et al., 2020) and MolBERT (Fabian et al., 2020) leverage the self-attention mechanism to capture complex relationships in molecular data, treating chemical structures as a form of language with atoms and bonds as vocabulary elements.

Transformer-based approaches excel at capturing long-range dependencies in molecular structures and generalizing from limited training data. Recent large language model (LLM) adaptations like MolT5 (Edwards et al., 2022) have demonstrated impressive capabilities in translating between different molecular representations and generating structures conditioned on textual descriptions of desired properties.

- **Diffusion Models**

Diffusion models represent a newer class of generative techniques that have gained prominence in drug discovery. These models learn to reverse a gradual noising process, generating complex data by iteratively denoising random samples. In the pharmaceutical context, models like EDM (Hoogeboom et al., 2022) and GCDM (Zhang et al., 2023) have shown exceptional promise for generating three-dimensional molecular conformations and protein structures.

The inherent ability of diffusion models to capture multimodal distributions makes them particularly suitable for modeling the complex energy landscapes associated with biomolecular structures. These models have demonstrated state-of-the-art performance in generating diverse, valid, and novel molecular entities while maintaining precise control over structural and physicochemical properties.

- **Reinforcement Learning for Molecular Design**

While not strictly a generative architecture in the traditional sense, reinforcement learning (RL) approaches have been successfully combined with generative models to optimize molecular structures toward specific objectives. Frameworks like REINVENT (Olivecrona et al., 2017) and GENTRL (Zhavoronkov et al., 2019) employ RL to guide molecular generation toward compounds with optimal property profiles, using carefully designed reward functions that incorporate multiple evaluation criteria.

The integration of RL with generative models addresses one of the key challenges in computational drug design: the need to simultaneously optimize for multiple, often competing, objectives such as potency, selectivity, metabolic stability, and synthetic accessibility.

Data Requirements and Sources for Generative AI in Drug Discovery

The performance of generative AI models in drug discovery is heavily dependent on the quality, quantity, and diversity of the training data. Several key data types and sources have emerged as particularly valuable for training pharmaceutical AI systems (Table 2).

Table 2. Key data types and sources for generative AI in drug discovery

Data Type	Description	Major Sources	Applications
Chemical Structures	Molecular representations (SMILES, graphs, 3D conformers)	ChEMBL, PubChem, ZINC, DrugBank	De novo molecule design, property prediction, QSAR modeling
Bioactivity Data	Target-ligand interaction data (binding affinities, IC50 values)	ChEMBL, BindingDB, PDBbind	Target prediction, virtual screening, activity prediction
Protein Structures	3D coordinates of protein structures	Protein Data Bank (PDB), AlphaFold DB	Structure-based design, protein-ligand docking, epitope prediction
ADMET Data	Absorption, distribution, metabolism, excretion, toxicity profiles	ADME DB, Tox21, ToxCast	Toxicity prediction, pharmacokinetic optimization
Omics Data	Genomic, transcriptomic, proteomic, metabolomic data	TCGA, GTEx, GEO, HPA	Target identification, biomarker discovery, patient stratification
Clinical Trial Data	Patient-level data from clinical studies	ClinicalTrials.gov, YODA, Project DataSphere	Trial design, patient selection, endpoint prediction
Patent Data	Chemical and biological information from patents	SureChEMBL, USPTO, EPO	Novelty assessment, IP landscape analysis, competitive intelligence

- **Data Preparation and Curation Challenges**

Despite the abundance of pharmaceutical data, several challenges persist in preparing high-quality datasets for AI model training:

1. **Data Heterogeneity**: Pharmaceutical data originates from diverse experimental setups, using different assay methodologies, conditions, and endpoints. Harmonizing these heterogeneous data sources requires sophisticated normalization and standardization procedures (Brown et al., 2018).

2. **Missing Values and Imbalanced Representations**: Bioactivity datasets often contain substantial missing values, with certain chemical scaffolds or targets overrepresented and others underrepresented. This imbalance can introduce biases in AI models and limit their generalizability to novel chemical spaces (Reker et al., 2020).
3. **Data Quality and Reproducibility Issues**: Experimental data in public repositories may contain errors, inconsistencies, or inadequate metadata. Ensuring data quality through rigorous validation, outlier detection, and quality control measures is essential for training reliable AI models (Fourches et al., 2010).
4. **Proprietary Data Barriers**: Many high-value pharmaceutical datasets remain proprietary, limiting the training data available to academic researchers and smaller organizations. This data asymmetry can create disparities in AI capabilities across the industry (Walters & Barzilay, 2021).
5. **Representational Challenges**: Effectively representing complex molecular structures and their properties in formats suitable for AI model consumption remains challenging. Various molecular featurization approaches, including fingerprints, descriptors, and graph-based representations, each have strengths and limitations for different applications (Wu et al., 2018).

Addressing these data challenges requires collaborative efforts across the pharmaceutical ecosystem, including precompetitive consortia for data sharing, standardized protocols for data generation and reporting, and advanced techniques for data augmentation and synthetic data generation.

APPLICATIONS OF GENERATIVE AI ACROSS THE DRUG DEVELOPMENT PIPELINE

Generative AI technologies have found applications throughout the drug development continuum, from early discovery to clinical development and post-approval monitoring. This section explores key applications across the pipeline, highlighting their potential to address traditional bottlenecks and enhance R&D productivity.

Target Identification and Validation

AI-Driven Target Discovery

Generative AI approaches are revolutionizing target identification by uncovering novel disease-associated proteins and biological pathways. Graph neural networks and transformer-based models trained on multimodal biological data (genomic, proteomic, metabolomic) can generate hypotheses about previously unrecognized disease mechanisms (Vamathevan et al., 2019).

For instance, BenevolentAI's target identification platform combines knowledge graph technology with generative AI to hypothesize novel targets for amyotrophic lateral sclerosis (ALS), leading to the discovery of a previously unexplored mechanism involving the RIPK1 protein (Brown et al., 2021). Similarly, Insitro's platform integrates high-throughput phenotypic screening with generative models to identify novel targets for metabolic and neurodegenerative diseases (Segal et al., 2021).

In Silico Target Validation

Traditional target validation relies heavily on time-consuming experimental techniques like gene knockouts and antibody inhibition studies. Generative AI accelerates this process through in silico target validation approaches, simulating the effects of target modulation on disease networks and predicting potential on- and off-target effects (Figure 3).

Figure 3. Workflow for AI-driven target validation, showing the integration of multi-omics data, network analysis, and predictive modeling to assess target druggability and disease relevance.

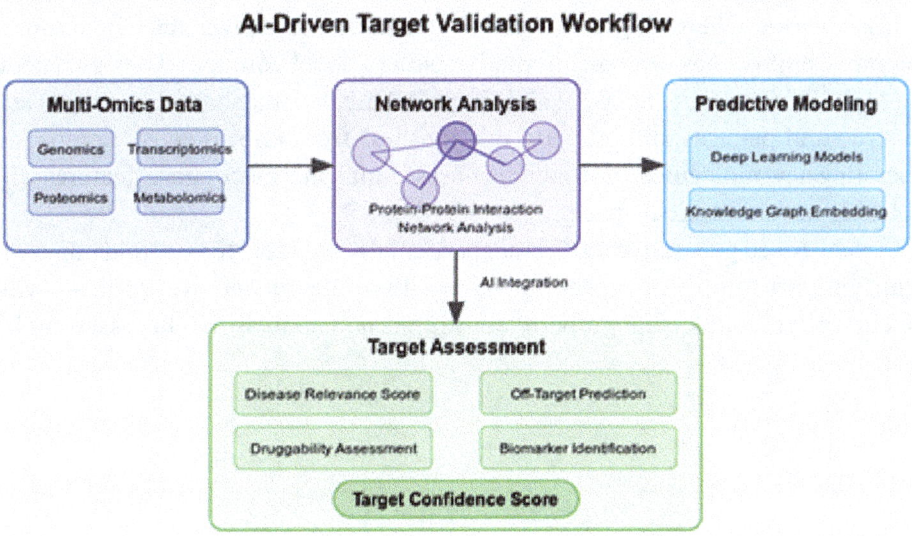

Deep generative models trained on perturbation datasets, such as those from the LINCS L1000 project, can predict the transcriptional responses to novel compound-target interactions, providing preliminary evidence of target engagement and downstream effects (Subramanian et al., 2017). These approaches enable rapid prioritization of targets based on predicted efficacy, safety profiles, and druggability, substantially reducing the time and resources required for target validation.

De Novo Molecule Design

Structure-Based Design

Structure-based de novo molecule design leverages 3D structural information about the target protein to generate novel ligands that optimally interact with the binding site. Generative AI architectures, particularly 3D-aware models like 3D-SBDD (Luo et al., 2021) and diffusion-based approaches, have demonstrated impressive capabilities in this domain.

These models can generate molecules that form specific interactions with key residues in the binding pocket while maintaining appropriate physicochemical properties for drug development. The integration of physics-based scoring functions with generative neural networks enables more accurate prediction of binding affinities and improves the success rate of computational design efforts.

Ligand-Based Design

In scenarios where target structural information is unavailable, ligand-based generative approaches offer an alternative path to novel compound design. Models like MolGPT (Bagal et al., 2021) and GraphINVENT (Bradshaw et al., 2020) learn the structural patterns and property relationships from known active compounds, generating new molecules that maintain the essential pharmacophoric features while exploring novel chemical space.

Ligand-based generative models are particularly valuable for scaffold hopping—identifying structurally diverse compounds with similar bioactivity profiles—which can circumvent intellectual property constraints and address liability issues in lead series.

Multi-Parameter Optimization

One of the most significant advantages of generative AI in drug design is the ability to simultaneously optimize multiple parameters. Traditional medicinal chemistry often encounters trade-offs between different properties, such as potency versus metabolic stability or solubility versus permeability.

Generative models equipped with multi-objective optimization capabilities, such as REINVENT (Blaschke et al., 2020) and GENTRL (Zhavoronkov et al., 2019), can navigate these complex trade-offs more effectively, generating compounds with balanced profiles across multiple dimensions of interest (Table 3).

Table 3. Multi-Parameter Optimization Objectives in Generative Drug Design

Property Category	Specific Parameters	Computational Assessment Methods
Target Engagement	Binding affinity, selectivity, kinetics	Docking, MM-GBSA, FEP+, ML-based scoring
Physicochemical	Solubility, lipophilicity, polar surface area	QSPR models, MD simulations, fragment-based predictions
ADME	BBB permeability, plasma protein binding, metabolic stability	QSAR models, ML classifiers, systems biology models
Safety	hERG inhibition, CYP450 interactions, hepatotoxicity	Toxicophore models, structural alerts, deep learning classifiers
Synthetic Accessibility	Synthetic complexity, retrosynthetic feasibility	SYBA, SCScore, reaction prediction models
Intellectual Property	Novelty, patent freedom-to-operate	Similarity searches, fragment analysis, automated patent mining

Lead Optimization

Structure-Activity Relationship (SAR) Exploration

Generative AI approaches excel at systematically exploring structure-activity relationships, a cornerstone of medicinal chemistry optimization. Models like Matched Molecular Pair Analysis (MMPA) augmented with deep learning (Pogány et al., 2018) can generate focused libraries of analogs, predicting the impact of specific structural modifications on activity and ADMET properties.

These approaches dramatically accelerate the design-make-test-analyze cycle in medicinal chemistry, enabling more efficient optimization campaigns and reducing the number of compounds that need to be synthesized and tested (Figure 4).

Figure 4. Comparison of traditional and AI-accelerated medicinal chemistry cycles, showing reduced timelines and increased efficiency in the design-make-test-analyze process.

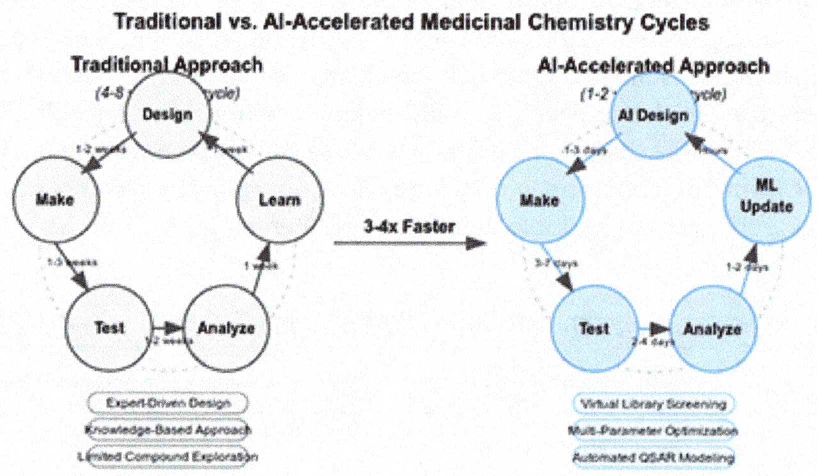

Predictive ADMET Modeling

Absorption, distribution, metabolism, excretion, and toxicity (ADMET) properties are critical determinants of a compound's developmental success. Generative models incorporating ADMET prediction capabilities, such as ADMETlab 2.0 (Xiong et al., 2021) and DeepPurpose (Huang et al., 2020), can prospectively optimize molecules for favorable pharmacokinetic profiles while maintaining target activity.

These approaches help identify and address potential liability issues early in the discovery process, reducing the risk of late-stage failures due to unfavorable ADMET properties. By incorporating mechanism-based toxicity predictions, these models can also guide the design of safer compounds with reduced off-target effects.

Synthetic Accessibility Assessment

A common limitation of computer-generated molecules is their synthetic inaccessibility. Modern generative frameworks address this challenge by incorporating synthetic accessibility scores (Ertl & Schuffenhauer, 2009) and retrosynthesis prediction models (Segler et al., 2018) into the generation process, ensuring that designed compounds can be readily synthesized.

More sophisticated approaches, such as SYNOPSIS (Grisoni et al., 2020) and Synthia™ (formerly Chematica), integrate reaction prediction models with generative design, creating closed-loop systems that simultaneously optimize for bioactivity and synthetic feasibility.

Clinical Development Applications

Patient Stratification and Biomarker Discovery

Generative models trained on multi-omics data can identify novel biomarkers and patient subpopulations likely to respond to specific therapeutic interventions. These approaches are particularly valuable for complex, heterogeneous diseases where traditional biomarkers may lack sensitivity or specificity.

Deep generative models, such as variational autoencoders trained on cancer genomics data, have successfully identified novel molecular signatures associated with treatment response, enabling more precise patient stratification for clinical trials (Way & Greene, 2018). Similar approaches have been applied to neurodegenerative and autoimmune disorders, revealing disease subtypes with distinct molecular pathologies and treatment responses.

Clinical Trial Design and Optimization

Generative AI approaches are transforming clinical trial design by optimizing protocol elements, inclusion/exclusion criteria, and endpoint selection. Models trained on historical trial data can generate optimized trial designs that maximize the probability of success while minimizing resource requirements and patient burden.

Advanced approaches, such as the Clinical Trial Optimizer developed by Unlearn. AI, employ generative models to create "digital twins" of patients, enabling smaller, more efficient trials through prognostic covariate adjustment (Fisher et al., 2021). These innovations are particularly valuable for rare diseases and precision medicine applications, where eligible patient populations may be limited.

Real-World Evidence Generation

Post-approval, generative AI facilitates the analysis of real-world data from electronic health records, claims databases, and patient registries. These approaches can identify previously unrecognized drug effects (both beneficial and adverse), optimal treatment sequences, and opportunities for label expansion.

Generative models trained on longitudinal patient data can simulate treatment trajectories under various scenarios, supporting comparative effectiveness research and health technology assessments without the need for additional clinical trials (Beaulieu-Jones et al., 2019).

CASE STUDIES AND BREAKTHROUGHS

AI-Designed Drug Candidates in Clinical Development

Several AI-designed drug candidates have now entered clinical development, providing tangible validation for generative approaches. Notable examples include:

- **Insilico Medicine's ISM001-055**

In 2021, Insilico Medicine announced that its AI-designed inhibitor of idiopathic pulmonary fibrosis (IPF) target had entered Phase I clinical trials. The compound, ISM001-055, was discovered using Insilico's GENTRL platform, which combines generative models with reinforcement learning for multi-parameter optimization.

The development timeline for this novel DDR1 kinase inhibitor was remarkably compressed, with only 18 months from target identification to preclinical candidate nomination, compared to the industry average of 3-5 years (Zhavoronkov et al., 2019). This acceleration demonstrates the transformative potential of generative AI in early drug discovery, particularly for novel targets with limited prior chemical matter.

- **Exscientia's EXS-21546**

Exscientia's AI-designed A2A receptor antagonist for cancer immunotherapy, EXS-21546, entered Phase I clinical trials in 2021. The compound was designed using Exscientia's Centaur Chemist™ platform, which employs active learning and generative design to efficiently explore chemical space.

The development of EXS-21546 required significantly fewer compounds to be synthesized and tested compared to traditional approaches, with only 136 compounds made during the discovery phase, compared to the industry average of 2,500+

(Jayatunga et al., 2022). This efficiency gain directly translates to reduced resource requirements and accelerated development timelines.

Computational Advances Enabled by Generative AI

- **AlphaFold2 and Protein Structure Prediction**

DeepMind's AlphaFold2 represents a landmark achievement in applying deep learning to protein structure prediction. The system uses a transformer-based architecture augmented with structural constraints to predict protein tertiary structures with unprecedented accuracy, often achieving results comparable to experimental methods like X-ray crystallography (Jumper et al., 2021).

The public release of the AlphaFold Protein Structure Database, containing predicted structures for nearly all human proteins, has democratized access to structural information and accelerated structure-based drug design efforts across the industry. This breakthrough addresses a long-standing bottleneck in drug discovery, where the scarcity of experimental protein structures limited the application of structure-based approaches.

- **RNA Drug Design**

Generative AI is also transforming RNA-targeted drug discovery, an emerging frontier in pharmaceutical research. Models like REMAP (He et al., 2020) and RNA-NET (Townshend et al., 2021) can predict RNA secondary structures and design small molecules that selectively bind to specific RNA motifs.

These approaches are particularly valuable for targeting "undruggable" proteins through their messenger RNA precursors and for developing therapeutics against RNA viruses like SARS-CoV-2. The integration of sequence-based and structure-based generative models enables more precise design of RNA-binding ligands with improved specificity and reduced off-target effects.

- **Industry Adoption and Impact**

The pharmaceutical industry has embraced generative AI through various mechanisms, including internal capability development, strategic partnerships, and acquisitions. Major pharmaceutical companies, including AstraZeneca, Pfizer, Merck, and Bayer, have established dedicated AI drug discovery units and formed strategic collaborations with AI-focused biotechnology companies.

These investments have begun to yield tangible results, with multiple AI-contributed drug candidates now advancing through clinical development. The impact extends beyond individual projects to fundamental changes in R&D operating models, with AI becoming increasingly integrated into decision-making processes throughout the development pipeline.

Economic analyses suggest that generative AI could reduce preclinical development timelines by 30-50% and decrease associated costs by 25-33%, potentially translating to billions of dollars in savings across the industry (Paul et al., 2021). However, realizing these benefits requires significant organizational changes, including workforce transformation, infrastructure investments, and cultural shifts toward data-centric operating models.

SOLUTIONS AND RECOMMENDATIONS

Despite its transformative potential, generative AI in drug development faces several significant challenges that must be addressed to fully realize its promise.

Data Quality and Availability

- **The Challenge of High-Quality Training Data**

The performance of generative AI models is fundamentally constrained by the quality, quantity, and diversity of available training data. In the pharmaceutical context, several data-related challenges persist:

1. **Experimental Variability**: Bioactivity data often exhibits significant inter-laboratory and inter-assay variability, introducing noise that can confound model training. Standardization efforts like MIABE (Minimum Information About a Bioactive Entity) aim to address this issue but remain incompletely implemented (Orchard et al., 2011).
2. **Positive Results Bias**: The scientific literature and public databases are skewed toward positive results, with inactive compounds and failed experiments under-reported. This reporting bias creates an incomplete picture of structure-activity relationships and can lead generative models to overestimate the probability of success for certain molecular features (Dahlin & Walters, 2014).
3. **Confidentiality Constraints**: Much of the highest-quality pharmaceutical data remains proprietary, limiting the training data available to academic researchers and smaller organizations. While precompetitive data-sharing initiatives like the

COVID Moonshot project (Chodera et al., 2020) have demonstrated the value of collaborative approaches, broader implementation remains challenging.

Data Augmentation and Synthetic Data Generation

To address data limitations, researchers have developed various data augmentation and synthetic data generation techniques:

1. **Transfer Learning and Few-Shot Learning**: Approaches that leverage pre-training on large, general chemical datasets before fine-tuning on smaller, specific datasets have shown promise for overcoming data scarcity in specialized domains (Stokes et al., 2020).
2. **Physics-Informed Data Augmentation**: Incorporating physical constraints and domain knowledge into data augmentation procedures can generate synthetically enriched datasets that maintain physical realism while expanding coverage of chemical space (Xu et al., 2021).
3. **Generative Models for Data Enhancement**: Using generative models themselves to create synthetic training data represents a bootstrapping approach to addressing data limitations. However, care must be taken to avoid reinforcing biases present in the initial training data (Arús-Pous et al., 2020).

Interpretability and Trustworthiness

- **Black Box Nature of Deep Learning Models**

The opacity of many deep learning models presents a significant challenge for adoption in the risk-averse pharmaceutical industry. Drug developers typically seek mechanistic understanding of structure-activity relationships to guide optimization efforts and support regulatory submissions.

Several approaches have emerged to enhance the interpretability of generative models:

1. **Attention Visualization**: For transformer-based models, attention mechanisms can be visualized to highlight which molecular features influence the model's predictions, providing insights into learned structure-activity relationships (Karpov et al., 2020).
2. **Latent Space Navigation**: For VAEs and similar models, structured exploration of the latent space can reveal meaningful chemical transformations and property relationships, aiding in interpretable molecular design (Jin et al., 2020).

3. **Explainable AI (XAI) Techniques**: Methods like SHAP (SHapley Additive exPlanations) and LIME (Local Interpretable Model-Agnostic Explanations) can be applied to generative models to provide post-hoc explanations of their outputs, enhancing transparency and trustworthiness (Lundberg & Lee, 2017).
   - **Validation and Experimental Feedback**

The gap between computational predictions and experimental reality remains a significant challenge. Generated molecules may look promising in silico but fail when synthesized and tested. Establishing reliable validation protocols and efficient experimental feedback loops is essential for improving model performance over time.

Recent advances in this area include:

1. **Active Learning Frameworks**: Systems that intelligently select the most informative compounds for experimental testing, maximizing the information gain from limited experimental resources (Reker et al., 2019).
2. **Automated Synthesis and Testing**: Integration of generative design with automated synthesis and high-throughput testing creates closed-loop systems that can rapidly validate predictions and refine models based on experimental results (Baranczak et al., 2017).
3. **Confidence Calibration**: Techniques to ensure that model confidence estimates accurately reflect prediction uncertainty, enabling more reliable prioritization of generated compounds (Scalia et al., 2020).

Regulatory Considerations

The application of generative AI in drug development raises several regulatory questions regarding validation, reproducibility, and documentation requirements. Regulatory agencies like the FDA and EMA are developing frameworks for evaluating AI-generated evidence, but many aspects remain under discussion.

Key considerations include:

1. **Model Validation and Verification**: Regulatory agencies will likely require comprehensive validation of AI models used in drug development, including demonstrations of performance across diverse datasets, robustness to data perturbations, and documentation of training procedures (Mak & Pichika, 2019).
2. **Explainability Requirements**: For safety-critical applications, regulators may require a certain level of explainability from AI systems, allowing human experts to understand and verify the rationale behind model predictions and generations (Amann et al., 2020).

3. **Software Validation**: AI systems used in regulated drug development processes will need to comply with software validation requirements, such as those outlined in FDA's 21 CFR Part 11 for electronic records and signatures (Artificial Intelligence/Machine Learning (AI/ML)-Based Software as a Medical Device (SaMD) Action Plan, 2021).
4. **Standardization Needs**: The development of industry standards for AI validation, documentation, and reporting would facilitate regulatory assessments and promote consistency across applications. Organizations like the Alliance for Artificial Intelligence in Healthcare (AAIH) are working toward such standardization efforts.

FUTURE RESEARCH DIRECTIONS

Looking beyond current applications, generative AI has the potential to catalyze paradigm shifts in pharmaceutical R&D, fundamentally transforming how drugs are discovered, developed, and delivered to patients.

Autonomous Drug Discovery Systems

The ultimate vision for AI in drug discovery is the development of fully autonomous systems capable of executing the entire discovery process with minimal human intervention. Such systems would integrate multiple AI modalities—generative models, predictive algorithms, active learning, and automated experimentation—into closed-loop platforms that continuously learn and improve from experimental feedback.

Early prototypes of autonomous discovery systems, such as Recursion Pharmaceuticals' MAP platform and Insilico Medicine's PHARMA system, have demonstrated the feasibility of this approach for specific applications. As these systems mature, they could dramatically accelerate the discovery of novel therapeutics while reducing costs and resource requirements.

The development of autonomous discovery systems raises important questions about the changing role of human scientists in pharmaceutical R&D. Rather than replacing human expertise, these systems are likely to augment human capabilities, allowing scientists to focus on creative problem-solving, hypothesis generation, and strategic decision-making while AI handles routine tasks and explores vastly larger solution spaces.

Adaptive Clinical Trials Powered by AI

In clinical development, generative AI could enable more adaptive, patient-centric trial designs that continuously evolve based on accumulating data. Digital twins of patients, generated through AI models trained on multi-omics and clinical data, could enable in silico trial simulations that predict outcomes for diverse patient populations under various treatment regimens.

These approaches could significantly reduce the time and cost of clinical development while improving success rates through:

1. **Optimized patient selection**: AI-driven identification of patients most likely to respond to treatment based on molecular and clinical profiles.
2. **Adaptive dosing regimens**: Personalized dosing schedules optimized in real-time based on individual patient responses.
3. **Surrogate endpoints**: AI-validated digital biomarkers that provide earlier indications of efficacy, potentially shortening trial duration.
4. **Synthetic control arms**: Generated patient populations that reduce the need for placebo controls in certain contexts, particularly for rare diseases.

Integration with Other Cutting-Edge Technologies

The transformative potential of generative AI in drug development will be further amplified through integration with other emerging technologies:

1. **Quantum Computing**: As quantum computing matures, it could enable more accurate simulation of molecular systems and accelerate certain types of AI training, potentially unlocking new capabilities in structure-based drug design and molecular property prediction (Cao et al., 2018).
2. **Automated Synthesis Platforms**: Integration of generative AI with robotic chemistry platforms, such as those developed by Strateos and Emerald Cloud Lab, could create end-to-end automated discovery systems that design, synthesize, and test compounds without human intervention (Bédard et al., 2018).
3. **Organ-on-a-Chip Technology**: Combining generative AI with microfluidic organ models could enable more predictive assessment of compound efficacy and toxicity, potentially reducing reliance on animal models and improving translation to human outcomes (Low et al., 2021).
4. **Blockchain and Federated Learning**: These technologies could enable more collaborative AI development while preserving data privacy and security, facilitating the creation of larger, more diverse training datasets through precompetitive consortia (Kuo et al., 2020).

Ethical and Societal Implications

The rapid advancement of AI in drug development also raises important ethical and societal questions that must be addressed:

1. **Access and Equity**: Ensuring that AI-driven innovations benefit patients globally, regardless of socioeconomic status or geographic location, requires thoughtful policies around intellectual property, pricing, and technology transfer.
2. **Workforce Transformation**: As AI automates certain aspects of pharmaceutical R&D, the industry must manage workforce transitions through reskilling, education, and the development of new roles that leverage complementary human-AI capabilities.
3. **Accountability and Governance**: Establishing clear frameworks for accountability in AI-driven drug development decisions, particularly when adverse events occur, will be essential for maintaining public trust an

CONCLUSION

This chapter has explored the transformative potential of generative AI in drug development, guided by a detailed review of the traditional drug discovery process, its challenges, and the integration of AI-driven innovations. Drug development is a long, expensive, and uncertain journey—often taking more than a decade and billions of dollars to bring a single treatment to market. Despite heavy investments, the success rate remains low, and many promising ideas never make it past early testing. In this context, generative AI has emerged as a game-changer. Unlike traditional tools that analyze existing data, generative AI has the ability to create—designing entirely new molecules, suggesting potential drug targets, and even helping tailor clinical trials to the right patients. Throughout this chapter, we've explored how these AI models work and where they're already making an impact across the drug development pipeline. We also looked at the challenges that come with adopting such powerful technologies. Concerns around data quality, explainability, and regulatory approval are real and must be addressed thoughtfully. Trust, transparency, and collaboration between researchers, developers, and regulators will be key to making the most of what generative AI has to offer. Looking to the future, it's clear that generative AI isn't just another tool—it could fundamentally reshape how we discover and develop new medicines. With more accessible data, smarter algorithms, and a shared commitment to innovation, we're entering a new chapter in pharmaceutical science. Ultimately, this technology holds the promise to speed up discovery, lower costs, and bring better treatments to patients faster. But realizing that promise will require not just advanced models, but also responsible leadership and a human-centered approach.

REFERENCES

Amann, J., Blasimme, A., Vayena, E., Frey, D., & Madai, V. I. (2020). Explainability for artificial intelligence in healthcare: A multidisciplinary perspective. *BMC Medical Informatics and Decision Making*, *20*(1), 310. DOI: 10.1186/s12911-020-01332-6 PMID: 33256715

Arús-Pous, J., Patronov, A., Bjerrum, E. J., Tyrchan, C., Reymond, J. L., Chen, H., & Engkvist, O. (2020). SMILES-based deep generative scaffold decorator for de-novo drug design. Journal of Cheminformatics, 12(1), 38. Artificial Intelligence/Machine Learning (AI/ML)-Based Software as a Medical Device (SaMD) Action Plan. (2021). U.S. Food and Drug Administration. https://www.fda.gov/media/145022/downloadDOI: 10.1186/s13321-020-00441-8

Bagal, V., Aggarwal, R., Vinod, P. K., & Priyakumar, U. D. (2021). MolGPT: Molecular generation using a transformer-decoder model. *Journal of Chemical Information and Modeling*, *62*(9), 2064–2076. DOI: 10.1021/acs.jcim.1c00600 PMID: 34694798

Baranczak, P. J., Shangari, N. G., Palacios, D. S., Kratz, J. M., & O'Shea, K. (2017). Automated chemistry: A vision for the future. *Journal of Medicinal Chemistry*, *60*(20), 8353–8358. DOI: 10.1021/acs.jmedchem.7b00641

Beaulieu-Jones, B. K., Finlayson, S. G., Chivers, C., Chen, I., McDermott, M., Kandola, J., Dalca, A. V., & Beam, A. L. (2019). Trends in the adoption of statistical and machine learning methods in biomedical research. *BMC Medical Research Methodology*, *19*(1), 162. DOI: 10.1186/s12874-019-0799-4 PMID: 31340753

Bédard, A. C., Adamo, A., Aroh, K. C., Russell, M. G., Bedermann, A. A., Torosian, J., Yue, B., Jensen, K. F., & Jamison, T. F. (2018). Reconfigurable system for automated optimization of diverse chemical reactions. *Science*, *361*(6408), 1220–1225. DOI: 10.1126/science.aat0650 PMID: 30237351

Blaschke, T., Arús-Pous, J., Chen, H., Margreitter, C., Tyrchan, C., Engkvist, O., Papadopoulos, K., & Patronov, A. (2020). REINVENT 2.0: An AI tool for de novo drug design. *Journal of Chemical Information and Modeling*, *60*(12), 5918–5922. DOI: 10.1021/acs.jcim.0c00915 PMID: 33118816

Bradshaw, J., Kusner, M. J., Paige, B., Segler, M. H., & Hernández-Lobato, J. M. (2020). A generative model for electron paths. arXiv preprint arXiv:1805.10970. https://arxiv.org/abs/1805.10970

Brown, N., Fiscato, M., Segler, M. H., & Vaucher, A. C. (2018). GuacaMol: Benchmarking models for de novo molecular design. *Journal of Chemical Information and Modeling*, *59*(3), 1096–1108. DOI: 10.1021/acs.jcim.8b00839 PMID: 30887799

Brown, P., Tan, A.-C., El-Esawi, M. A., Liehr, T., Blanck, O., Gladue, D. P., Almeida, G. M. F., Cernava, T., Sorzano, C. O., Yeung, A. W. K., Engel, M. S., Chandrasekaran, A. R., Muth, T., Staege, M. S., Daulatabad, S. V., Widera, D., Zhang, J., Meule, A., Honjo, K., & Zhou, Y.RELISH Consortium. (2021). Large expert-curated database for benchmarking document similarity detection in biomedical literature search. *Database : The Journal of Biological Databases and Curation*, *2019*, baz085. Advance online publication. DOI: 10.1093/database/baz085 PMID: 33326193

Cao, Y., Romero, J., & Aspuru-Guzik, A. (2018). Potential of quantum computing for drug discovery. IBM Journal of Research and Development, 62(6), 6:1-6:20. DOI: 10.1147/JRD.2018.2888987

Chithrananda, S., Grand, G., & Ramsundar, B. (2020). ChemBERTa: Large-scale self-supervised pretraining for molecular property prediction. arXiv preprint arXiv:2010.09885. https://arxiv.org/abs/2010.09885

Chodera, J., Lee, A. A., London, N., & von Delft, F. (2020). Crowdsourcing drug discovery for pandemics. *Nature Chemistry*, *12*(7), 581–581. DOI: 10.1038/s41557-020-0496-2 PMID: 32555379

Cook, D., Brown, D., Alexander, R., March, R., Morgan, P., Satterthwaite, G., & Pangalos, M. N. (2014). Lessons learned from the fate of AstraZeneca's drug pipeline: A five-dimensional framework. *Nature Reviews. Drug Discovery*, *13*(6), 419–431. DOI: 10.1038/nrd4309 PMID: 24833294

Dahlin, J. L., & Walters, M. A. (2014). The essential roles of chemistry in high-throughput screening triage. *Future Medicinal Chemistry*, *6*(11), 1265–1290. DOI: 10.4155/fmc.14.60 PMID: 25163000

De Cao, N., & Kipf, T. (2018). MolGAN: An implicit generative model for small molecular graphs. arXiv preprint arXiv:1805.11973. https://arxiv.org/abs/1805.11973

DiMasi, J. A., Grabowski, H. G., & Hansen, R. W. (2016). Innovation in the pharmaceutical industry: New estimates of R&D costs. *Journal of Health Economics*, *47*, 20–33. DOI: 10.1016/j.jhealeco.2016.01.012 PMID: 26928437

Dobson, C. M. (2004). Chemical space and biology. *Nature*, *432*(7019), 824–828. DOI: 10.1038/nature03192 PMID: 15602547

Edwards, C., Lai, T., Ros, K., Honke, G., & Ji, H. (2022). Translation between molecules and natural language. arXiv preprint arXiv:2204.11817. https://arxiv.org/abs/2204.11817 DOI: 10.18653/v1/2022.emnlp-main.26

Ertl, P., & Schuffenhauer, A. (2009). Estimation of synthetic accessibility score of drug-like molecules based on molecular complexity and fragment contributions. *Journal of Cheminformatics*, *1*(1), 8. DOI: 10.1186/1758-2946-1-8 PMID: 20298526

Fabian, B., Edlich, T., Gaspar, H., Segler, M., Meyers, J., Fiscato, M., & Ahmed, M. (2020). Molecular representation learning with language models and domain-relevant auxiliary tasks. arXiv preprint arXiv:2011.13230. https://arxiv.org/abs/2011.13230

Fisher, C. K., Smith, A. M., & Walsh, J. R. (2021). Machine learning for comprehensive forecasting of Alzheimer's Disease progression. *Scientific Reports*, *11*(1), 1–13. DOI: 10.1038/s41598-021-99494-4 PMID: 33414495

Fourches, D., Muratov, E., & Tropsha, A. (2010). Trust, but verify: On the importance of chemical structure curation in cheminformatics and QSAR modeling research. *Journal of Chemical Information and Modeling*, *50*(7), 1189–1204. DOI: 10.1021/ci100176x PMID: 20572635

Gómez-Bombarelli, R., Wei, J. N., Duvenaud, D., Hernández-Lobato, J. M., Sánchez-Lengeling, B., Sheberla, D., Aguilera-Iparraguirre, J., Hirzel, T. D., Adams, R. P., & Aspuru-Guzik, A. (2018). Automatic chemical design using a data-driven continuous representation of molecules. *ACS Central Science*, *4*(2), 268–276. DOI: 10.1021/acscentsci.7b00572 PMID: 29532027

Grisoni, F., Neuhaus, C. S., Gabernet, G., Müller, A. T., Hiss, J. A., & Schneider, G. (2020). Designing anticancer peptides by constructive machine learning. *ChemMedChem*, *15*(4), 300–305. DOI: 10.1002/cmdc.201900599 PMID: 29679519

Guimaraes, G. L., Sanchez-Lengeling, B., Outeiral, C., Farias, P. L. C., & Aspuru-Guzik, A. (2017). Objective-reinforced generative adversarial networks (ORGAN) for sequence generation models. arXiv preprint arXiv:1705.10843. https://arxiv.org/abs/1705.10843

He, S., Guo, F., Zou, Q., & Ding, H. (2020). MRMD2.0: A Python tool for machine learning with feature ranking and reduction. *Current Bioinformatics*, *15*(10), 1213–1221. DOI: 10.2174/2212392XMTA2bMjko1

Hoogeboom, E., Satorras, V. G., Vignac, C., & Welling, M. (2022). Equivariant diffusion for molecule generation in 3D. arXiv preprint arXiv:2203.17003. https://arxiv.org/abs/2203.17003

Huang, K., Fu, T., Glass, L. M., Zitnik, M., Xiao, C., & Sun, J. (2020). DeepPurpose: A deep learning library for drug-target interaction prediction. *Bioinformatics (Oxford, England)*, *36*(22-23), 5545–5547. DOI: 10.1093/bioinformatics/btaa1005 PMID: 33275143

Hughes, J. P., Rees, S., Kalindjian, S. B., & Philpott, K. L. (2011). Principles of early drug discovery. *British Journal of Pharmacology*, *162*(6), 1239–1249. DOI: 10.1111/j.1476-5381.2010.01127.x PMID: 21091654

Jayatunga, M. K., Jung, S., & Chen, J. (2022). AI in small-molecule drug discovery: A coming wave. *Nature Reviews. Drug Discovery*, *21*(3), 175–176. DOI: 10.1038/d41573-022-00025-1 PMID: 35132242

Jin, W., Barzilay, R., & Jaakkola, T. (2020). Hierarchical graph-to-graph translation for molecules. arXiv preprint arXiv:1907.11223. https://arxiv.org/abs/1907.11223

Jumper, J., Evans, R., Pritzel, A., Green, T., Figurnov, M., Ronneberger, O., Tunyasuvunakool, K., Bates, R., Žídek, A., Potapenko, A., Bridgland, A., Meyer, C., Kohl, S. A. A., Ballard, A. J., Cowie, A., Romera-Paredes, B., Nikolov, S., Jain, R., Adler, J., & Hassabis, D. (2021). Highly accurate protein structure prediction with AlphaFold. *Nature*, *596*(7873), 583–589. DOI: 10.1038/s41586-021-03819-2 PMID: 34265844

Kadurin, A., Nikolenko, S., Khrabrov, K., Aliper, A., & Zhavoronkov, A. (2017). druGAN: An advanced generative adversarial autoencoder model for de novo generation of new molecules with desired molecular properties in silico. *Molecular Pharmaceutics*, *14*(9), 3098–3104. DOI: 10.1021/acs.molpharmaceut.7b00346 PMID: 28703000

Karpov, P., Godin, G., & Tetko, I. V. (2020). Transformer-CNN: Swiss knife for QSAR modeling and interpretation. *Journal of Cheminformatics*, *12*(1), 17. DOI: 10.1186/s13321-020-00423-w PMID: 33431004

Kuo, T. T., Gabriel, R. A., Cidambi, K. R., & Ohno-Machado, L. (2020). EXpectation Propagation LOgistic REgRession on permissioned blockCHAIN (ExplorerChain): Decentralized privacy-preserving online healthcare analytics. *IEEE Journal of Biomedical and Health Informatics*, *24*(8), 2278–2287. DOI: 10.1109/JBHI.2020.2969648 PMID: 31841426

Low, L. A., Mummery, C., Berridge, B. R., Austin, C. P., & Tagle, D. A. (2021). Organs-on-chips: Into the next decade. *Nature Reviews. Drug Discovery*, *20*(5), 345–361. DOI: 10.1038/s41573-020-0079-3 PMID: 32913334

Lundberg, S. M., & Lee, S. I. (2017). A unified approach to interpreting model predictions. *Advances in Neural Information Processing Systems*, *30*, 4765–4774.

Luo, S., Guan, J., Ma, J., & Peng, J. (2021). A 3D-based graph convolution network for predicting protein-ligand binding affinity. *bioRxiv*. DOI: 10.1101/2021.04.16.440230

Macarron, R., Banks, M. N., Bojanic, D., Burns, D. J., Cirovic, D. A., Garyantes, T., Green, D. V., Hertzberg, R. P., Janzen, W. P., Paslay, J. W., Schopfer, U., & Sittampalam, G. S. (2011). Impact of high-throughput screening in biomedical research. *Nature Reviews. Drug Discovery*, *10*(3), 188–195. DOI: 10.1038/nrd3368 PMID: 21358738

Mak, K. K., & Pichika, M. R. (2019). Artificial intelligence in drug development: Present status and future prospects. *Drug Discovery Today*, *24*(3), 773–780. DOI: 10.1016/j.drudis.2018.11.014 PMID: 30472429

Mullard, A. (2016). Parsing clinical success rates. *Nature Reviews. Drug Discovery*, *15*(7), 447–447. DOI: 10.1038/nrd.2016.136 PMID: 27357012

Olivecrona, M., Blaschke, T., Engkvist, O., & Chen, H. (2017). Molecular de-novo design through deep reinforcement learning. *Journal of Cheminformatics*, *9*(1), 48. DOI: 10.1186/s13321-017-0235-x PMID: 29086083

Orchard, S., Al-Lazikani, B., Bryant, S., Clark, D., Calder, E., Dix, I., Engkvist, O., Forster, M., Gaulton, A., Gilson, M., Glen, R., Grigorov, M., Hammond-Kosack, K., Harland, L., Hopkins, A., Larminie, C., Lynch, N., Mann, R. K., Murray-Rust, P., & Hermjakob, H. (2011). Minimum information about a bioactive entity (MIABE). *Nature Reviews. Drug Discovery*, *10*(9), 661–669. DOI: 10.1038/nrd3503 PMID: 21878981

Paul, D., Sanap, G., Shenoy, S., Kalyane, D., Kalia, K., & Tekade, R. K. (2021). Artificial intelligence in drug discovery and development. *Drug Discovery Today*, *26*(1), 80–93. DOI: 10.1016/j.drudis.2020.10.010 PMID: 33099022

Pogány, P., Arad, N., Genway, S., & Pickett, S. D. (2018). De novo molecule design by translating from reduced graphs to SMILES. *Journal of Chemical Information and Modeling*, *59*(3), 1136–1146. DOI: 10.1021/acs.jcim.8b00626 PMID: 30525594

Reker, D., Bernardes, G. J., & Rodrigues, T. (2019). Computational advances in combating colloidal aggregation in drug discovery. *Nature Chemistry*, *11*(5), 402–418. DOI: 10.1038/s41557-019-0234-9 PMID: 30988417

Reker, D., Hoyt, E. A., Bernardes, G. J., & Rodrigues, T. (2020). Adaptive optimization of chemical reactions with minimal experimental information. *Cell Reports. Physical Science*, *1*(10), 100247. DOI: 10.1016/j.xcrp.2020.100247

Scalia, G., Grambow, C. A., Pernici, B., Li, Y. P., & Green, W. H. (2020). Evaluating scalable uncertainty estimation methods for deep learning-based molecular property prediction. *Journal of Chemical Information and Modeling*, *60*(6), 2697–2717. DOI: 10.1021/acs.jcim.9b00975 PMID: 32243154

Scannell, J. W., Blanckley, A., Boldon, H., & Warrington, B. (2012). Diagnosing the decline in pharmaceutical R&D efficiency. *Nature Reviews. Drug Discovery*, *11*(3), 191–200. DOI: 10.1038/nrd3681 PMID: 22378269

Scannell, J. W., & Bosley, J. (2016). When quality beats quantity: Decision theory, drug discovery, and the reproducibility crisis. *PLoS One*, *11*(2), e0147215. DOI: 10.1371/journal.pone.0147215 PMID: 26863229

Segal, C., Homza, A., Tu, R., & Xing, E. P. (2021). Leveraging multi-task learning to classify diseases from histology data: A comparison of deep learning architectures. arXiv preprint arXiv:2107.05984. https://arxiv.org/abs/2107.05984

Segler, M. H., Preuss, M., & Waller, M. P. (2018). Planning chemical syntheses with deep neural networks and symbolic AI. *Nature*, *555*(7698), 604–610. DOI: 10.1038/nature25978 PMID: 29595767

Stokes, J. M., Yang, K., Swanson, K., Jin, W., Cubillos-Ruiz, A., Donghia, N. M., MacNair, C. R., French, S., Carfrae, L. A., Bloom-Ackermann, Z., Tran, V. M., Chiappino-Pepe, A., Badran, A. H., Andrews, I. W., Chory, E. J., Church, G. M., Brown, E. D., Jaakkola, T. S., Barzilay, R., & Collins, J. J. (2020). A deep learning approach to antibiotic discovery. *Cell*, *180*(4), 688–702. DOI: 10.1016/j.cell.2020.01.021 PMID: 32084340

Subramanian, A., Narayan, R., Corsello, S. M., Peck, D. D., Natoli, T. E., Lu, X., Gould, J., Davis, J. F., Tubelli, A. A., Asiedu, J. K., Lahr, D. L., Hirschman, J. E., Liu, Z., Donahue, M., Julian, B., Khan, M., Wadden, D., Smith, I. C., Lam, D., & Golub, T. R. (2017). A next generation connectivity map: L1000 platform and the first 1,000,000 profiles. *Cell*, *171*(6), 1437–1452. DOI: 10.1016/j.cell.2017.10.049 PMID: 29195078

Townshend, R. J., Eismann, S., Watkins, A. M., Rangan, R., Karelina, M., Das, R., & Dror, R. O. (2021). Geometric deep learning of RNA structure. *Science*, *373*(6558), 1047–1051. DOI: 10.1126/science.abe5650 PMID: 34446608

Vamathevan, J., Clark, D., Czodrowski, P., Dunham, I., Ferran, E., Lee, G., Li, B., Madabhushi, A., Shah, P., Spitzer, M., & Zhao, S. (2019). Applications of machine learning in drug discovery and development. *Nature Reviews. Drug Discovery*, *18*(6), 463–477. DOI: 10.1038/s41573-019-0024-5 PMID: 30976107

Walters, W. P., & Barzilay, R. (2021). Applications of deep learning in molecule generation and molecular property prediction. *Accounts of Chemical Research, 54*(2), 263–270. DOI: 10.1021/acs.accounts.0c00699 PMID: 33370107

Way, G. P., & Greene, C. S. (2018). Extracting a biologically relevant latent space from cancer transcriptomes with variational autoencoders. *Pacific Symposium on Biocomputing, 23*, 80–91. DOI: 10.1142/9789813235533_0008 PMID: 29218871

Wu, Z., Ramsundar, B., Feinberg, E. N., Gomes, J., Geniesse, C., Pappu, A. S., Leswing, K., & Pande, V. (2018). MoleculeNet: A benchmark for molecular machine learning. *Chemical Science (Cambridge), 9*(2), 513–530. DOI: 10.1039/C7SC02664A PMID: 29629118

Xiong, G., Wu, Z., Yi, J., Fu, L., Yang, Z., Hsieh, C., Yin, M., Zeng, X., Wu, C., Lu, A., Chen, X., Hou, T., & Cao, D. (2021). ADMETlab 2.0

Zhavoronkov, A., Ivanenkov, Y. A., Aliper, A., Veselov, M., Aladinskiy, V., Aladinskaya, A., Terentiev, V., Polykovskiy, D., Kuznetsov, M., Asadulaev, A., Volynkin, V., Zholus, A., Shayakhmetov, R., Zhebrak, A., Minaeva, L., Zagribelnyy, B., Lee, L. H., Soll, R., Madge, D., & Aspuru-Guzik, A. (2019). Deep learning enables rapid identification of potent DDR1 kinase inhibitors. *Nature Biotechnology, 37*(9), 1038–1040. DOI: 10.1038/s41587-019-0224-x PMID: 31477924

ADDITIONAL READING

Budinich, M., Blaschke, T., & Segler, M. H. S. (2024). REINVENT 4: Modern AI-driven generative molecule design. *Journal of Cheminformatics, 16*(1), 45. Advance online publication. DOI: 10.1186/s13321-024-00812-5 PMID: 38627862

Liu, X., Lu, Z., Wang, T., & Liu, F. (2024). Large language models facilitating modern molecular biology and novel drug development. *Frontiers in Pharmacology, 15*, 1458739. Advance online publication. DOI: 10.3389/fphar.2024.1458739 PMID: 39776586

KEY TERMS AND DEFINITIONS

Generative AI: A branch of artificial intelligence that creates new data instances—such as molecules or protein structures—rather than simply interpreting existing data. In pharmaceutical research, it is used for de novo drug design and multi-objective molecular optimization.

Reinforcement Learning (RL): A machine learning approach where agents learn to make decisions by receiving rewards or penalties. In drug discovery, RL guides generative models to design compounds with desired properties through reward-based optimization.

De Novo Molecule Design: The process of generating entirely new molecular structures from scratch using AI models. It aims to discover novel drug candidates with optimized properties, often without requiring prior structural knowledge of known compounds.

Multi-Parameter Optimization: An approach in drug design where several properties—such as potency, toxicity, solubility, and synthesizability—are optimized simultaneously. Generative AI frameworks are tailored to handle such complex, competing objectives.

ADMET: An acronym for Absorption, Distribution, Metabolism, Excretion, and Toxicity—key pharmacokinetic and safety parameters that influence drug viability. AI models predict ADMET properties early to reduce late-stage failures.

Synthetic Accessibility: A measure of how easily a designed compound can be synthesized in the lab. AI models incorporate synthetic accessibility scores or retrosynthesis predictions to ensure practicality of molecule synthesis.

Bioactivity Data: Information about how biological targets respond to chemical compounds, including binding affinity and IC50 values. Such data fuels training for predictive and generative models in AI-driven drug discovery.

Protein Structures: 3D models of proteins used to inform structure-based drug design. AI tools leverage this structural data to design ligands that precisely fit target binding sites, improving efficacy.

Target Identification: The process of discovering biological molecules, such as proteins, that can be modulated to treat disease. Generative AI models analyze omics data and biological networks to propose novel therapeutic targets.

Data Curation: The process of cleaning, standardizing, and validating datasets used in AI model training. High-quality data curation is essential for ensuring accuracy, reproducibility, and generalizability in generative drug design.

Chapter 6
AI-Driven Smart Manufacturing and Automation in Pharmaceutical Production

Arshi Naim
https://orcid.org/0000-0003-1325-6964
Business Management, European Global Institute of Innovation and Technology, Malta

Anandhavalli Muniasamy
https://orcid.org/0000-0001-8940-3954
Department of Informatics and Computer Systems, College of Computer Science, King Khalid University, Saudi Arabia

Mohammad Ibrahim Khan
International Medical University, Malyasia

Mohammad Faiz Khan
Ministry of Interiors, Security Forces Hospital, Saudi Arabia

ABSTRACT

Artificial Intelligence (AI) is transforming pharmaceutical manufacturing by enabling smart automation, optimizing production processes, and ensuring regulatory compliance. This chapter explores the role of AI-driven technologies in enhancing efficiency, quality control, and decision-making within pharmaceutical production. It provides an overview of Industry 4.0 advancements, highlighting key AI applications

DOI: 10.4018/979-8-3373-2043-4.ch006

such as predictive maintenance, digital twins, and robotics. A case study illustrates real-world AI implementation, emphasizing benefits and challenges. Additionally, the chapter discusses AI-driven solutions, best practices for integration, and regulatory considerations. Finally, future directions and emerging trends in AI-powered pharmaceutical manufacturing are examined.

INTRODUCTION

The pharmaceutical industry is undergoing a transformative revolution catalyzed by the rapid advancement of artificial intelligence (AI) and automation technologies. The convergence of AI with Industry 4.0 paradigms—such as the Internet of Things (IoT), cyber-physical systems, cloud computing, and big data analytics—has set the foundation for what is now being termed as "Pharma 4.0" (Rüßmann et al., 2015). Within this context, smart manufacturing and automation are no longer optional innovations but critical imperatives for pharmaceutical companies seeking to enhance productivity, maintain regulatory compliance, ensure quality, and accelerate time-to-market.

Traditionally, pharmaceutical manufacturing has been characterized by batch-based processes, manual interventions, and complex regulatory workflows. These conventional methodologies, while reliable, are increasingly proving insufficient in a global landscape that demands agility, personalization, and cost-effectiveness. AI technologies such as machine learning (ML), deep learning (DL), natural language processing (NLP), and reinforcement learning are now being employed to optimize manufacturing processes, monitor equipment health, predict production anomalies, and enable real-time quality assurance (Blanco-González et al., 2023).

Smart manufacturing in the pharmaceutical domain refers to the integration of intelligent algorithms with real-time data streams from manufacturing systems. These technologies enable predictive maintenance, adaptive process control, and dynamic scheduling of operations. Automation, in turn, enhances operational efficiency and minimizes human error, especially in highly sensitive operations such as drug synthesis, formulation, and packaging. By leveraging AI and automation, pharmaceutical firms can achieve consistent product quality, reduced operational downtime, and better resource utilization (Dunjko & Briegel, 2018).

Historical Context and Technological Evolution

The roots of automation in the pharmaceutical sector can be traced back to the early implementation of programmable logic controllers (PLCs) and supervisory control and data acquisition (SCADA) systems in the 1980s. While these systems enabled a certain degree of automation, they lacked the cognitive abilities and decision-making capabilities of modern AI systems. Over time, as data collection became more sophisticated, the pharmaceutical industry began to realize the untapped potential of data-driven insights.

With the advent of AI and big data, the ability to analyze vast volumes of manufacturing data and extract actionable insights has fundamentally changed operational strategies. AI-powered systems can learn from historical data to forecast demand, optimize material use, and maintain compliance with Good Manufacturing Practices (GMP). The shift from rule-based automation to intelligent automation marks a paradigm shift in how pharmaceutical operations are conceived and executed (Topol, 2019).

Moreover, the regulatory landscape is also adapting to these changes. Agencies such as the U.S. Food and Drug Administration (FDA) and the European Medicines Agency (EMA, 2023) are now exploring frameworks that accommodate AI-enabled manufacturing systems. Initiatives like the FDA's Emerging Technology Program aim to support innovation by providing guidance on the adoption of advanced technologies in drug manufacturing (FDA, 2023).

Drivers of AI-Driven Smart Manufacturing

Several factors are accelerating the adoption of AI and automation in pharmaceutical production:

1. **Complexity of Drug Development**: The increasing complexity of modern therapeutics—such as biologics, cell and gene therapies—demands more sophisticated manufacturing processes. These require real-time monitoring and control systems that can adapt to subtle variations in process conditions.
2. **Globalization and Competition**: Pharmaceutical companies are under pressure to reduce costs while maintaining high-quality standards. AI-enabled automation can optimize resource allocation, minimize waste, and reduce operational costs.
3. **Personalized Medicine**: The rise of personalized medicine calls for flexible and adaptive manufacturing setups that can handle small-batch production with high precision. AI facilitates this by enabling real-time analytics and process customization.
4. **Regulatory Compliance and Quality Control**: Ensuring compliance with GMP and other regulatory standards is paramount in pharmaceuticals. AI tools can assist in documentation, traceability, and continuous quality verification.

5. **Pandemic Preparedness**: The COVID-19 pandemic exposed vulnerabilities in pharmaceutical supply chains and manufacturing systems. AI and automation offer resilience by enabling remote monitoring, digital twins, and rapid reconfiguration of production lines (Li et al., 2017).

Research Gap

Despite the growing interest and several pilot projects showcasing the potential of AI in pharmaceutical manufacturing, its adoption remains fragmented and inconsistent across the industry. Several critical research and implementation gaps persist:

- **Lack of Standardization**: There is a lack of standardized frameworks for integrating AI systems within existing manufacturing infrastructures. This results in interoperability challenges and fragmented data ecosystems.
- **Data Quality and Availability**: AI systems require large, high-quality datasets for training. In many manufacturing environments, data is siloed, unstructured, or of insufficient granularity to support advanced analytics.
- **Explainability and Trust in AI**: Black-box AI models often lack transparency, making it difficult for regulatory bodies and stakeholders to trust AI-generated decisions. Explainable AI (XAI) is still in its infancy in this domain.
- **Skilled Workforce**: There is a gap in interdisciplinary talent that combines domain expertise in pharmaceutical sciences with AI and data science capabilities. This impedes the smooth adoption of AI-based solutions.
- **Regulatory Uncertainty**: While regulatory bodies are becoming more open to AI, the lack of clear guidelines and frameworks specific to smart manufacturing continues to be a barrier.

Addressing these gaps is crucial for mainstreaming AI and automation in pharmaceutical production. Further research is needed to develop robust, explainable, and scalable AI models that can operate within the stringent regulatory and operational constraints of the pharmaceutical industry.

Objectives of the Chapter

This chapter aims to present a comprehensive overview of how AI-driven smart manufacturing and automation are transforming pharmaceutical production. The specific objectives include:

1. **To explore the evolution of AI technologies in pharmaceutical manufacturing**

This includes a historical review of automation and the transition to intelligent systems, highlighting key milestones and technological breakthroughs.

2. **To identify the core components of AI-driven smart manufacturing systems**

Components such as machine learning algorithms, data acquisition systems, digital twins, and robotic process automation (RPA) will be discussed in depth.

3. **To analyze real-world case studies and industry applications**

The chapter will examine how leading pharmaceutical firms have implemented AI and automation in production, quality assurance, and supply chain management.

4. **To discuss challenges and limitations in the current landscape**

Emphasis will be placed on data governance, ethical issues, explainability, and regulatory compliance in AI-driven environments.

5. **To propose a framework for implementing AI-based smart manufacturing in pharmaceuticals**

The chapter will offer a structured roadmap covering assessment, planning, integration, validation, and scaling of AI solutions.

6. **To identify future research directions and policy implications**

Based on the identified gaps, the chapter will outline areas for future inquiry, including the development of AI governance frameworks, cross-industry collaborations, and the role of public-private partnerships.

AI and automation are redefining the contours of pharmaceutical manufacturing, ushering in a new era of precision, efficiency, and adaptability. However, these advancements come with their own set of challenges that must be addressed through targeted research, cross-disciplinary collaboration, and policy innovation. This chapter endeavors to provide an in-depth exploration of these transformative technologies, while also charting a path forward for their responsible and effective integration into pharmaceutical production systems.

BACKGROUND

The pharmaceutical industry, historically reliant on traditional and often rigid manufacturing paradigms, is experiencing an inflection point. This transformation is being propelled by the convergence of multiple technological forces, particularly artificial intelligence (AI), machine learning (ML), robotics, and data analytics. To fully appreciate the disruptive impact of AI-driven smart manufacturing and automation in pharmaceuticals, it is essential to understand the background landscape in which these innovations are taking place.

The Transition from Traditional to Smart Manufacturing

Conventional pharmaceutical production has largely operated within batch-based manufacturing frameworks. These models, though time-tested, often suffer from inefficiencies such as production downtime, human error, delayed quality control, and resource waste (Gandu et al., 2023). Moreover, the batch approach limits scalability and adaptability, particularly when dealing with personalized therapies and novel drug formulations that require rapid changes in process parameters.

Smart manufacturing aims to overcome these limitations by integrating AI, sensor networks, and real-time data analysis to enable dynamic decision-making and adaptive control of production systems. Smart systems continuously learn from data, adjust process variables in real-time, and predict equipment or material failures before they occur (Prabu et al., 2025). This shift from reactive to predictive operations underpins the core philosophy of Industry 4.0 in the pharmaceutical domain, also referred to as "Pharma 4.0".

Key Technologies Enabling Smart Pharmaceutical Manufacturing

Smart manufacturing in the pharmaceutical industry is rapidly advancing, powered by the integration of cutting-edge digital technologies with traditional production processes. Artificial Intelligence (AI) lies at the heart of this transformation, enabling manufacturers to make faster, more accurate decisions, improve quality control, reduce waste, and enhance operational efficiency. However, AI does not function in isolation; rather, it relies on a suite of core enabling technologies that form the foundation for AI's implementation in a manufacturing environment. These include Cyber-Physical Systems (CPS), digital twins, advanced robotics and automation, big data analytics, and cloud computing. Each of these technologies plays a unique and essential role in building an intelligent and responsive manufacturing ecosystem.

1. Cyber-Physical Systems (CPS)

Cyber-Physical Systems represent the backbone of smart manufacturing. These systems tightly integrate computational elements with physical processes through embedded sensors, actuators, and communication networks. In the context of pharmaceutical manufacturing, CPS acts as the central nervous system, continuously monitoring critical process parameters such as temperature, pressure, pH levels, mixing speed, humidity, and more.

CPS ensures real-time data collection and processing by interfacing with equipment across the manufacturing line. For instance, in a bioreactor used for the fermentation of biologic drugs, sensors embedded within the CPS track variables like nutrient concentration, gas flow rates, and cell density. These inputs are then analyzed by AI algorithms to determine whether conditions need to be adjusted. If necessary, CPS can autonomously alter the environment—adjusting the temperature, for example, or modifying agitation speed—to maintain optimal conditions for production.

By implementing closed-loop control mechanisms, CPS can instantly respond to deviations, effectively minimizing human intervention and reducing process variability. This autonomous adaptability is essential for maintaining consistent product quality in a highly regulated industry. According to Lee et al. (2015), CPS enhances the resilience and responsiveness of manufacturing systems by linking cyber intelligence directly with physical operations.

2. Digital Twins

Digital twins are another transformative technology at the core of smart manufacturing. A digital twin is a dynamic, digital replica of a physical process, product, or system. It continuously receives data from its physical counterpart through CPS and IoT devices, enabling real-time monitoring, simulation, and prediction.

In pharmaceutical production, digital twins serve multiple strategic functions. They are extensively used to simulate complex processes, such as chemical reactions, fermentation, or freeze-drying, without risking disruption to actual manufacturing lines. This allows operators and engineers to conduct "what-if" analyses—testing different parameters or process changes virtually before applying them in real life. These simulations provide insights into the potential effects on yield, purity, cycle time, and other critical quality attributes (CQAs).

Moreover, digital twins play a vital role in facilitating continuous improvement and innovation. For example, if a new formulation is being considered or a process is being transferred to a different facility, the digital twin can help ensure that these changes are properly validated and optimized before any physical implementation occurs.

Digital twins also improve traceability and regulatory compliance. Since every change and its corresponding outcome can be tracked within the simulation environment, they offer a robust digital audit trail—an invaluable feature in the strictly regulated pharmaceutical landscape. As noted by Fuller et al. (2020), the integration of AI into digital twins further elevates their capability to not just simulate current conditions but to proactively optimize and control manufacturing performance.

3. Advanced Robotics and Automation

Automation has long been a part of pharmaceutical manufacturing, especially for high-volume tasks such as pill counting or packaging. However, the advent of AI-driven robotics is expanding the scope of automation into more sensitive and complex areas such as aseptic filling, chemical synthesis, and sterile material handling.

Modern robotic systems are increasingly being deployed in cleanroom environments, where human presence must be minimized to reduce contamination risks. These robots, guided by AI and machine vision, can carry out tasks like vial filling, syringe assembly, and precise reagent dispensing with high accuracy and repeatability.

4. Big Data and Cloud Computing

The vast amount of data generated across production stages—raw material inspection, in-process testing, and final product release—presents a significant opportunity for optimization. Cloud platforms allow centralized storage and processing of this data, enabling predictive analytics and cross-functional insights that would be infeasible with siloed on-premises systems.

In the era of smart pharmaceutical manufacturing, Big Data and Cloud Computing serve as foundational enablers of artificial intelligence (AI) integration. Modern pharmaceutical operations generate immense volumes of data at every stage of the product lifecycle—from raw material procurement and in-process monitoring to quality assurance and post-market surveillance. Traditionally, much of this data resided in disparate, siloed systems, limiting its utility for real-time decision-making or predictive analytics. The advent of cloud computing and big data technologies has fundamentally transformed this landscape.

Big data encompasses structured and unstructured data streams, including process control data, laboratory results, sensor readings, environmental monitoring, equipment logs, and even external data such as regulatory updates or supply chain disruptions. Harnessing these vast and varied data sources is critical to training and deploying robust AI models. For instance, predictive models that forecast equipment failures or deviations in product quality rely on historical process data enriched with real-time inputs.

Cloud computing provides the infrastructure needed to store, manage, and analyze these massive datasets. Cloud platforms enable centralized, scalable, and secure data management, allowing multiple stakeholders—ranging from manufacturing teams and quality control units to regulatory affairs—to access and act upon unified datasets. Moreover, cloud-based AI tools can process this data in real-time, supporting advanced analytics like anomaly detection, root cause analysis, and batch release prediction.

The synergy between big data and cloud computing facilitates cross-functional integration, improves operational transparency, and accelerates continuous process verification (CPV). It also supports compliance with Good Manufacturing Practice (GMP) guidelines by enhancing traceability and documentation. As pharmaceutical manufacturers continue to embrace AI, cloud-enabled big data analytics will remain a cornerstone of intelligent, agile, and compliant manufacturing ecosystems.

Applications of AI in Pharmaceutical Manufacturing

AI technologies have shown considerable potential in improving both upstream and downstream manufacturing processes.

Process Optimization and Control

AI algorithms can be used to optimize process parameters dynamically. For instance, ML models trained on historical process data can identify optimal settings for drug formulation or fermentation processes (Kamble et al., 2020). AI-based control systems adapt to process drift and maintain consistent output quality, reducing the need for manual intervention.

Predictive Maintenance

One of the earliest and most impactful applications of AI in manufacturing is predictive maintenance. AI models analyze sensor data to predict machine failures and schedule maintenance proactively. This approach drastically reduces unplanned downtime and enhances overall equipment effectiveness (Choudhary et al., 2019).

Real-Time Quality Monitoring

Real-time release testing (RTRT) is a regulatory concept that aligns well with AI-based quality monitoring. AI systems continuously monitor critical quality attributes (CQAs) and can make real-time decisions about batch quality without needing off-line lab testing (Vora et al., 2023).

Anomaly Detection and Root Cause Analysis

AI-powered systems are capable of flagging abnormal trends and deviations from standard process behavior. These systems can also perform root cause analysis by evaluating complex multivariate data, which may be infeasible for human operators to analyze in real time.

Strategic Advantages for Pharmaceutical Enterprises

The strategic benefits of adopting AI and automation in manufacturing go far beyond operational efficiency. Some of the key advantages include:

- **Shorter Time to Market**: Smart systems reduce production cycle times and enable faster scale-up from lab to commercial production.
- **Sustainability**: AI-driven systems optimize energy consumption, reduce waste, and support environmentally sustainable practices (Bahrin et al., 2016).
- **Regulatory Compliance**: Automated and traceable workflows simplify compliance with regulations such as FDA 21 CFR Part 11 (FDA, 2023), which governs electronic records and signatures.
- **Improved Supply Chain Resilience**: AI tools can model supply chain risks, optimize inventory, and enhance demand forecasting—critical in an increasingly global and uncertain market.

Industry Adoption: Current Landscape

While many pharmaceutical companies are in the exploratory or pilot phases of AI adoption, a few have already made significant strides. For example:

- **Pfizer** has used AI to optimize its mRNA vaccine production by employing predictive modeling to adjust synthesis parameters in real-time.
- **Novartis** has partnered with technology firms to develop AI-enabled manufacturing facilities that leverage digital twins and real-time analytics.
- **GSK** has integrated AI platforms into its drug development and production lines to improve process efficiency and quality management.

These examples indicate a growing recognition of AI's potential, although full-scale adoption remains limited due to technological, regulatory, and organizational challenges.

Challenges Hindering Large-Scale Adoption

Despite its promise, several barriers are impeding the large-scale implementation of AI-driven automation in pharmaceutical production:

- **Data Integrity and Integration**: Legacy systems often lack the infrastructure for seamless data sharing, hindering AI model development.
- **Cultural Resistance**: Workforce resistance to technological change remains a critical obstacle, especially in organizations with established manual processes.
- **Validation Complexity**: AI systems require new approaches for validation, including lifecycle management and continuous performance monitoring, as traditional validation models may not suffice (Schmidt, et al., 2020).
- **Cybersecurity Risks**: With increased connectivity comes increased vulnerability. AI-enabled systems must be protected against data breaches, intellectual property theft, and operational sabotage.

These challenges underscore the need for interdisciplinary efforts involving data scientists, process engineers, regulatory bodies, and business leaders to ensure the safe and effective deployment of AI in manufacturing. The background of AI-driven smart manufacturing in the pharmaceutical industry reveals a landscape that is both ripe with opportunity and fraught with complexity. Technological advancements have made it feasible to integrate AI into various stages of drug production, yet adoption remains inconsistent. As the industry matures, a concerted effort is required to address technical limitations, regulatory uncertainties, and organizational inertia. The next sections of this chapter will delve deeper into the models, methodologies, and case studies that illustrate successful implementations, while also proposing frameworks for broader adoption.

AI-DRIVEN SMART MANUFACTURING AND AUTOMATION IN PHARMACEUTICAL PRODUCTION

AI in Pharmaceutical Manufacturing

Artificial Intelligence (AI) is transforming the pharmaceutical manufacturing landscape by enhancing production speed, precision, and compliance. AI-enabled smart manufacturing integrates advanced technologies such as robotics, machine learning (ML), digital twins, and predictive analytics to create interconnected systems capable of autonomous decision-making. These innovations are driving a shift from traditional batch processing to continuous, intelligent manufacturing systems that are adaptable and resilient.

AI technologies are particularly advantageous in managing high-volume, data-intensive pharmaceutical operations. With the increase in data from quality control (QC), sensor readings, supply chain systems, and manufacturing equipment, AI models provide real-time analytics that support quality assurance (QA), maintenance prediction, and cost reduction. Automation, combined with AI, reduces human error, ensures repeatability, and optimizes production environments.

According to Accenture (2023), the adoption of AI and machine learning in the pharmaceutical sector has grown by over 35% in the last two years, indicating its critical role in meeting growing global healthcare demands and regulatory scrutiny. AI has become a catalyst for improving throughput, reducing production cycle time, and ensuring adherence to Good Manufacturing Practices (GMP).

Figure 1 shows the overview of AI-Driven Smart Manufacturing and Automation in Pharmaceutical Production covered in this section.

Figure 1. Overview of AI-Driven Smart Manufacturing and Automation in Pharmaceutical Production

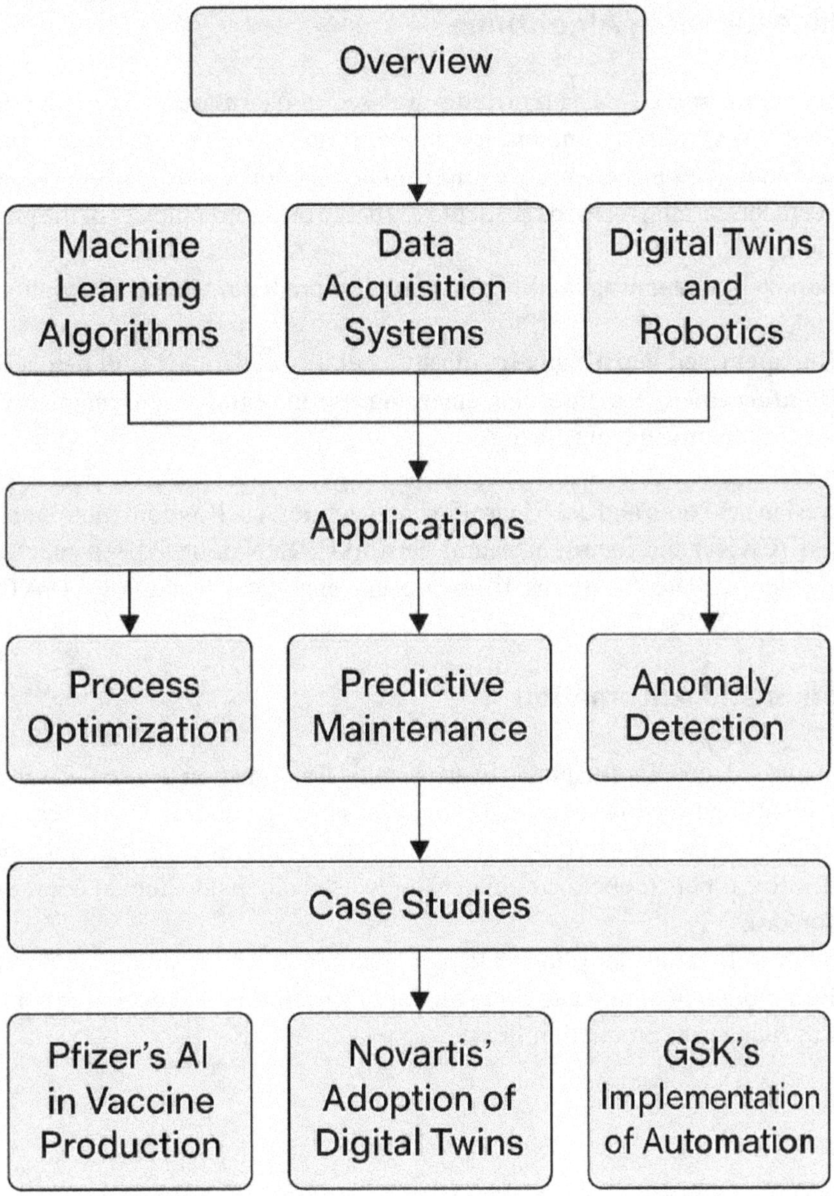

KEY TECHNOLOGIES ENABLING AI-DRIVEN MANUFACTURING

Machine Learning Algorithms

Machine Learning (ML) algorithms are used in pharmaceutical production for a range of tasks, from optimizing formulations and predicting batch outcomes to detecting anomalies and ensuring equipment health. Supervised, unsupervised, and reinforcement learning methods are deployed based on the complexity of the problem.

- **Supervised learning** is commonly used for predicting process deviations and yields.
- **Unsupervised learning** helps cluster operational data for fault detection.
- **Reinforcement learning** has emerging use in optimizing dynamic systems for continuous manufacturing.

Bayesian networks and deep learning architectures, such as convolutional neural networks (CNNs) and recurrent neural networks (RNNs), have been successfully implemented to detect patterns from process analytical technology (PAT) data (Kausik et al., 2025).

Robotics and Automation

AI-powered robots are central to pharmaceutical automation, particularly in sterile environments and repetitive tasks. Robotics systems guided by vision recognition and feedback loops are used for pill sorting, vial filling, packaging, and labeling. Collaborative robots (cobots) are increasingly used alongside human operators for precision tasks.

Moreover, robotics helps in reducing contamination risks in aseptic processes. AI-driven motion planning and force feedback systems are enhancing robot adaptability to changes in production lines.

Digital Twins and Simulation

A digital twin is a virtual replica of a physical manufacturing process or system. In pharmaceutical manufacturing, digital twins are employed for simulating drug production pipelines, optimizing facility design, and training operators without disrupting actual production.

By continuously feeding real-time data from physical sensors into the virtual model, digital twins provide predictive insights into process behavior and can simulate changes without risking compliance. According to a 2024 Gartner report, 50% of pharmaceutical manufacturers plan to adopt digital twins for at least one stage of their production by 2026.

APPLICATIONS OF AI IN SMART PHARMACEUTICAL MANUFACTURING

Process Optimization

AI enables real-time monitoring and optimization of critical process parameters (CPPs) and critical quality attributes (CQAs). Techniques such as multivariate data analysis (MVDA) and support vector machines (SVMs) are used to maintain quality by design (QbD) standards.

Examples include:

- Optimizing granulation parameters in solid dosage manufacturing.
- Predicting ideal mixing times and temperatures in API synthesis.
- Enhancing bioreactor yield in biologics through ML-based process controls.

Real-time feedback control systems (e.g., using reinforcement learning) allow for dynamic adjustment of variables such as pH, viscosity, and temperature to ensure consistent product quality (Vespoli et al., 2025).

Predictive Maintenance

Machine downtime can lead to substantial financial losses. AI-powered predictive maintenance leverages IoT sensors and ML models to anticipate failures before they occur. Time-series forecasting, decision trees, and neural networks are used to predict wear-and-tear in centrifuges, compressors, and HVAC systems.

Recent advancements include federated learning for predictive analytics, where models learn collaboratively across devices while maintaining data privacy, reducing regulatory concerns (Walter, 2025).

Quality Control and Defect Detection

AI-based visual inspection systems are revolutionizing quality assurance. Computer vision algorithms identify minute defects in tablets, blister packs, and labels with higher precision and speed than human inspectors. Natural language processing (NLP) is also being employed in parsing batch manufacturing records and lab reports for compliance audits.

Generative adversarial networks (GANs) have been used to simulate defective product scenarios for training defect detection algorithms under limited-data conditions (Singh et al., 2020).

Supply Chain Automation

AI models forecast demand, manage inventory, and optimize supply chain logistics. Reinforcement learning and deep Q-learning are increasingly used to optimize raw material procurement, warehouse operations, and transportation scheduling. Integration with blockchain further enhances transparency and traceability.

An example includes the implementation of AI-powered supply chain control towers by leading manufacturers to identify bottlenecks and reroute logistics in real-time (IDC Health Insights, 2024).

CASE STUDIES OF AI-DRIVEN MANUFACTURING

Pfizer – AI in Vaccine Production

During the COVID-19 pandemic, Pfizer collaborated with IBM and other tech providers to implement AI in its mRNA vaccine production. AI models were used to:

- Predict equipment malfunctions.

- Optimize cold chain logistics.
- Monitor quality attributes of lipid nanoparticles.

Pfizer's adoption of real-time release testing (RTRT) through AI-enabled spectroscopy reduced testing time by 30% while maintaining regulatory compliance (Pfizer Annual Report, 2023).

The urgency brought on by the COVID-19 pandemic necessitated innovative responses from global pharmaceutical companies. Pfizer, in partnership with BioNTech, developed one of the world's first approved mRNA COVID-19 vaccines. However, producing this vaccine at scale posed significant manufacturing challenges—especially around the unique characteristics of mRNA-based formulations, which are highly sensitive to environmental conditions and require precision handling. To meet global demand, Pfizer collaborated with IBM and other technology providers to implement artificial intelligence in key areas of its vaccine production.

One of the key implementations was the use of AI models to predict equipment malfunctions before they occurred. By leveraging machine learning algorithms trained on historical performance and real-time sensor data, Pfizer could identify patterns indicative of potential failures. These predictive maintenance systems enabled preemptive servicing of critical equipment such as bioreactors, filtration units, and chromatography columns.

This proactive approach not only minimized unplanned downtimes but also reduced the risk of batch failures, which can be extremely costly in high-speed vaccine manufacturing. Given the scale and speed of production required, even brief equipment failures could lead to significant delays. AI helped Pfizer ensure higher levels of equipment availability and efficiency throughout the production process.

Cold chain logistics was another area where AI played a vital role. The Pfizer-BioNTech vaccine required storage at ultra-low temperatures (approximately -70°C), making its distribution a complex logistical challenge. AI-powered logistics platforms were used to track, monitor, and optimize the movement of vaccines through the supply chain. These platforms integrated real-time temperature and location data from sensors embedded in shipping containers, allowing AI models to flag deviations or predict where a shipment might be at risk due to environmental conditions or delays.

Through AI-driven optimization, Pfizer reduced waste caused by spoilage, improved delivery timelines, and ensured the integrity of the vaccines reaching healthcare facilities. This precision was especially critical in the early phases of vaccine rollout, when every dose mattered.

Pfizer also integrated AI into its quality control processes. A key innovation was the adoption of real-time release testing (RTRT) using AI-enabled spectroscopy. Instead of relying solely on traditional laboratory-based batch testing, Pfizer deployed inline spectroscopic sensors capable of analyzing lipid nanoparticles—the tiny carriers used to deliver mRNA molecules into human cells.

AI algorithms were used to interpret complex spectral data, enabling real-time monitoring of critical quality attributes (CQAs) such as particle size, uniformity, and encapsulation efficiency. These capabilities allowed Pfizer to detect deviations instantly and adjust the process without interrupting production.

According to the Pfizer Annual Report (2023), the use of AI-enhanced RTRT led to a 30% reduction in testing time while maintaining compliance with regulatory standards. This significantly accelerated batch release and contributed to faster global vaccine distribution.

Novartis – Digital Twins for Biologics Manufacturing

Novartis has implemented digital twin technology in its biologics production facility in Switzerland. The system:

- Simulates fermentation and purification processes.
- Predicts the effect of parameter changes on yields.
- Enables virtual validation of process changes.

With AI algorithms integrating sensor data, Novartis achieved a 20% reduction in process deviations and a 15% increase in bioreactor productivity (Novartis Technology Brief, 2023).

While vaccines represented the cutting edge of response to the pandemic, biologics—complex drugs derived from living organisms—have continued to grow in importance. Novartis, a leader in biologics, has made substantial strides in digital transformation, particularly through the use of digital twin technology in its state-of-the-art biologics production facility in Switzerland.

A digital twin is a virtual replica of a physical system that mirrors real-world behavior using real-time data. In the context of biologics manufacturing, digital twins simulate every aspect of the production process—from fermentation to purification—using mathematical models, sensor data, and AI algorithms.

Novartis' digital twin integrates data from various sensors embedded throughout the manufacturing line. These include temperature probes, pressure sensors, pH meters, and bioreactor monitors. Machine learning models analyze this data to predict the behavior of the system under different conditions.

The digital twin allows Novartis to simulate changes in fermentation parameters such as agitation speed, nutrient feed rates, or temperature settings. Before making actual changes on the manufacturing floor, engineers can test different scenarios virtually, significantly reducing the risk of unintended consequences. The ability to predict how changes will affect product yield, impurity levels, and overall quality has transformed process development and scale-up.

This virtual validation of process changes saves time and resources and accelerates the regulatory approval process. Novartis can demonstrate to regulators that new process conditions have been extensively modeled and validated in silico before real-world implementation.

By integrating AI into its digital twin systems, Novartis achieved tangible operational gains. According to the Novartis Technology Brief (2023), the use of digital twins led to a 20% reduction in process deviations, helping ensure more consistent batch quality. Furthermore, bioreactor productivity improved by 15%, allowing the facility to produce more product using the same physical infrastructure.

These improvements are particularly significant in biologics, where production costs are high, and any variability can compromise safety and efficacy. AI has enabled Novartis to increase throughput, maintain high quality standards, and reduce the time and cost associated with bringing biologics to market.

GlaxoSmithKline (GSK) – Automation in Fill-Finish Operations

GSK's Singapore facility introduced a fully automated fill-finish line powered by AI-driven robotics and ML algorithms. The implementation featured:

- Automated inspection of sterile vials.
- AI-powered scheduling systems for production planning.
- Predictive alarms for temperature and pressure anomalies.

According to GSK's internal review, the implementation resulted in a 40% reduction in human error and a 25% increase in overall throughput (GSK Innovation Report, 2023).

While upstream production processes have seen notable innovations, downstream operations such as fill-finish—where drugs are placed into final containers—are equally critical. GlaxoSmithKline (GSK) has focused its AI efforts on modernizing these operations in its Singapore facility, transforming them through robotics and machine learning.

At GSK, fill-finish operations are now largely handled by a fully automated system that uses AI-powered robots. These robots manage the entire process, from the sterile filling of vials to labeling, capping, and packaging. The automation not only speeds up the process but also reduces human involvement, which is a significant source of contamination risk in sterile environments.

One of the most impactful features is the integration of computer vision systems for automated inspection. These systems use deep learning algorithms to analyze images of each vial for defects, such as cracks, particulate contamination, or improper seals. Unlike traditional visual inspection, which is time-consuming and prone to human error, AI-driven inspection is consistent and highly accurate.

The facility also employs AI for production scheduling and predictive monitoring. Machine learning algorithms analyze historical data and real-time operational variables to optimize production schedules, balancing equipment availability, material supply, and workforce efficiency. Predictive alarms are set to monitor temperature and pressure anomalies in storage tanks and pipelines, ensuring early intervention and minimizing risk.

According to the GSK Innovation Report (2023), the AI-driven automation has led to a 40% reduction in human error and a 25% increase in overall throughput. These gains underscore how automation, when combined with AI, can dramatically enhance operational efficiency, product safety, and workforce productivity.

Despite its potential, AI adoption in pharmaceutical manufacturing faces several challenges:

- **Regulatory Constraints**: Stringent validation and audit trails required by FDA and EMA must be maintained. Regulatory bodies are still evolving their stance on black-box AI systems.
- **Data Integrity**: The quality, granularity, and consistency of data directly influence model performance.
- **Integration Complexity**: Legacy systems and infrastructure pose hurdles to AI integration.
- **Talent Gap**: There is a shortage of skilled professionals who understand both AI and pharmaceutical manufacturing intricacies.

Nevertheless, the future is promising. Emerging technologies such as explainable AI (XAI), federated learning, and edge computing are addressing many current limitations. Government initiatives like the FDA's Emerging Technology Program (ETP) are accelerating the validation and deployment of AI systems.

SOLUTIONS AND RECOMMENDATIONS

As AI-driven smart manufacturing continues to redefine pharmaceutical production, organizations face unique challenges that require targeted, strategic solutions. These recommendations are structured across five core domains—technological integration, data governance, regulatory alignment, workforce development, and collaborative innovation—to support sustainable and scalable adoption of AI in pharmaceutical manufacturing environments.

Technological Integration and Infrastructure Development

Establishing a Scalable AI Infrastructure

Pharmaceutical manufacturers must invest in scalable, modular infrastructures capable of integrating AI solutions with existing manufacturing execution systems (MES), laboratory information management systems (LIMS), and enterprise resource planning (ERP) platforms. This includes enabling real-time data ingestion from IoT-enabled devices and supporting hybrid-cloud architectures for processing large volumes of sensor data and analytics.

Solution:

- Adopt microservices-based architectures to allow flexibility in AI model deployment and updates.
- Implement edge AI systems for on-premise, real-time analytics, especially in GMP-critical operations where latency and data control are crucial.

Digital Twin and Cyber-Physical Integration

AI deployment should be reinforced by cyber-physical systems and digital twins to ensure that simulations, training, and predictive modeling are accurate and production-relevant. Advanced process control (APC) techniques powered by AI algorithms can be embedded within digital twin ecosystems to proactively resolve operational bottlenecks.

Recommendation:

- Pilot digital twin applications at the unit operation level (e.g., bioreactors, chromatography) before scaling to plant-wide systems.
- Integrate high-resolution temporal data streams (e.g., PAT, SCADA) into virtual models for enhanced simulation fidelity.

Data Governance and Quality Assurance

Establishing Robust Data Governance Frameworks

High-quality, clean, and annotated datasets are prerequisites for effective AI model training. Pharmaceutical firms must implement comprehensive data governance strategies to ensure the reliability, traceability, and security of all data sources, especially those associated with process monitoring and quality control.

Recommendation:

- Form data governance committees to oversee lifecycle management of data assets.
- Use AI-specific metadata tagging, data lineage tracking, and audit logging to maintain data integrity across systems.

Leveraging FAIR Principles for AI Readiness

FAIR (Findable, Accessible, Interoperable, and Reusable) data principles can significantly enhance the usability of pharmaceutical data in AI applications. Manufacturers should prioritize standardizing terminologies, data formats, and ontologies to facilitate algorithm training, validation, and deployment.

Solution:

- Use open data standards such as Allotrope Data Format (ADF) or AnIML to structure analytical and production data.
- Partner with data custodians and AI vendors to create semantic data layers for interoperability.

Regulatory and Ethical Compliance

Promoting Explainable and Transparent AI (XAI)

Regulatory bodies such as the FDA, EMA, and ICH increasingly expect AI models used in production to be interpretable. Black-box algorithms present a significant risk in regulated environments, particularly when involved in critical decisions related to batch release, process deviation handling, or QC failure prediction.

Recommendation:

- Incorporate XAI frameworks such as SHAP (SHapley Additive exPlanations) and LIME (Local Interpretable Model-Agnostic Explanations) during model development.
- Document model logic and outputs clearly for audit purposes and compliance readiness.

Accelerating Regulatory Harmonization and Sandboxes

Regulators must collaborate internationally to develop shared AI validation frameworks. Regulatory sandboxes—controlled environments that allow companies to experiment with new technologies under regulatory oversight—can provide essential flexibility.

Solution:

- Encourage public-private partnerships to co-develop AI risk assessment and performance validation protocols.
- Introduce pre-market guidance documents and post-market surveillance practices tailored to AI systems in pharma.

Workforce Development and Upskilling

Building Interdisciplinary Talent Pools

AI-driven pharmaceutical manufacturing demands professionals who possess a hybrid skill set: domain expertise in pharma processes, data science acumen, and regulatory knowledge. Upskilling and reskilling existing employees through targeted programs is vital for fostering adoption readiness.

Recommendation:

- Develop in-house AI academies or collaborate with academic institutions to offer certification programs.
- Implement cross-training workshops between data engineers and process scientists.

Organizational Change Management

Cultural readiness is a crucial determinant in the successful deployment of AI systems. Resistance to technological disruption often stems from fear of redundancy or workflow shifts. Leaders must create environments that emphasize continuous learning and innovation.

Solution:

- Deploy change management frameworks such as ADKAR (Awareness, Desire, Knowledge, Ability, and Reinforcement).
- Include frontline operators in AI pilot initiatives to encourage ownership and trust in AI outputs.

Collaborative Innovation and Ecosystem Development

Public-Private Consortia and Research Hubs

The complexity and regulatory sensitivity of pharmaceutical manufacturing necessitate collaborative models to drive innovation. Shared R&D platforms, data exchange mechanisms, and joint validation efforts are essential for de-risking AI adoption.

Recommendation:

- Engage with AI-focused consortia such as the Manufacturing USA Institutes or IMI (Innovative Medicines Initiative).
- Leverage testbeds and co-innovation labs to simulate, test, and refine AI models before real-world deployment.

Open Innovation with AI Startups and Academia

Startups and academic labs often pioneer disruptive AI technologies that larger firms may find risky to develop in-house. Strategic collaborations can infuse agility and creativity into conservative manufacturing environments.

Solution:

- Establish AI venture arms or innovation incubators focused on smart manufacturing.
- Sponsor academic grants or doctoral fellowships on pharmaceutical AI applications.

The convergence of AI and pharmaceutical manufacturing holds transformative potential—redefining operational excellence, quality assurance, and patient-centric delivery. However, this transformation demands more than just technological tools; it requires a holistic realignment of infrastructure, policies, human capital, and collaborative ethos. The solutions and recommendations outlined herein provide a pragmatic roadmap for researchers, policymakers, and industry leaders to ensure that AI's integration into pharmaceutical production is not only efficient but ethical, sustainable, and resilient.

FUTURE RESEARCH DIRECTIONS

Future Research Directions

As artificial intelligence (AI) continues to disrupt pharmaceutical manufacturing, future research must evolve beyond isolated automation solutions toward holistic, adaptive ecosystems. While current implementations of AI offer valuable productivity and quality gains, several unresolved issues—ranging from model generalizability to ethical AI deployment—demand deeper exploration. Future research must adopt an interdisciplinary, multi-stakeholder approach to tackle the complexities inherent in regulated, high-stakes pharmaceutical environments.

This section outlines key research trajectories that hold the potential to refine, reimagine, and revolutionize AI-driven smart manufacturing in the pharmaceutical industry.

Development of Generalizable and Transferable AI Models

Cross-Platform Model Interoperability

Current AI models in pharmaceutical manufacturing are often tailored to specific datasets, facilities, or equipment. This lack of generalizability restricts cross-platform adoption, complicating efforts to scale AI systems enterprise-wide. Future research should prioritize developing AI models that are transferable across various production environments without compromising accuracy or regulatory compliance.

Research Opportunity:

- Investigate domain adaptation techniques to enable AI models trained in one production environment to adapt with minimal retraining in another.
- Develop hybrid modeling approaches combining physics-informed machine learning (PIML) with data-driven models to enhance interpretability and transferability.

Integration of Quantum AI in Pharmaceutical Manufacturing

Quantum computing has recently emerged as a game-changer in pharmaceutical R&D, especially for molecular simulations. However, its application in manufacturing—especially via quantum machine learning (QML)—remains largely unexplored.

Hybrid Quantum-Classical Algorithms for Process Optimization

Quantum-enhanced optimization algorithms could be used to manage complex process variables, such as multi-scale granulation, fluid dynamics in bioreactors, or energy-efficient lyophilization.

Research Opportunity:

- Develop and test QML algorithms for real-time optimization of pharmaceutical unit operations.
- Establish simulation platforms for benchmarking classical vs. quantum-assisted models.

AI-Powered Autonomous Pharmaceutical Facilities (Industry 5.0)

While Industry 4.0 focuses on automation and data exchange, Industry 5.0 emphasizes human-machine collaboration, resilience, and sustainability. The vision of autonomous pharmaceutical manufacturing facilities—powered by AI, robotics, and edge computing—presents a fertile area for research.

Human-AI Collaboration Models

There is a growing need to design human-AI interfaces that allow for seamless decision-making while preserving operator oversight, especially in GMP-compliant processes.

Research Opportunity:

- Explore reinforcement learning techniques to create adaptive control systems that incorporate real-time human feedback.
- Study cognitive load, user trust, and interpretability in human-AI collaboration in high-risk pharmaceutical scenarios.

Sustainable and Green AI for Pharmaceutical Production

As pharmaceutical companies pursue carbon-neutral goals, AI's role in minimizing resource consumption and environmental impact becomes vital. However, AI systems themselves often have a substantial energy footprint.

AI for Sustainable Resource Allocation

Advanced AI algorithms can support real-time optimization of water, solvents, and energy use, aligning manufacturing outcomes with sustainability goals.

Research Opportunity:

- Study life cycle assessment (LCA)-based AI models that evaluate environmental impacts across drug manufacturing stages.
- Research energy-efficient AI model architectures (e.g., TinyML) suitable for edge deployment in resource-sensitive pharmaceutical settings.

AI-Augmented Predictive Maintenance and Lifecycle Modeling

Predictive maintenance using AI is currently limited to simple anomaly detection via sensor data. More sophisticated AI tools are needed to forecast the entire lifecycle of equipment, facilities, and processes.

Digital Twins with Predictive Lifecycle Modeling

Digital twin frameworks must evolve to include predictive degradation models, real-time fatigue analysis, and spare part logistics—all powered by AI.

Research Opportunity:

- Integrate AI-based lifecycle cost estimation tools into plant-level digital twins.
- Use survival analysis and Bayesian networks to enhance predictive failure models.

Ethical AI and Algorithmic Bias in Pharmaceutical Manufacturing

Most discussions around AI ethics focus on patient data or clinical AI. However, biases can also exist in manufacturing—especially in datasets reflecting legacy equipment performance or operator behavior.

Auditing and Mitigating Bias in Manufacturing AI

Bias in process models can affect quality control predictions, resource allocations, or even maintenance schedules, leading to operational inequities.

Research Opportunity:

- Develop fairness metrics and bias detection algorithms specifically for manufacturing data.
- Investigate regulatory frameworks for ethical AI in pharmaceutical production beyond patient-facing applications.

Federated Learning for Collaborative Model Training

Pharmaceutical firms are often reluctant to share proprietary manufacturing data due to IP and regulatory concerns. Federated learning (FL) offers a decentralized training paradigm where local AI models are trained collaboratively without centralizing sensitive data.

Secure, Privacy-Preserving Collaborative AI

Federated AI could enable collaborative process optimization across manufacturing sites or organizations while preserving privacy.

Research Opportunity:

- Test differential privacy techniques and homomorphic encryption in federated learning for pharmaceutical manufacturing use cases.
- Examine trust mechanisms and model validation strategies for multiparty FL networks.

Advanced AI for In-Line Quality Control and Adaptive Manufacturing

In-line quality control (QC) using AI can reduce cycle time, minimize rejects, and increase yield. The future lies in adaptive manufacturing systems that adjust control parameters based on real-time quality feedback.

Real-Time Adaptive Process Control

Research is needed to implement deep reinforcement learning (DRL) for multivariable process control, allowing continuous learning and adaptation without process interruptions.

Research Opportunity:

- Build DRL-based control systems for continuous manufacturing units such as twin-screw extruders or continuous mixers.
- Study convergence guarantees and safety envelopes for AI in critical control loops.

Integration of AI with Blockchain for Traceability

Counterfeit drugs and data falsification in production remain persistent threats. Integrating AI with blockchain can provide immutable records, enhance traceability, and detect anomalies in production data streams.

AI-Blockchain Convergence for GMP Compliance

This convergence can enable real-time validation of AI model decisions and data provenance, fostering transparency and trust in autonomous systems.

Research Opportunity:

- Develop smart contracts that trigger alerts based on AI-driven quality or process deviations.
- Investigate decentralized identity (DID) systems for secure equipment-to-equipment communications.

The road ahead for AI-driven smart manufacturing in the pharmaceutical sector is rich with possibility but paved with complexity. Future research must be simultaneously ambitious and responsible, blending cutting-edge technological advances with robust ethical, regulatory, and practical considerations. By exploring the domains highlighted above—from federated learning to quantum AI and sustainable design—researchers can co-create an AI-powered pharmaceutical future that is not only smarter but also safer, more transparent, and more inclusive.

CONCLUSION

Artificial Intelligence (AI) is no longer a peripheral innovation in pharmaceutical production; it has become a transformative force redefining how drugs are developed, manufactured, and delivered. From the earliest stages of digital automation to the current paradigm of smart manufacturing, AI technologies have matured into critical components of pharmaceutical supply chains, quality assurance processes, and adaptive production ecosystems. As this chapter has demonstrated, AI-driven smart manufacturing and automation offer unprecedented opportunities to optimize operations, ensure regulatory compliance, and achieve consistent, scalable, and patient-centric pharmaceutical outputs.

Reaffirming the Need for AI in Pharmaceutical Manufacturing

The pharmaceutical industry faces unparalleled challenges: the need for faster drug development, rising operational costs, supply chain fragility, and stringent regulatory demands. Traditional manufacturing models—largely linear and batch-based—are ill-equipped to handle this complexity. In this context, the convergence of AI, machine learning (ML), robotics, Internet of Things (IoT), and real-time analytics offers a responsive, data-driven alternative that promises flexibility, agility, and resilience.

AI-driven solutions enable real-time monitoring and predictive maintenance, facilitate adaptive process control, and support continuous quality verification—features that are essential for Good Manufacturing Practice (GMP) compliance. These systems are also integral to realizing the goals of Industry 4.0 and the emerging paradigm of Industry 5.0, which emphasizes not only automation but also personalization, ethical AI integration, and human-machine collaboration.

Strategic Benefits and Transformation Milestones

Throughout this chapter, various use cases and models have highlighted how AI has revolutionized key manufacturing processes, such as:

- **Predictive Analytics:** Used for raw material assessment and supply chain forecasting.
- **Process Analytical Technology (PAT):** Enhanced by ML algorithms to enable in-line and at-line monitoring of critical quality attributes (CQAs).
- **Digital Twins:** Creating virtual replicas of manufacturing lines, allowing for simulations, optimizations, and pre-emptive troubleshooting.
- **Autonomous Robotics:** Used for precise, repetitive tasks in sterile environments, reducing human error and contamination risks.
- **Computer Vision:** Automating quality control in packaging and tablet inspections.
- **Natural Language Processing (NLP):** Parsing regulatory documents and standard operating procedures (SOPs) to ensure compliance and faster approvals.

Such applications underscore the fact that AI is no longer an experimental novelty but an operational necessity. The pharmaceutical organizations that have invested early in AI infrastructure—both technological and human—are already seeing tangible returns in terms of reduced downtimes, enhanced production efficiency, improved traceability, and stronger regulatory positioning.

Addressing Gaps and Challenges

However, despite the promises and progress, AI-driven smart manufacturing is not without its caveats. Multiple challenges remain that limit the full-scale, global implementation of AI in pharmaceutical production:

- **Data Silos and Standardization Issues:** Pharmaceutical manufacturing data is often fragmented across legacy systems, laboratories, and production units. Integrating these into a coherent AI model demands significant investment in data cleaning, ontology alignment, and interoperability frameworks.
- **Regulatory Ambiguity:** Regulatory agencies are still evolving their frameworks around AI in manufacturing. Concerns about algorithm explainability, validation, audit trails, and accountability must be addressed through active dialogue between developers, manufacturers, and regulators.
- **Talent Gaps and Change Management:** Successfully deploying AI requires multidisciplinary expertise—data scientists, pharmacists, automation engineers, and regulatory experts. Moreover, transitioning from manual to AI-assisted operations requires structured change management programs, including staff retraining and role redesign.
- **Cybersecurity Risks:** With increased digitalization comes the threat of cyberattacks. AI-driven manufacturing platforms must be secured with multilayered cybersecurity protocols, especially in light of sensitive patient data and proprietary formulations.

Recognizing and resolving these barriers is essential to foster widespread AI adoption. Research-based strategies, institutional collaboration, and policy reforms will be critical in this regard.

Synthesis of Key Case Studies

The three case studies examined in this chapter have underscored the real-world applicability and ROI of AI technologies in pharmaceutical manufacturing:

- **Pfizer's Use of AI for COVID-19 Vaccine Production:** By leveraging AI models for production scaling, quality control, and predictive maintenance, Pfizer demonstrated how AI could shorten timelines and ensure consistency at an unprecedented scale.
- **Novartis' Smart Manufacturing Initiative:** Novartis has adopted AI-powered data lakes and digital twins to streamline its production work-flows and reduce operational costs, setting a benchmark for global pharma automation.
- **GSK's Use of Robotics and AI for Adaptive Production:** GSK's combination of AI and collaborative robotics enables continuous process optimization, yielding both higher throughput and reduced human error.

These real-world examples affirm that AI is not just a theoretical framework—it is being actively deployed, delivering tangible results across continents and therapeutic areas.

The Promise of Ethical, Inclusive, and Sustainable AI

Looking ahead, the role of AI will expand from optimization to stewardship. Ethical AI principles—such as fairness, transparency, and accountability—must be built into manufacturing algorithms. As pharmaceutical companies increasingly collaborate on AI-driven platforms, global data governance protocols will be necessary to prevent misuse and ensure equitable innovation.

In addition, sustainability will become a central metric in AI implementation. Green AI models that reduce energy consumption, minimize waste, and optimize resource use will align with broader Environmental, Social, and Governance (ESG) mandates. These considerations are vital not only for compliance but also for brand reputation and consumer trust.

Furthermore, the idea of inclusive AI must gain momentum. Models must be trained and validated using diverse datasets to avoid systemic bias that can lead to skewed predictions in global production scenarios.

Aligning with Future Research and Innovation Landscapes

In the "Future Research Directions" section, this chapter outlined several compelling areas for exploration, including:

- Quantum machine learning for process simulation and real-time control.
- Federated learning for collaborative model development across pharma companies.

- Explainable AI (XAI) for regulatory compliance and operational transparency.
- Blockchain integration for tamper-proof data trails and anti-counterfeit measures.
- Hybrid edge-cloud architectures for low-latency, resilient operations.

These avenues not only represent technological innovation but also strategic levers that pharmaceutical companies can employ to future-proof their operations.

In the coming decade, we expect to see AI-driven platforms that are self-correcting, ethically governed, and seamlessly integrated across R&D, production, logistics, and post-market surveillance. Such a holistic approach will redefine what pharmaceutical manufacturing means—not just in terms of processes, but in terms of outcomes and impact.

Final Reflections and the Path Forward

The integration of AI into pharmaceutical manufacturing is not just about technological augmentation—it is a paradigm shift that touches upon every aspect of drug production, from raw material sourcing to patient delivery. As AI becomes more intelligent, contextual, and autonomous, it will redefine the roles of humans, the nature of workflows, and the structure of pharmaceutical ecosystems.

Policymakers, academic researchers, manufacturers, and technologists must work in tandem to shape this future. Regulatory frameworks must evolve to accommodate dynamic, self-improving systems. Educational institutions must nurture a new generation of AI-literate pharmaceutical professionals. Industry leaders must invest in not only tools but also in trust—ensuring that the AI systems they deploy are transparent, fair, and aligned with both regulatory norms and ethical standards.

The journey toward fully autonomous pharmaceutical manufacturing is long and complex, but the foundations have been laid. As this chapter has shown, the technology exists, the use cases are proven, and the potential is immense. The challenge now is not just to build smarter factories, but to create resilient, ethical, and human-centric systems that will define the next era of pharmaceutical excellence.

REFERENCES

Accenture. (2023). *AI in Pharma Manufacturing: Trends and Market Insights.* Accenture Insights.

Bahrin, M. A. K., Othman, M. F., Azli, N. H. N., & Talib, M. F. (2016). Industry 4.0: A review on industrial automation and robotic. *Jurnal Teknologi, 78*(6), 137–143. DOI: 10.11113/jt.v78.9285

Blanco-González, A., Cabezón, A., Seco-González, A., Conde-Torres, D., Antelo-Riveiro, P., Piñeiro, Á., & Garcia-Fandino, R. (2023, June 18). The Role of AI in Drug Discovery: Challenges, Opportunities, and Strategies. *Pharmaceuticals (Basel, Switzerland), 16*(6), 891. DOI: 10.3390/ph16060891 PMID: 37375838

Choudhary, A., Harding, J. A., & Tiwari, M. K. (2019). Data mining in manufacturing: A review based on the kind of knowledge. *Journal of Intelligent Manufacturing, 30*(4), 1393–1410. DOI: 10.1007/s10845-017-1318-0

Dunjko, V., & Briegel, H. J. (2018). Machine learning & artificial intelligence in the quantum domain: A review of recent progress. *Reports on Progress in Physics, 81*(7), 074001. DOI: 10.1088/1361-6633/aab406 PMID: 29504942

European Medicines Agency. (2023). *EMA Reflection Paper on Artificial Intelligence in Medicines Regulation.* https://www.ema.europa.eu

FDA. (2023). Emerging Technology Program. U.S. Food and Drug Administration. https://www.fda.gov/drugs/pharmaceutical-quality-resources/emerging-technology-program

Fuller, A., Fan, Z., Day, C., & Barlow, C. (2020). Digital twin: Enabling technologies, challenges and open research. *IEEE Access : Practical Innovations, Open Solutions, 8*, 108952–108971. DOI: 10.1109/ACCESS.2020.2998358

Gandu, Sravanthi, & Gandla, Kumaraswamy & Vaishnavi, M & Repudi, Lalitha. (. (2023). A review on implementation of automation in the pharmaceutical industries. *World Journal of Advanced Research and Reviews., 18*, 606–615. DOI: 10.30574/wjarr.2023.18.2.0858

Gartner. (2024). *Digital Twin Adoption in Pharma Manufacturing*. Gartner Research.

GSK. (2023). *Innovation and Automation Annual Report.* GlaxoSmithKline plc

IDC Health Insights. (2024). *AI Control Towers in Pharma Supply Chains.* IDC Reports.

Kamble, S. S., Gunasekaran, A., Gawankar, S. A., & Dhone, N. C. (2020). A performance measurement system for industry 4.0 enabled smart manufacturing system in SMMEs—A review and empirical investigation. *International Journal of Production Economics, 229*, 107853. DOI: 10.1016/j.ijpe.2020.107853

Kausik, S. K., Rashid, A. B., Baki, R. F., & Maktum, M. M. J. (2025). Machine learning algorithms for manufacturing quality assurance: A systematic review of performance metrics and applications. *Array (New York, N.Y.), 26*, 100393. DOI: 10.1016/j.array.2025.100393

Lee, J., Bagheri, B., & Kao, H. A. (2015). A Cyber-Physical Systems Architecture for Industry 4.0-Based Manufacturing Systems. *Manufacturing Letters, 3*, 18–23. DOI: 10.1016/j.mfglet.2014.12.001

Li, Jian-qiang & Yu, F. & Deng, Genqiang & Luo, Chengwen & Ming, Zhong & Yan, Qiao. (2017). Industrial Internet: A Survey on the Enabling Technologies, Applications, and Challenges. IEEE Communications Surveys & Tutorials. PP. 1-1. .DOI: 10.1109/COMST.2017.2691349

Novartis. (2023). *Technology Brief: Smart Manufacturing and Digital Twins*. Novartis AG.

Pfizer. (2023). *Annual Sustainability and Innovation Report*. Pfizer Inc.

Prabu, S., Senthilraja, R., Jayapoorani, S., & Arun, M. (2025). AI-Driven Predictive Maintenance for Smart Manufacturing Systems Using Digital Twin Technology. *International Journal of Computational and Experimental Science and Engineering., 11*. Advance online publication. DOI: 10.22399/ijcesen.1099

Rüßmann, M., Lorenz, M., Gerbert, P., Waldner, M., Justus, J., Engel, P., & Harnisch, M. (2015). Industry 4.0: The future of productivity and growth in manufacturing industries.

Schmidt, P., Biessmann, F., & Teubner, T. (2020). Transparency and trust in artificial intelligence systems. *Journal of Decision Systems, 29*(4), 260–278. Advance online publication. DOI: 10.1080/12460125.2020.1819094

Singh, R., Garg, R., Patel, N., & Braun, M. (2020)... *Generative Adversarial Networks for Synthetic Defect Generation in Assembly and Test Manufacturing., 1-5*, 1–5. Advance online publication. DOI: 10.1109/ASMC49169.2020.9185242

Topol, E. (2019). *Deep Medicine: How Artificial Intelligence Can Make Healthcare Human Again*. Basic Books.

Vespoli, S., Mattera, G., Marchesano, M. G., Nele, L., & Guizzi, G. (2025). Adaptive manufacturing control with deep reinforcement learning for dynamic WIP management in Industry 4.0. *Computers & Industrial Engineering*, *202*, 110966. DOI: 10.1016/j.cie.2025.110966

Vora, L. K., Gholap, A. D., Jetha, K., Thakur, R. R. S., Solanki, H. K., & Chavda, V. P. (2023, July 10). Artificial Intelligence in Pharmaceutical Technology and Drug Delivery Design. *Pharmaceutics*, *15*(7), 1916. DOI: 10.3390/pharmaceutics15071916 PMID: 37514102

Walter, Holmes. (2025). Integrating Federated Learning in Drug Development: Balancing Data Privacy and Predictive Accuracy.

ADDITIONAL READING

Khalid, S. (2025). Optimization of pharmaceutical processes using artificial intelligence. *Clinical Medicine and Health Research Journal*, *5*(1), 1134–1144. DOI: 10.18535/cmhrj.v5i1.447

Mohammed, Z. A., Mohammed, M., Mohammed, S., & Syed, M. (2024). Artificial intelligence: Cybersecurity threats in pharmaceutical. *International Advanced Research Journal in Science. Engineering and Technology*, *11*, 11801. Advance online publication. DOI: 10.17148/IARJSET.2024.11801

Pandey, P., & Pal, R. (2023). Artificial intelligence (AI) and robotics used in pharmaceutical industry.

KEY TERMS AND DEFINITIONS

Artificial Intelligence (AI): Computational systems that simulate human intelligence to perform tasks like learning, reasoning, and decision-making.

Smart Manufacturing: A data-driven manufacturing approach that leverages AI, IoT, and automation to enhance efficiency and adaptability.

Pharmaceutical Automation: The use of robotics and automated systems to perform repetitive tasks in drug manufacturing, reducing human intervention and error.

Digital Twin: A virtual replica of physical manufacturing processes used for simulation, monitoring, and optimization in real-time.

Process Analytical Technology (PAT): A framework for designing, analyzing, and controlling manufacturing through timely measurements of critical quality parameters.

Machine Learning (ML): A subset of AI that enables systems to learn from data and improve performance without explicit programming.

Internet of Things (IoT): A network of interconnected devices that collect and exchange real-time data to support smart operations in manufacturing.

Predictive Maintenance: AI-enabled technique that forecasts equipment failures and schedules maintenance to prevent unplanned downtimes.

Cyber-Physical Systems (CPS): Integrated systems where physical processes are monitored and controlled by computer-based algorithms.

Regulatory Compliance: Adherence to legal and industry-specific guidelines (e.g., GMP, FDA, EMA) essential in pharmaceutical production.

Natural Language Processing (NLP): A branch of AI that allows machines to understand and interpret human language for tasks like SOP analysis and documentation.

Autonomous Robotics: Robotic systems powered by AI to perform tasks independently in sterile and high-precision environments.

Supply Chain Optimization: Application of AI to forecast demand, manage inventories, and streamline logistics in pharmaceutical supply chains.

Explainable AI (XAI): AI models designed to provide transparent reasoning behind decisions, important for regulatory scrutiny and trust.

Federated Learning: A collaborative ML technique that trains models across decentralized data sources without exchanging the data itself.

Edge AI: AI deployed on local devices near the data source, enabling real-time analytics without relying on centralized cloud processing.

Sustainability in Pharma: The integration of AI tools to reduce energy use, minimize waste, and promote eco-friendly manufacturing practices.

Industry 4.0: The fourth industrial revolution characterized by automation, data exchange, and cyber-physical systems in manufacturing.

Industry 5.0: The evolution of Industry 4.0 that emphasizes human-centricity, personalization, and ethical AI integration.

Blockchain in Pharma: A decentralized technology used to enhance transparency, traceability, and anti-counterfeiting in drug production and distribution.

Chapter 7

Supply Chain Optimization-based Drug Polymer Analysis Using AI Model for Synthesis and Characterization

Lubin Balasubramanian
SRM Institute of Science and Technology, India

G. Balamurugan
SRM Institute of Science and Technology, India

Nagamany Abirami
Sri Venkateshwaraa College of Engineering and Technology, India

U. Muruganantham
Manakula Vinayagar Institute of Technology, India

S. Magesh
https://orcid.org/0000-0003-2876-7337
Dr. M. G. R Educational and Research Institute, India

R. Manikandan
https://orcid.org/0000-0001-6116-2132
SASTRA University, India

ABSTRACT

Research on drug creation and development is crucial for chemical scientists and pharmaceutical businesses. On the other hand, drug design and discovery are hampered by limited efficacy, off-target delivery, time consumption, and excessive cost. Using the available three-dimensional structures, molecular docking can be utilised to anticipate the strength of the binding of small-molecule binders and their chemical derivatives to a macromolecular target. In process of finding as well as developing new drugs, artificial intelligence as well as machine learning technol-

DOI: 10.4018/979-8-3373-2043-4.ch007

ogies are essential. This chapter proposes novel technique in drug polymer-based synthesis and characterisation analysis with supply chain optimisation using artificial intelligence with machine learning algorithm. Then, the supply chain optimisation is based on drug synthesis and structure analysis using particle adversarial reinforcement Markov binary optimisation model. The experimental analysis has been carried out for various drug-polymer structure datasets in terms of prediction accuracy, random precision, and Recall.

INTRODUCTION

This chapter presents an AI- and ML-driven approach to improving drug discovery through polymer-based synthesis and optimized supply chains. The processes used to manufacture pharmaceuticals have undergone significant change. The focus shifted to Process Analytical Technology (PAT) and Quality by Design (QbD) tools to enhance the overall quality of production process. These technologies provide a science-based method to guarantee product quality through process understanding. Pharmaceutical manufacturing quality faults are regulated and monitored since they might have significant repercussions. Regulatory bodies frequently examine the process's control and robustness when evaluating a product's approval. Years of work and money could be at risk if necessary quality standards are not met, particularly since regulatory bodies could not approve process modifications without convincing proof (Staszak, M et al., 2022). Therefore, modern manufacturing systems attempt to give robots human knowledge in response to the growing complexity of production processes and the growing need for high-quality and efficient goods.

Pharmacogenomic tests, on the other hand, also aid in the formulation of drugs and the decision on dosages for individual patients. Patients' genomic profiles are used to make these decisions since their genetic makeup may cause them to metabolize particular medications differently, which could result in adverse side effects. Individual differences in drug-metabolising enzyme genes, including cytochrome P450 (CYP450), lead to such drug responses. Testing based on pharmacogenomics provides safe and optimum use of medications in heart disease treatment along with cancer adjuvant therapy and psychiatry while treating HIV and other infectious conditions and dermatological diseases (Nangia, A. K., 2024). Drug discovery complexity grows from processing requirements and regulatory agency guidelines that provide detailed specifications. The expensive ongoing research for developing new drugs takes an extensive period. A new medication requires ten to fifteen years of scientific evaluation and experimental testing before manufacturing.

Laboratory investigations of existing compounds become impractical because potential new medicine candidates exceed research capacity. New in silico screening techniques for large drug libraries have emerged in information and communication technologies and increased computing power for the past 10 years. This stage before preclinical research lowers financial burden and expands the area available for drug discovery. The pharmaceutical business may benefit from integrating AI and ML in manufacturing (Gupta, R. et al., 2021). AI-assisted manufacturing techniques can help create more robust production processes and offer financial benefits. AI can improve manufacturing efficiency, resulting in more output and lower waste. To significantly improve production operations, machine learning algorithms ensure that specific tasks are carried out more accurately and help identify areas where manufacturing processes can be further reduced. Prominent pharmaceutical companies have already incorporated or purchased AI technologies. AI can be used to forecast maintenance, increase industrial reuse, eliminate material waste, and carry out quality control. In addition to managing shortages and production line problems, ML may help anticipate and prevent over and undersupply. AI might offer chances to reduce waste and increase production efficiency (Zhao, X. et al., 2022). For instance, CNC (computer numerical control) can automate a process that relies on human intervention to enter or handle data.

In addition to ensuring that tasks are carried out with extreme precision, machine learning algorithms also assess the procedure to identify areas for simplification. This lowers material waste, speeds up production, and guarantees that the product's essential quality standards are consistently met (Carracedo-Reboredo, P et al., 2021). Digital marketing has replaced traditional methods of marketing medicinal items. Even the way that customers purchase medications has changed from traditional in-store to online. AI may help thoroughly analyze a product's essential needs from the viewpoint of consumers and market demands, which supports decision-making through prediction tools. In addition to increasing sales, AI can forecast sales, saving money by preventing excess inventory or clientele loss from shortages. AI can support the development of creative marketing strategies that raise revenue and brand recognition. Applications of AI and sophisticated analytics are revolutionizing markets and companies by enabling increased productivity and efficiency. AI has the potential to significantly impact pharmaceutical sales and marketing, which mostly rely on human skills like knowledge and reasoning (Martinelli, D. D., 2022).

BACKGROUND

ML methods and their application in the pharmaceutical sector have grown due to the recent enormous expansion in computing power. Developing computer platforms with a distributed architecture provides nearly limitless storage access and a significant boost in processing power needed for sophisticated AI systems to learn. Additionally, it makes it possible to process a wide variety of massive data sets, which forms the foundation for creating trustworthy machine learning systems. Global competitiveness is strengthened through information technology implementation that enables the business process to rebuild supplier-user collaboration and supply chain waste removal, and it streamlines operations for both time savings and enhanced quality. Much scholarly research has focused on inventory management (Zhuang, Z. et al., 2024). The Work (Jayaraman, A. et al., 2024) designed a system method incorporating an original management mode with BP neural network and genetic algorithm to enhance hospital drug inventory operations. The author (Garg S et al., 2024) developed a decision support system (DSS) that assists SMEs with data collection and exploitation while helping them make decisions when faced with business ambiguity for inventory management and sourcing applications. To help farmers manage their fresh agricultural product inventories at several links, including supermarkets, distribution centers, professional cooperatives, and other markets, Work (Zhao J et al., 2024) established an integrated model. Several models for inventory control issues were put forth in work (Wyrembek M et al., 2025).

Deterministic single, multi, and stochastic product approaches have been widely investigated to solve the inventory routing problem (IRP). A new two-stage hybrid method was proposed by (Parvatikar, P P et al., 2023) to present a generalized IRP solution. To optimize routing, location, and inventory decisions in multi-level supply chains, location routing problems and fuel feeding were introduced (Li S et al., 2024). In a different approach, (Zhang Y et al., 2023) integrated money movement modeling into system dynamics framework of beer division game to design a cash flow-based (CFB) function. For centralized and decentralized supply chain management (SCM), (Güleryüz C et al., 2025) developed a multi-objective genetic algorithm optimization framework based on NSGA and bullwhip effect modeling. Research into improving inventory management in stochastic systems is growing. However, modern supply chains are enormous and complex, exposing them to many risks. Supply chain processes can mitigate risks of this disruption with an integrated planning method and eliminate or minimize the impact of unexpected disruptions to the supply chain. For example, under random supply disruption, (He S et al., 2025) examined a coordinated location inventory problem in a stochastic supply chain system (SCS). At the same time, (Benavides-Hernández J et al., 2024) proposed a multi-item economic production quantity model with shortages for a vendor-managed inventory system involving one vendor and multiple retailers in an uncertain environment. In parallel research, highly effective advanced computational approaches have been demonstrated to solve large-scale, complex problems. A third example is the DeepVS system, which performed outstandingly by testing 95,000 decoys against 40 receptors and 2,950 ligands (Bai X et al., 2024). Thus, it shows the capability of using computational models and data-driven methods to make more efficient decisions and optimize the process, wherever feasible, in supply chain management and any highly complex environment. In predictive modeling, (Mohammadpour A et al., 2025) analyzed weekly gas consumption forecasts for three buildings using ARMA, SARMA, and a genetic algorithm-optimized regression wavelet neural network (REGWANN). The machine learning (ML) model reduced error rates by 22.6%, 17.7%, and 57% for the three buildings over five years. Similarly, (Mubashir T et al., 2023) used six years of sales data to predict demand for five Industry 4.0 products, comparing statistical forecasting methods—ETS and SARIMAX—with ML models like Random Forest, XGBoost, and LSTM. Among these, the ML models, particularly LSTM, showed superior demand prediction accuracy, achieving significantly lower RMSE values.

1. Drug Polymer-Based Synthesis And Characterization Analysis

First, the stock solutions needed for membrane formulation were prepared for the synthesis process. The k-carrageenan solution was prepared by dissolving k-carrageenan in distilled water, while the chitosan solution was dissolved in distilled water with 5% acetic acid. In this case, 500 mg of each polymer was dissolved in 20 mL of distilled water and stirred continuously for 2 h by a magnetic stirrer. The membrane preparation was done using glycerol (G) as a plasticizer. They added glycerol, k-carrageenan, and chitosan to their stock solutions, after which PVA/PVP polymers and MTX were added. The mixture was stirred using magnetic stirrer, then poured into sterile Petri dishes to air dry and later analyzed. In the same way, membranes prepared using Span 80 as a plasticizer were employed.

2. FT–IR Spectrum

The Infrared spectra were obtained in the 400–4000 cm^{-1} region with an optical resolution of 4 cm^{-1}, and 20 scans per analysis, using Shimadzu IRTracer-ATR spectrometer. The ATR accessory used for all analyses was an ATR accessory equipped with a single reflection diamond ATR crystal mounted on a ZnSe plate.

Thermogravimetric Analysis (TGA)

A Mettler TOLEDO TGA/DSC3+ analyzer was used in a synthetic air environment with a flow rate of 20mL/min over a 25-400 °C temperature range for conducting a TG/DTG experiment. Since samples were placed in an aluminum pan, they were heated at 10 °C per minute. Calibration standards of indium (12.29 mg), aluminum (5.52 mg), gold (41.01 mg), and palladium (26.67 mg) were used to calibrate the TGA/DSC3+.

UV–VIS Spectrophotometry

Samples in 200–400 nm range were analysed by double beam An T90 + UV-Vis Spectrophotometer. UV–VIS data interval was 1.00 nm, scan rate was 100.0 nm min−1.

Membranes Characterisation

The following tests were employed to characterize the membranes physicochemically: biodegradation rate, water vapor permeability, and swelling ratio.

Swelling Ratio (*SR* (%))

Ten mm × ten mm of membranes were incubated in phosphate-buffered saline (PBS, pH 7.4) at 37 °C to determine their swelling behavior. The samples were taken out of the solution at 24-hour mark, blotted with filter paper to remove any surface-adsorbed water, and weighed. The following formula (1) was used to determine swelling ratio of water absorbed:

$$SR\left(\%\right) = \frac{W_s - W_d}{W_d} \times 100 \tag{1}$$

3. Biodegradation Rate

The membranes' biodegradation rate (MR (%)) was investigated by tracking the samples' weight loss over time. Wet samples of every membrane, measuring 10 mm by 10 mm and having a defined weight (W0), were placed in an incubator set at 37 °C and submerged in a lysozyme/PBS solution containing 3 mg/mL. Samples were removed and weighed (Wt) at pre-established intervals after the remaining incubation medium was blotted out. During the observation period, the biodegradation kinetics were taken into account as mass loss by equation (2)

$$MR\left(\%\right) = \frac{W_t}{W_0} \times 100 \quad (2)$$

MOLECULAR DRUG-TARGET INTERACTION ANALYSIS USING NAÏVE CONVOLUTIONAL REGRESSIVE VECTOR NEURAL NETWORKS (NCRVNN)

Figure 1 shows the suggested procedure flowchart. The specifics of each step are listed below. The target proteins are connected to medication molecules, creating a network of pharmacological targets. To obtain positive datasets from network, all drug-target pairs are considered positive samples in gold standard dataset. For the negative sample, we have remaining drug-target pairs in network. Created datasets are unbalanced since scale of non-interaction pairs is significantly greater than that of interaction pairs. We randomly chose negative samples from the remaining drug-target pairings in the network until negative samples equaled the positive samples to address bias brought on by unbalanced data sets.

Figure 1. Proposed molecular drug-target interaction analysis

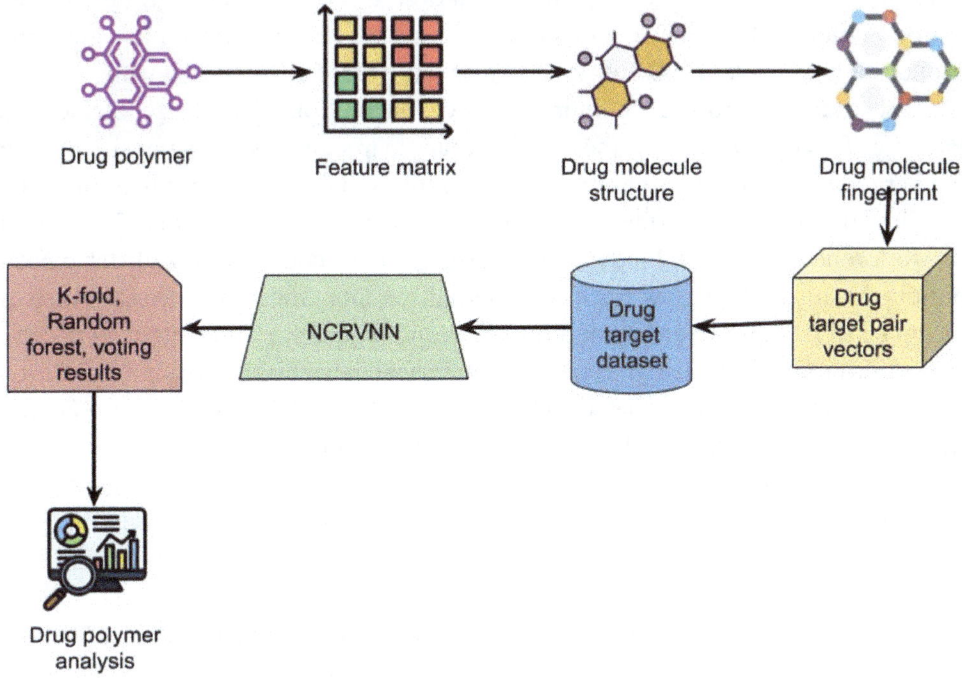

Based on the information collected from the protein sequence, the frequency of amino acids is computed. The following formula (3) is used to calculate this method:

$$g(m,n) = \frac{H(m,n)}{H(n)}, m \in \{1,2,\ldots,21\}, n \in \{W_1, W_2, \cdots, W_L\} \tag{3}$$

The graph attention mechanism assigns attention coefficients to neighboring nodes to obtain more significant neighboring features for constructed drug–target structure data. It is necessary to fuse forecast results of various viewpoints since they contain disparate information. This work uses an adaptive weighting technique to combine the losses of several perspectives and create an optimization objective function.

The first subgroup (red color) clarifies that the spectra belong to the same group at an acidic pH regardless of the different excitation; there is no discernible peak shift. On the other hand, under basic pH conditions, the PL peak for second and third subgroups is somewhat shifted towards a higher wavelength. However, the shift is not particularly noticeable—less than 1 nm. The first and second groups are dispersed throughout a small area, but third group is surprisingly dispersed over a large area. This might be because a very small pH shift at 240–280 nm excitation causes the emergence of new spectral characteristics, and the most incredible PL intensity was also recorded at 260 nm excitation. It is clear that the group with the maroon-colored ellipse has many variations, and PL research should use the same excitation wavelength (260 nm) to look into any potential PL mechanisms.

Three crucial parameters comprise Naïve Convolution: Kernel size, Stride, and Padding. This option controls the output feature map's dimension. After subtracting the kernel width from the input width, the result will be added with two times the Padding, divided by the stride width, total result will be added with one. The neural network relies heavily on hidden dense layers. Three sequential models have been built in this research project. Each contains a different number of neurons in each of its thick layers. Input layers are part of the second sequential model network design. In the pre-processing stage, the dataset's numerical data must be normalized. Seven characteristics were concatenated and normalized. Several thick layers come behind it. The second classification deep model consists of four dense layers containing 32, 24, 12, and 8 neurons. Deep models in the third category consist of six dense layers, with varying numbers of neurons in each layer.64 neurons make up first dense layer, 64 neurons make up second, 32 neurons make up the third, and 24 neurons make up fourth. There are 12 in the fifth tier and 8 in the sixth.

First, we provide a set of training samples. So, one of a fundamental ideas behind linear separable SVM is that we can separate the training sample set of different categories using an appropriate partition hyperplane in sample space such that M is the training sample set. Nevertheless, suppose we ignore all spatial dimensions. In their natural context, we often refer to a linear function as portions of hyperplanes in n-dimensional space, which are straight lines in the case of two-dimensional space and planes in the case of n-dimensional space. For example, we look at a simple example of two-dimensional space. “O” stands for positive classes, and “X” for negative classes in the example. The samples are linearly detachable, but it is apparent from a graphical point of view that many lines can partition the samples in addition to this straight line. Linear separable SVM represents data with lines with most considerable intervals and the ability to split the data accurately.

Calculating interval in sample space is essential since maximum interval is desired. Division of hyperplane in sample space is described by linear equation that follows (4):

$$W^T x + b = 0 \tag{4}$$

Assume that the training samples can be accurately classified by the hyperplane, meaning that the following formula holds true for the training samples by eqn (5)

$$w^t x_i + b \geq 1, y = 1$$

$$w^t + b < 1, y = -1 \tag{5}$$

The maximum interval hypothesis is the name given to the formula above. When presented as a negative sample, it signifies that the sample is positive. The value of 1 or -1 that is stated here is merely for calculational convenience; any constant might be used in theory.

Particle Adversarial Reinforcement Markov Binary Optimization (PARMBO) Model

A particle can travel at the same speed as in the prior iteration. In contrast to the typical PSO method, which only permits particles to travel faster or slower rates, this concept allows particles to move at three alternative speeds: slower, faster, and constant. The main advantage to velocity pausing is that adding a third movement option can help maintain a balance between exploitation and exploration and prevent premature convergence within standard PSO. Mathematically, velocity pausing concept is written as follows (6):

$$V_i\left(t+1\right) = \begin{cases} V_i(t) & \text{if rand} < \alpha \\ w\,V_i(t) & \text{Otherwise} \\ +c_1 r_3\left(\text{ Pbest }_i(t) - X_i(t)\right) & \\ +c_2 r_4\left(\text{ gbest }^t(t) - X_i(t)\right) & \end{cases} \tag{6}$$

In our case, an refers to the velocity pausing parameter, and ViðtÞ and Viðt þ 1Þ are velocities of particle i at iterations t and t þ 1. If pausing parameter an>1, all particles will change their velocities at every iteration as exactly as traditional PSO algorithm does. This is undesirable because there can be no velocity halting. On the other hand, a very low value of a will operate so that particles will not move more or less quickly but will only move with a constant speed. Therefore, selecting the best value for a balanced velocity pausing scenario is necessary for optimum performance.

The discriminator network was entrusted with differentiating between synthetic and genuine traffic samples and giving the generator feedback to enhance the caliber of the traffic it produced. With several layers and activation functions selected to capture intricacy of network traffic data, discriminator and generator networks were built as deep neural networks.

Gradient backpropagation was utilized to iteratively update discriminator and generator networks during the GAN training process, optimizing each network's loss function. Training and validation sets were created from the dataset. Adam optimizer was used to update the network's parameters, carefully adjusting the momentum and learning rate parameters to guarantee steady training convergence. Regularisation strategies like weight decay and dropout were used to enhance method generalization abilities and reduce the chance of overfitting. To ensure the model successfully learned distribution of typical network traffic and gradually enhanced its anomaly detection skills, training was carried out over several epochs, with the model's performance assessed at each epoch.

Superscript (k) indicates k extra historical steps that are being conditioned on function. Markov property states that with every action agent may choose, every state X is sufficient statistic (in predicting next state and expected reward). The assumption that every action is available in every state is widely held, but in this case, that assumes that every state must also be adequate in identifying a range of actions the agent can perform. Usually, the behavior of an RL agent is determined by a (Markov) policy π: X $\rightarrow$ Pr(A). The agent aims to learn an optimal policy π $*$ that maximizes value at each state. It is worth mentioning that practically all RL algorithms rely on the assumption that optimal policy is stationary and Markov. Thus, it only depends on state. If decision process is Markov, this assumption is only appropriate.

A prespecified weighting scheme w(x) is typically chosen, which indicates how important it is for each ground state x to its abstract state z, having a set of x's weights for each z summing to one. A w-weighted sum of ground dynamics can then be used to define the abstract transition dynamics Tφ (and similarly for reward): P x0∈z 0 P x∈z T(x 0 |a, x)w(x) = Tφ(z 0 |a, z) =. This approach assumes that Tφ and Rφ are independent of the policy and timestep and that abstract decision process is Markov by construction. However, this is oversimplifying the situation. Abstract transition dynamics are not Markov; instead, they vary according to the degree of history conditioning: Pr(zA|at = a0, zt = zB, at−1 = a1, zt−1 = zA) = 1, but Tφ(zA|at = a0, zt = zB) = 0.5. The dynamics of ground MDP are entirely deterministic (and Markov). This approach assumes that Tφ and Rφ are independent of the policy and timestep and that abstract decision process is Markov by construction. However, this is oversimplifying the situation. Abstract transition dynamics are not Markov; instead, they vary according to the degree of history conditioning: Pr(zA|at = a0, zt = zB, at−1 = a1, zt−1 = zA) = 1, but Tφ(zA|at = a0, zt = zB) = 0.5. On the other hand, the dynamics of the ground MDP are entirely deterministic (and Markov).

SOLUTIONS AND RECOMMENDATIONS

Experimental setup: PaDEL was used in ChemDes to extract drug characteristics. As a comprehensive set of molecular descriptors capturing different chemical and structural properties, PasDel was a good candidate. Extracted features were 265 topological descriptors representing molecular connectivity and shape and 489 E-state descriptors containing atomic contributions to molecular properties. In addition, molecular shape and branching were measured via 3 Kappa descriptors. Basic properties such as molecular weight and hydrogen bond donor/acceptor counts were described, and fifteen molecular property descriptors were calculated. Six quantum chemical descriptors were included to describe the molecular energy and electron distribution. A set of 42 Basak descriptors was used to extend the topological information, 6 BCUT descriptors for molecular diversity, 96 Burden descriptors for weighted atomic properties, 56 connectivity descriptors for molecular path analysis, and 120 constitutional descriptors for fundamental count-based molecular characteristics. All features found in BioTriangle were used to represent target proteins in a complete characterization. The most essential features for further reduction and analysis were selected by applying dimensionality reduction. This leads the obtained dimensionality-reduced vector for medications and target proteins to be a single 100-dimensional feature vector. Moreover, using a grid search to get the final parameter necessary for prediction in an ensemble method gives results that are more stable and reliable than just using the parameters of an individual method.

One of the standard hyperparameter optimizations is via grid search, wherein final specifications are discovered using a method. It was used to try out every possible combination of hyperparameters in the parameter space. The best possible combination of parameters is chosen as an ensemble model's final parameters.

Dataset description: Yamanishi_08 is one of the industry standards for drug-target interaction (DTI) prediction. The dataset was generated from reputable databases DrugBank, SuperTarget, BRENDA, and KEGG BRITE. The DTI sub-datasets are also categorized into four types according to different target protein classes: nuclear receptors (NR), G protein-coupled receptors (GPCR), ion channels (IC), and enzymes (E). These divisions guarantee complete representativeness of various input drug-target interactions across different biological systems. Also, drug chemical structures and protein sequences from the targets were brought from these databases. All examples around DRUG NAMES D00542 and TARGET NAMES 10369 were carefully collected for the dataset, which included considerable and credible drug-target chemical structures and protein sequence pairs for accurate DTI prediction. Upon meticulously tallying these datasets, we have determined that there are 90, 635, 1476, and 2926 known drug-target interaction pairs in that order. Consequently, four datasets used to construct positive samples for studies yield 5127 interacting pairs. Table 1 lists the specific number of recognized medications, targets, and interactions.

Table 1. Experimental drug-target benchmark datasets utilized in this study

Datasets	Drugs	Interaction	Targets
Enzyme	445	2926	664
Ion Channel	210	1476	204
GPCR	223	635	95
Nuclear Receptor	54	90	26

Table 2. Comparative analysis of various drug-polymer structure datasets

Techniques	Dataset	Prediction accuracy	F- 1 score	Random Precision	Recall	NSE
LS-SVM	**Nuclear receptors**	70	74	71	69	70
	GPCR	75	77	74	72	68
	Ion channels	80	79	76	75	67
	Enzymes	85	83	84	82	60

continued on following page

Table 2. Continued

Techniques	Dataset	Prediction accuracy	F- 1 score	Random Precision	Recall	NSE
GENTRL	Nuclear receptors	78	75	73	72	77
	GPCR	82	79	77	75	70
	Ion channels	87	82	83	80	68
	Enzymes	90	89	86	87	66
NCRVNN_PARMBO	Nuclear receptors	83	85	82	80	63
	GPCR	87	88	85	84	58
	Ion channels	92	90	87	86	53
	Enzymes	97	95	94	93	46

Table 2 shows Comparative analysis of various drug-polymer structure datasets. A comparison has been made between existing LS-SVM, GENTRL, and proposed FCGNBBPS_CMEAGANN regarding prediction accuracy, F- 1 SCORE, random precision, Recall, and NSE.

Figure 2. Comparative analysis for various drug-polymer structure datasets - LS-SVM

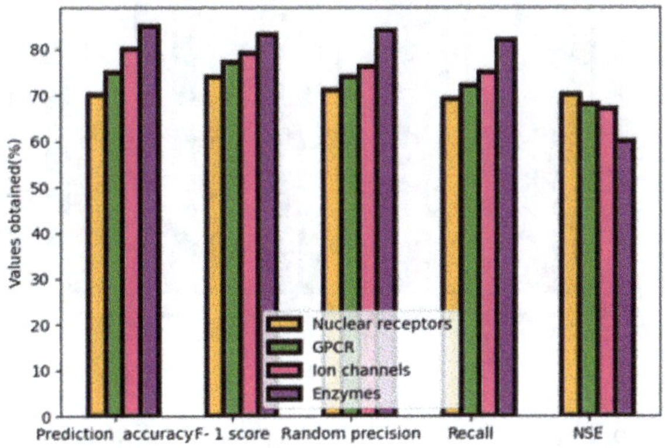

Figure 3. Comparative analysis for various drug-polymer structure datasets - GENTRL

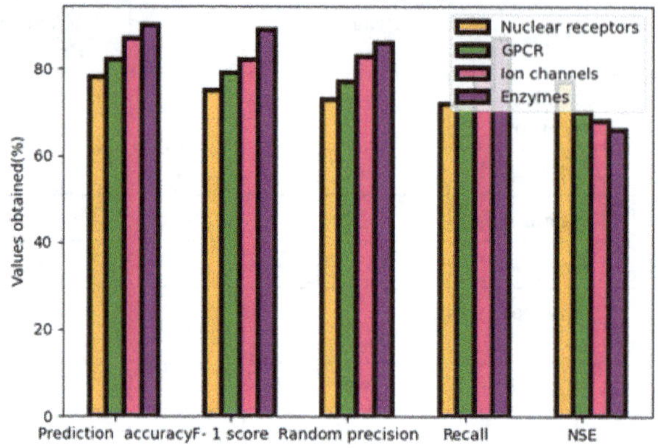

Figure 4. Comparative analysis for various drug-polymer structure datasets - proposed FCGNBBPS_CMEAGANN

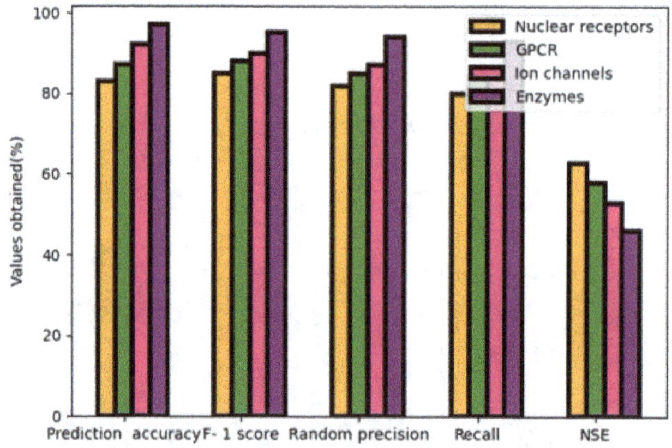

Finally, Figures 2,3, and 4 shows how existing methods perform on different drug-polymer structure datasets based on performance metrics such as Random Precision, Recall, F1-Score, Prediction Accuracy, and Normalized Squared Error (NSE). On the Nuclear Receptors (NR) dataset, the best existing LS-SVM model gets a Random Precision of 71%, Recall of 69%, F1-Score of 74%, and Prediction Accuracy of 70%, as well as NSE of 70%. However, the random precision in the GENTRL model is 73%, the Recall is 72%, the F1-Score is 75%, the prediction accuracy is 78%, and the NSE is 77%. Nevertheless, the proposed method produced significantly better results: random precision at 82%, recall at 80%, F1 score at 85%, prediction accuracy at 83%, and NSE at 63%. In the GPCR dataset, through the same procedure, LS-SVM presented a Random Precision of 74%, Recall of 72%, F1-Score of 77%, Prediction Accuracy of 75%, and NSE of 68%. The results from GENTRL were better, with Random Precision of 77%, Recall of 75%, F1-Score of 79%, Prediction Accuracy of 82% and NSE of 70%. On the other hand, the proposed technique also achieved a Prediction Accuracy of 87%, Recall of 84%, F1-Score of 88%, Random Precision of 85%, and NSE of 58%. For the Ion Channels (IC) dataset, the LS-SVM obtained Random Precision of 76%, Recall of 75%, F1 Score of 79%, Prediction Accuracy of 81%, and NSE of 67%. Using the GENTRL model increased the metrics, with a random precision of 83%, Recall of 80%, F1 Score of 82%, prediction accuracy of 87%, and NSE of 68%. Regarding the proposed method, it had the highest performance with Random Precision of 87%, Recall of 86%, F1 Score of 90%, Prediction Accuracy of 92%, and NSE value of 53%. Finally, for the Enzymes dataset, LS-SVM recorded its best result with a Random Precision of 84%, Recall of 82%, F1-Score of 83%, Prediction Accuracy of 85%, and NSE of 60%. The GENTRL model predictions improved with a Random Precision of 86%, Recall of 87%, F1-Score of 89%, Prediction Accuracy of 90%, and NSE of 66%. The proposed technique achieved outstanding results, with a Random Precision of 94%, Recall of 93%, F1-Score of 95%, Prediction Accuracy of 97%, and NSE of 46%, demonstrating its superior performance compared to other methods.

FUTURE RESEARCH DIRECTIONS

Data balance processing has been shown to have a significant impact on performance. Based on the conditional generative countermeasure network, this study's small-sample ML data categorization demonstrated a higher generalization rate than traditional data processing methods. The data feature extraction problem was transformed into a linear solution by mapping sample data into Hilbert space. A sample data feature matrix was then created, and each data feature matrix's entropy and the sample data matrix's mutual entropy were calculated. These results were used to modify the target relative entropy. Additionally, using a combination of molecular descriptors and the phase equilibrium concept, a machine-learning model was constructed to predict the solubility of APIs in polymers with high accuracy and efficiency.

The few-shot learning framework employed computational chemistry for screening molecular descriptors and thermodynamic theory for data augmentation. Findings demonstrated that ML method could effectively guide development of pharmaceutical formulations by accurately predicting API-polymer phase diagrams, expanding data on API solubility in polymers, and reproducing relationship between API solubility and interaction methods between API and polymer.

CONCLUSION

This study suggests a revolutionary approach to drug polymer-based production, characterisation analysis, and supply chain optimization using artificial intelligence and machine learning algorithms. Based on their synthesis and characterization models, a molecular drug target interaction study employing naïve convolutional regressive vector neural networks has assessed the drug structure here. Once the supply chain optimization is based on drug synthesis and structural analysis, Markov binary optimization model with particle adversarial reinforcement is used. We, therefore, propose a universal model for predicting the guest-host binding energy using input features conforming to a neural network and a set of quantitative structural activity connections. Pharmacophore-like structures, pharmacokinetic properties, and different chemical spaces of natural products constantly lead to their research for novel bioactive chemicals with economic potential. Physico-chemical variation of bioactive chemicals and their lower toxicity makes them more valuable relative to developing novel medications.

REFERENCES

Bai, X., Xu, Y., & Liu, Y. (2024). Therapeutic effects of DOX-loaded hydrogel MOF nanocarriers on triple negative breast cancer and derivative design via reinforcement learning. *Scientific Reports*, *14*(1), 23946. DOI: 10.1038/s41598-024-75466-2 PMID: 39397066

Benavides-Hernández, J., & Dumeignil, F. (2024). From characterisation to discovery: Artificial intelligence, machine learning and high-throughput experiments for heterogeneous catalyst design. *ACS Catalysis*, *14*(15), 11749–11779. DOI: 10.1021/acscatal.3c06293

Carracedo-Reboredo, P., Liñares-Blanco, J., Rodríguez-Fernández, N., Cedrón, F., Novoa, F. J., Carballal, A., Maojo, V., Pazos, A., & Fernandez-Lozano, C. (2021). A review on machine learning approaches and trends in drug discovery. *Computational and Structural Biotechnology Journal*, *19*, 4538–4558. DOI: 10.1016/j.csbj.2021.08.011 PMID: 34471498

Garg, S., Arora, K., Singh, S., & Nagarajan, K. (2024). Artificial Intelligence and Machine Learning in Drug Discovery and Development. In *Artificial Intelligence in the Age of Nanotechnology* (pp. 42–61). IGI Global.

Güleryüz, C., Sumrra, S. H., Hassan, A. U., Mohyuddin, A., Waheeb, A. S., Awad, M. A., Jalfan, A. R., Noreen, S., Kyhoiesh, H. A. K., & El Azab, I. H. (2025). A machine learning and DFT assisted analysis of benzodithiophene based organic dyes for possible photovoltaic applications. *Journal of Photochemistry and Photobiology A Chemistry*, *460*, 116157. DOI: 10.1016/j.jphotochem.2024.116157

Gupta, R., Srivastava, D., Sahu, M., Tiwari, S., Ambasta, R. K., & Kumar, P. (2021). Artificial intelligence to deep learning: Machine intelligence approach for drug discovery. *Molecular Diversity*, *25*(3), 1315–1360. DOI: 10.1007/s11030-021-10217-3 PMID: 33844136

He, S., Barón, A., Munteanu, C. R., de Bilbao, B., Casañola-Martin, G. M., Chelu, M., Musuc, A. M., Bediaga, H., Ascencio, E., Castellanos-Rubio, I., Arrasate, S., Pazos, A., Insausti, M., Rasulev, B., & González-Díaz, H. (2025). Drug Release Nanoparticle System Design: Data Set Compilation and Machine Learning Modeling. *ACS Applied Materials & Interfaces*, *17*(3), 5290–5306. DOI: 10.1021/acsami.4c16800 PMID: 39800937

Jayaraman, A., & Olsen, B. (2024). Convergence of artificial intelligence, machine learning, cheminformatics, and polymer science in macromolecules. *Macromolecules*, *57*(16), 7685–7688. DOI: 10.1021/acs.macromol.4c01704

Li, S., Zhang, H., Holby, E. F., Zelenay, P., & Kort-Kamp, W. J. (2024). Machine learning-guided design, synthesis, and characterisation of atomically dispersed electrocatalysts. *Current Opinion in Electrochemistry*, *48*, 101578. DOI: 10.1016/j.coelec.2024.101578

Martinelli, D. D. (2022). Generative machine learning for de novo drug discovery: A systematic review. *Computers in Biology and Medicine*, *145*, 105403. DOI: 10.1016/j.compbiomed.2022.105403 PMID: 35339849

Mohammadpour, A., Dolatabadi, M., Bontempi, E., & Shahsavani, E. (2025). Synthesis and characterisation of novel lignocellulosic biomass-derived activated carbon for dye removal: Machine learning optimization, mechanisms, and antibacterial properties. *Biomass and Bioenergy*, *192*, 107490. DOI: 10.1016/j.biombioe.2024.107490

Mubashir, T., Tahir, M. H., Mahmoud, M. H. H., Shafiq, Z., Ashraf, M., El Azab, I. H., & Janjua, M. R. S. A. (2023). Designing of symmetric and asymmetric small molecule acceptors for organic solar cells: A farmwork based on Machine learning, virtual screening, and structural analysis. *Journal of Photochemistry and Photobiology A Chemistry*, *444*, 114977. DOI: 10.1016/j.jphotochem.2023.114977

Nangia, A. K. (2024). Importance of Structural Databases, Molecular Pharmacophores, Supramolecular Heterosynthons, and Artificial Intelligence–Machine Learning–Neural Network Tools in Drug Discovery. *Crystal Growth & Design*, *24*(16), 6888–6910. DOI: 10.1021/acs.cgd.4c00422

Parvatikar, P. P., Patil, S., Khaparkhuntikar, K., Patil, S., Singh, P. K., Sahana, R., Kulkarni, R. V., & Raghu, A. V. (2023). Artificial intelligence: Machine learning approach for screening large database and drug discovery. *Antiviral Research*, *220*, 105740. DOI: 10.1016/j.antiviral.2023.105740 PMID: 37935248

Staszak, M., Staszak, K., Wieszczycka, K., Bajek, A., Roszkowski, K., & Tylkowski, B. (2022). Machine learning in drug design: Use of artificial intelligence to explore the chemical structure–biological activity relationship. *Wiley Interdisciplinary Reviews. Computational Molecular Science*, *12*(2), e1568. DOI: 10.1002/wcms.1568

Wyrembek, M., Baryannis, G., & Brintrup, A. (2025). Causal machine learning for supply chain risk prediction and intervention planning. *International Journal of Production Research*, 1–20. DOI: 10.1080/00207543.2025.2458121

Zhang, Y., Fan, M., Xu, Z., Jiang, Y., Ding, H., Li, Z., Shu, K., Zhao, M., Feng, G., Yong, K.-T., Dong, B., Zhu, W., & Xu, G. (2023). Machine-learning screening of luminogens with aggregation-induced emission characteristics for fluorescence imaging. *Journal of Nanobiotechnology*, *21*(1), 107. DOI: 10.1186/s12951-023-01864-9 PMID: 36964565

Zhao, J., Wang, J., & Anderson, N. (2024). Machine learning applications in forest and biomass supply chain management: A review. *International Journal of Forest Engineering*, *35*(3), 371–380. DOI: 10.1080/14942119.2024.2380230

Zhao, X., Sun, Y., Zhang, R., Chen, Z., Hua, Y., Zhang, P., Guo, H., Cui, X., Huang, X., & Li, X. (2022). Machine learning modeling and insights into the structural characteristics of drug-induced neurotoxicity. *Journal of Chemical Information and Modeling*, *62*(23), 6035–6045. DOI: 10.1021/acs.jcim.2c01131 PMID: 36448818

Zhuang, Z., & Barnard, A. S. (2024). Property Prediction for Complex Compounds Using Structure-Free Mendeleev Encoding and Machine Learning. *Journal of Chemical Information and Modeling*, *64*(24), 9205–9214. DOI: 10.1021/acs.jcim.4c01343 PMID: 39665625

ADDITIONAL READING

Bao, Z., Kim, J., Le Devedec, F., Clasky, A., & Allen, C. (2025). Polymer microparticles in an evolving drug delivery landscape: Challenges and the role of machine learning. *International Journal of Pharmaceutics*, *125906*, 125906. Advance online publication. DOI: 10.1016/j.ijpharm.2025.125906 PMID: 40578461

Patalas-Maliszewska, J., Szmołda, M., & Łosyk, H. (2024). Integrating Artificial Intelligence into the Supply Chain in Order to Enhance Sustainable Production—A Systematic Literature Review. *Sustainability (Basel)*, *16*(16), 7110. DOI: 10.3390/su16167110

Swarnkar, S., Dixit, R., Prajapati, T., Sinha, U., Rathore, Y., & Bhosle, S.Suman Kumar Swarnkar. (2024). Integrating Artificial Intelligence and Data Analytics for Supply Chain Optimization in the Pharmaceutical Industry. *Journal of Electrical Systems.*, *20*(3s), 682–690. DOI: 10.52783/jes.1358

KEY TERMS AND DEFINITIONS

Biodegradation Rate (MR): The rate at which a membrane or material breaks down over time in a biological environment, typically measured by mass loss in a lysozyme solution.

Drug Polymer-Based Synthesis: The formulation of drug delivery systems using biopolymers like chitosan and k-carrageenan to improve drug stability, release, and bioavailability.

Infrared Spectroscopy (FT–IR): An analytical technique used to identify the functional groups in a compound or polymer by measuring the absorbance of infrared radiation.

Pharmacogenomics: The study of how an individual's genetic makeup affects their response to drugs. It is used to personalize medicine, optimize dosages, and reduce adverse drug reactions.

Process Analytical Technology (PAT): A system for designing, analyzing, and controlling pharmaceutical manufacturing processes through real-time measurements to ensure final product quality.

Quality by Design (QbD): A scientific, risk-based approach to pharmaceutical development that emphasizes product and process understanding and control, ensuring quality is built into the manufacturing process from the start.

UV–VIS Spectrophotometry: An analytical technique that measures the absorbance of ultraviolet or visible light by a sample, commonly used to assess the optical properties and concentration of drug-polymer formulations.

Supply Chain Optimization: The application of advanced technologies such as AI and ML to streamline production, inventory management, and logistics in pharmaceutical manufacturing, aiming to reduce costs, minimize waste, and ensure timely delivery of high-quality products.

Swelling Ratio (SR): A measure of how much a polymer membrane can absorb water or fluid, calculated as the percentage increase in weight after incubation in a solution.

Thermogravimetric Analysis (TGA): A technique used to assess the thermal stability and composition of a material by measuring changes in weight as a function of temperature.

Chapter 8
AI in Hospital Administration and Formulary Design:
Optimizing Resource Allocation and Patient Flow

Kanagaraj Rengaramanujam
https://orcid.org/0000-0002-0244-7645
Verland Foundation, USA

Anandhavalli Muniasamy
https://orcid.org/0000-0001-8940-3954
College of Computer Science, King Khalid University, Saudi Arabia

ABSTRACT

Artificial Intelligence (AI) is transforming hospital administration by improving resource allocation, patient flow, and formulary design. This chapter explores how AI technologies—such as machine learning, predictive analytics, and data-driven tools—enhance hospital efficiency, scheduling, and medication optimization. A real-world case study highlights AI's impact, while practical recommendations address implementation strategies and integration challenges. Future directions consider AI's role in personalized medicine, cost reduction, and ethical concerns, offering a roadmap for advancing healthcare management.

DOI: 10.4018/979-8-3373-2043-4.ch008

INTRODUCTION

1.1 The Evolving Landscape of Healthcare Administration

The modern healthcare ecosystem is undergoing a profound transformation, driven by digital innovation, demographic shifts, and increasing clinical complexity. Hospital administrators are tasked with the challenge of maintaining operational efficiency, patient safety, and cost control in an environment marked by growing patient volumes, workforce shortages, and budgetary constraints (Badwan et al., 2023). In parallel, the pharmaceutical arm of hospital operations—particularly formulary design and medication management—must address rising drug costs, variability in prescribing patterns, and the growing demand for precision therapeutics (Ramezani, 2023).

Despite major strides in health information systems, most hospitals still depend on reactive and often fragmented decision-making processes. Administrative and pharmaceutical workflows are typically siloed, leading to suboptimal resource utilization, medication errors, and reduced patient satisfaction. The COVID-19 pandemic further exposed systemic vulnerabilities, including ICU bed shortages, delayed admissions, and global disruptions in medication supply chains (Iyengar et al., 2020). These challenges underscore the urgent need for intelligent, data-driven systems capable of real-time decision-making and adaptive resource planning.

1.2 Artificial Intelligence as a Healthcare Enabler

Artificial Intelligence (AI) encompasses a range of computational techniques that enable machines to simulate human-like cognitive processes such as learning, reasoning, and decision-making (Russell & Norvig, 2021). Within healthcare, AI applications span a wide spectrum—from clinical decision support and diagnostic imaging to administrative automation and pharmaceutical analytics. Key AI methodologies relevant to hospital operations include machine learning (ML), natural language processing (NLP), deep learning (DL), and reinforcement learning (RL) (Topol, 2019).

In hospital administration, AI-powered systems can forecast admission trends, predict patient length of stay (LOS), optimize staffing levels, and manage ICU capacities (Jiang et al., 2017). Similarly, in formulary management, AI tools analyze medication usage patterns, detect adverse drug interactions, and recommend evidence-based alternatives, thereby promoting cost-effectiveness and medication safety (Rajkomar et al., 2019).

Rather than functioning as standalone technologies, AI systems are increasingly being integrated into hospital information systems (HIS), electronic health records (EHRs), and pharmacy benefit management (PBM) platforms, enabling cross-functional automation and real-time decision support.

1.3 Optimizing Hospital Resource Allocation Using AI

One of the most compelling applications of AI in hospital management is its ability to optimize resource allocation in dynamic, high-pressure environments. Machine learning models trained on historical and real-time data can predict patient inflow, bed occupancy rates, and critical care demands with impressive accuracy (Shah et al., 2019). Reinforcement learning algorithms have been shown to optimize staff scheduling and equipment deployment by continuously learning from system feedback (Komorowski et al., 2018).

For instance, AI systems deployed in emergency departments (EDs) have demonstrated success in anticipating surges in patient volume, enabling administrators to pre-emptively reassign resources or expand capacity (Chenais et al., 2023). Similarly, predictive tools that estimate the LOS based on comorbidities and treatment pathways support discharge planning and reduce unnecessary bed blocking.

Moreover, robotic process automation (RPA) powered by AI is streamlining administrative functions such as claims processing, inventory control, and appointment scheduling—functions that traditionally consume significant staff time and are prone to error (Davenport & Kalakota, 2019).

1.4 AI and Intelligent Patient Flow Management

Patient flow refers to the movement of individuals through various points of care in the hospital, from admission to discharge. Poor patient flow leads to delays, overcrowding, and reduced quality of care. AI-enabled systems can model patient trajectories, identify flow bottlenecks, and recommend workflow redesigns (Gettman, 2023).

For example, time-series forecasting models can detect patterns in patient arrivals based on environmental, epidemiological, and seasonal factors (Muralitharan et al., 2021). AI dashboards integrated into hospital command centers provide real-time visualizations of patient locations, test completions, and bed statuses, supporting proactive clinical and operational decision-making (Goyal et al., 2023).

Furthermore, AI-based early warning systems can identify high-risk patients likely to require intensive care or prolonged hospitalization, allowing for resource planning and timely intervention. Such systems have been shown to improve care continuity, reduce readmissions, and enhance discharge throughput (Churpek et al., 2016).

1.5 Enhancing Formulary Design through AI

Formulary design is central to pharmaceutical governance in hospitals. Traditionally managed by pharmacy and therapeutics (P&T) committees, formularies are curated lists of approved medications aimed at promoting standardized, cost-effective treatment. However, manual formulary management is time-consuming and often lacks timely data to support dynamic adjustments.

AI tools offer a new paradigm in formulary design by analyzing large volumes of medication data, including utilization trends, cost analyses, and therapeutic outcomes. Machine learning algorithms can identify high-cost medications with low clinical benefit, recommend biosimilars or generics, and flag off-label prescribing patterns (He et al., 2019). NLP systems can extract safety signals from unstructured clinical notes and literature, supporting pharmacovigilance efforts (Wu et al., 2019).

More advanced AI platforms can simulate the budgetary impact of introducing new drugs and predict patient-level responses to specific therapies, paving the way for precision formulary decisions (Miotto et al., 2018). AI can also assist in medication reconciliation and adherence monitoring—key components of safe transitions of care.

1.6 Research Gap

While the transformative potential of AI in hospital administration and formulary design is well-documented, several critical research gaps persist:

- **Integration Deficits**: Existing studies often examine AI applications in silos, with limited exploration of integrated systems that coordinate hospital logistics with pharmaceutical management.
- **Data Fragmentation**: Most hospital systems suffer from data fragmentation, where patient, clinical, and pharmaceutical data reside in incompatible platforms, limiting the scope and accuracy of AI models.
- **Limited Implementation Evidence**: There is a lack of real-world, longitudinal studies evaluating the scalability and sustainability of AI tools in diverse hospital settings, especially in low- and middle-income countries (LMICs).
- **Ethical and Legal Ambiguity**: Questions surrounding algorithmic bias, transparency, data privacy, and liability remain unresolved, hindering institutional trust in AI systems (Amann et al., 2020).
- **Skills and Workforce Gaps**: Successful AI integration requires a digitally literate workforce capable of interpreting AI outputs and integrating them into clinical workflows—a capability that is currently lacking across many institutions.

These gaps present significant opportunities for future research, innovation, and policy-making to foster responsible and effective AI adoption in healthcare.

1.7 Objectives of the Chapter

The primary goal of this chapter is to explore how artificial intelligence can be leveraged to enhance hospital administration and formulary design. The specific objectives are:

- To analyze the role of AI in resource allocation within hospitals, including predictive analytics, staffing optimization, and logistics management.
- To evaluate AI applications in improving patient flow, focusing on early warning systems, discharge planning, and capacity forecasting.
- To examine how AI supports formulary design through medication data mining, cost-effectiveness modeling, and pharmacovigilance.
- To identify the technical, ethical, and operational barriers to AI implementation in hospital and pharmacy settings.
- To propose an integrated AI framework that bridges hospital operations with pharmaceutical governance.
- To offer recommendations for future research directions and institutional policies to guide AI deployment in healthcare.

1.8 Structure of the Chapter

The remaining sections of this chapter are structured to provide a comprehensive overview of AI applications in healthcare operations. Section 2 outlines the AI methodologies employed in this domain, while Section 3 highlights practical use cases in hospital administration. Section 4 delves into the role of AI in optimizing formularies, followed by Section 5, which discusses the challenges of implementation and related ethical concerns. Section 6 introduces a proposed integrated AI framework for hospital systems, and Section 7 concludes the chapter with key insights and strategic recommendations. Section 7 concludes with key insights and recommendations.

BACKGROUND

2.1 The Complexity of Hospital Administration

Hospitals represent some of the most complex operational environments in any sector. From managing patient inflows and discharges to coordinating multidisciplinary teams and clinical workflows, hospital administration must function like a finely tuned system. However, this complexity is often exacerbated by unpredictable patient volumes, resource limitations, and systemic inefficiencies (Tiwari et al., 2021). A single delay in a diagnostic test or bed assignment can create cascading effects throughout a facility, contributing to overcrowding, prolonged wait times, and increased healthcare costs.

Traditionally, hospital resource management relied on rule-based systems and manual inputs, which are insufficient for responding to dynamic, real-time variables (Green, 2003). Moreover, decisions made in administrative silos—such as staffing, inventory control, or discharge planning—rarely account for upstream or downstream implications, resulting in fragmented service delivery. These shortcomings highlight the need for adaptive systems that can synthesize multidimensional data, learn from evolving trends, and support proactive decision-making.

2.2 Challenges in Formulary Design and Medication Management

Formulary design is central to ensuring safe, effective, and economically viable medication use in hospitals. Yet, this process is not without its challenges. Pharmacy and therapeutics (P&T) committees are typically tasked with reviewing vast amounts of clinical literature, cost data, and utilization statistics to determine which medications should be included in the formulary. The sheer volume and variability of data—ranging from drug efficacy studies to pharmacoeconomic models—make this process time-consuming and prone to inconsistencies (Beis et al., 1999).

Additionally, drug pricing volatility, patent expirations, and the emergence of biosimilars further complicate formulary decisions. Without robust analytical support, hospitals may struggle to evaluate the trade-offs between therapeutic benefit and financial impact. Compounding the issue is the tendency to base formulary decisions on retrospective data, which may not reflect current patient needs, emerging resistance patterns, or personalized treatment considerations (Heindel et al., 2021).

An integrated, data-driven approach to formulary design—anchored in real-time utilization trends, clinical outcomes, and patient demographics—could significantly enhance both cost-efficiency and clinical value. This is where AI offers tremendous promise.

2.3 The Data Explosion in Healthcare and the Role of AI

Over the past decade, the proliferation of digital health technologies has led to an unprecedented explosion in healthcare data. Hospitals now collect and store petabytes of information, including structured data (e.g., lab results, vital signs) and unstructured data (e.g., clinical notes, discharge summaries). According to estimates, healthcare data is growing at an annual rate of over 36%, outpacing most other sectors (IDC, 2024).

This data deluge, while rich in potential insights, is often underutilized due to limitations in traditional data processing systems. Artificial Intelligence provides the necessary computational frameworks to harness this information. AI can identify hidden patterns, forecast future events, and support real-time decision-making across both clinical and administrative domains (Kaul et al., 2020).

For instance, unsupervised learning models can cluster patients with similar resource utilization profiles, aiding in personalized bed and medication planning. Meanwhile, supervised learning models can predict high-cost patients or those at risk of readmission, allowing for targeted interventions. These capabilities can greatly enhance hospital performance metrics, including average length of stay, readmission rates, and cost per case.

2.4 Global Case Studies of AI in Hospital Operations

Several hospitals across the globe have begun piloting AI tools to optimize operational efficiency. For example, the Cleveland Clinic has implemented predictive algorithms that estimate patient discharges, which has helped improve bed turnover rates and reduce emergency department congestion (Strome, 2020). In Singapore, AI has been used to dynamically assign ICU beds based on real-time acuity scores, resulting in more efficient triage and resource deployment (Ngiam & Khor, 2019).

Similarly, the University of Chicago Medicine introduced an AI system called eCART, which aggregates EHR data to predict patient deterioration. Although initially deployed for clinical purposes, its insights were also used by administrators to prioritize ICU transfers and streamline patient flow (UChicago Medicine, 2025). These case studies highlight that AI is not just a technological novelty but a strategic asset in hospital management. Figure 1 shows the AI in hospital management.

Figure 1. AI in hospital management

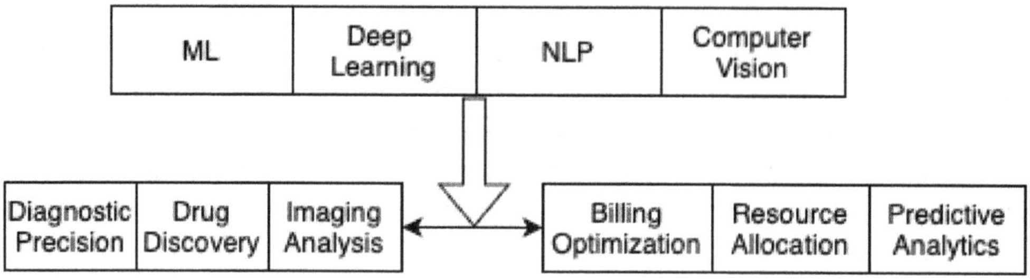

2.5 AI in Hospital Pharmacy and Drug Inventory Management

Artificial Intelligence is also gaining traction in pharmacy operations, particularly in inventory forecasting and medication safety. Hospitals typically manage inventories for thousands of drug formulations, many of which have different storage requirements, expiration periods, and usage trends. Overstocking leads to waste, while understocking jeopardizes patient care.

AI-based inventory management systems use historical dispensing data, seasonal demand trends, and supplier reliability scores to forecast medication needs with high accuracy (Almeman et al., 2024). These systems are especially useful during epidemics or mass casualty incidents when drug demand spikes unpredictably.

Additionally, AI is improving pharmacovigilance by mining adverse event reports, social media, and scientific publications to detect drug safety signals faster than traditional methods. Such tools can be integrated into hospital pharmacy dashboards to support formulary updates and clinical alerts (Denck et al., 2023).

In terms of compliance, AI can also assist in monitoring adherence to formulary protocols, flagging outlier prescriptions, and generating real-time alerts for potential therapeutic duplications or contraindications—functions that are increasingly important in high-volume hospitals with decentralized care teams.

2.6 Institutional Readiness and Implementation Barriers

While the benefits of AI in hospital operations and pharmacy management are increasingly evident, several barriers hinder large-scale adoption. Institutional readiness is a major concern. Many hospitals lack the IT infrastructure, data interoperability, and workforce training required to deploy and maintain AI systems (Morley et al.,

2020). Moreover, the absence of standardized AI governance frameworks leads to concerns over accountability, algorithmic transparency, and regulatory compliance.

Data quality is another limiting factor. AI models are only as good as the data they are trained on, and healthcare datasets often suffer from inconsistencies, missing values, and biases. Without rigorous data curation and continuous validation, AI systems may generate inaccurate or inequitable recommendations (Mittelstadt et al., 2016).

In addition, there is growing apprehension among healthcare professionals about "black-box" AI systems—those whose decision-making processes are not easily explainable. Addressing this will require the development of interpretable AI models, as well as clear guidelines on clinician–AI collaboration.

These concerns underscore the importance of developing tailored AI solutions that are not only technically robust but also ethically sound, context-sensitive, and aligned with institutional workflows.

AI IN HOSPITAL ADMINISTRATION AND FORMULARY DESIGN

The integration of AI into hospital administration and formulary design has revolutionized resource management, patient flow optimization, and drug utilization. This section provides an in-depth analysis of AI models that are instrumental in these domains, focusing on various applications and case studies that highlight their impact on improving hospital efficiency and patient outcomes. Figure 2 shows the Flowchart for the AI Workflow in Hospital Administration and Formulary Design.

Figure 2. Flowchart: AI workflow in hospital administration and formulary design

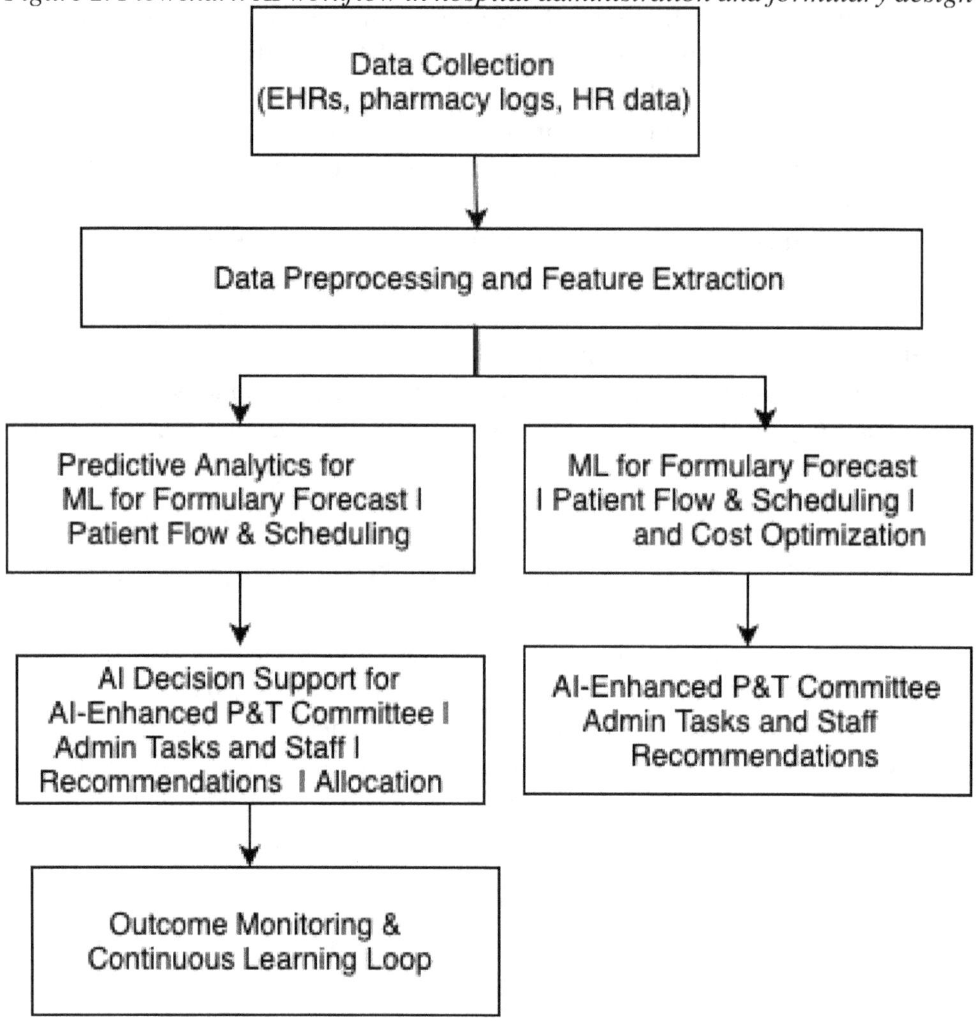

3.1 AI Models in Hospital Administration

3.1.1 Predictive Analytics for Patient Flow Management

Predictive analytics involves using historical data to forecast future events, which can be pivotal in managing patient flow within a hospital. AI-driven predictive models use machine learning algorithms to analyze vast datasets from hospital management systems, Electronic Health Records (EHRs), and other administrative sources to predict patient admissions, discharges, and emergency department (ED) visits.

For instance, machine learning models such as decision trees and ensemble methods (e.g., random forests) have been successfully deployed to predict peak admission times and potential bottlenecks in patient care (Peixoto et al., 2022). These models provide hospital administrators with the ability to anticipate spikes in patient volume, enabling them to adjust staffing levels, optimize bed occupancy, and streamline discharge planning processes. A study by Adhiya et al. (2024) utilized a machine learning model to predict the likelihood of patient readmission within 30 days. This model enabled the hospital to allocate resources more efficiently, reduce readmission rates, and improve overall patient care by focusing resources on high-risk patients.

3.1.2 Reinforcement Learning in Resource Allocation and Staff Scheduling

AI models based on reinforcement learning (RL) are particularly useful for real-time decision-making in hospital administration. In contrast to traditional algorithms, RL models dynamically adapt to ongoing changes in patient care needs and hospital operations. These models use feedback loops to continuously improve resource allocation strategies, such as staff scheduling, equipment allocation, and patient routing.

For example, RL algorithms have been applied to optimize shift planning for healthcare workers, ensuring that staff levels match patient demands across departments (Teng et al., 2022). This reduces the incidence of burnout, enhances employee satisfaction, and ensures that sufficient medical staff is available at critical times. RL has also been used in ED management to optimize patient triage and reduce wait times by allocating limited resources (e.g., ICU beds, operating rooms) based on real-time patient needs (Duma et al., 2023).

3.1.3 Natural Language Processing (NLP) for Administrative Automation

Natural Language Processing (NLP) plays a crucial role in automating administrative tasks, such as processing unstructured clinical notes, generating reports, and improving patient interaction systems. By analyzing textual data from patient records, hospital administrators can extract valuable insights that inform decision-making and improve patient care workflows.

In hospitals, NLP can be used to automate routine tasks such as appointment scheduling, processing discharge summaries, and managing patient queries. Furthermore, NLP algorithms can extract and classify symptoms, diagnoses, and treatments mentioned in clinical notes, which can then be used to inform administrative planning and resource allocation (Payal et al., 2022).

3.2 AI Models in Formulary Design

Formulary design is a critical aspect of hospital administration, where decisions on medication selection are made based on clinical efficacy, patient safety, and cost-effectiveness. AI models are transforming this process by providing data-driven insights that assist pharmacists and administrators in making informed decisions about drug formulary selection.

3.2.1 Machine Learning in Drug Utilization and Forecasting

Machine learning models are widely used to analyze historical prescription data and predict future drug demand. These models use time-series forecasting techniques such as Long Short-Term Memory (LSTM) networks and ARIMA models to anticipate the need for specific medications based on patient trends, seasonal patterns, and even regional disease outbreaks. For example, hospitals often struggle with balancing the inventory of high-cost medications, which can either lead to drug shortages or excessive stockpiling. By leveraging machine learning to forecast demand for specific drugs, hospitals can ensure that they maintain optimal stock levels while minimizing waste and the financial burden associated with overstocking (Fourkiotis et al., 2024).

3.2.2 AI for Pharmacoeconomic Modeling and Cost-Effectiveness Analysis

AI models such as decision trees, Markov models, and Monte Carlo simulations are increasingly used to perform pharmacoeconomic modeling and cost-effectiveness analysis. These models analyze the long-term financial implications of drug treatments, enabling hospitals to make more informed decisions about formulary inclusion based on the balance between clinical efficacy and treatment costs.

A particularly promising approach involves the integration of AI models with real-time clinical and economic data, allowing hospitals to continually assess the cost-effectiveness of therapies. Bayesian networks, for example, can incorporate uncertainty in drug costs, patient outcomes, and clinical guidelines to generate personalized cost-effectiveness recommendations (Baio et al., 2014).

3.2.3 Personalized Formulary Management Using AI and EHR Integration

With the widespread use of Electronic Health Records (EHRs), hospitals now have access to vast amounts of patient-level data, including diagnoses, demographics, medical histories, and genetic profiles. AI models can analyze this data to recommend personalized medication options tailored to individual patients. This approach ensures that formulary decisions are not based solely on population-level data but are instead customized to reflect the unique characteristics of each patient (Raza et al., 2022).

AI-driven formulary management systems can incorporate factors such as comorbidities, allergies, and treatment preferences to suggest medications that are both clinically appropriate and cost-effective. These personalized approaches help to reduce adverse drug reactions and improve patient outcomes by selecting the most suitable therapies for each individual.

3.3 Comparative Summary of AI Models in Hospital Administration and Formulary Design

Table 1 summarizes the key AI techniques used in hospital administration and formulary design.

Table 1. Comparative summary of ai models in hospital administration and formulary design

AI Technique	Hospital Administration Use	Formulary Design Use
Predictive Analytics	Patient flow prediction, resource allocation	Demand forecasting, medication usage analysis
Reinforcement Learning	Real-time staff scheduling and resource allocation	Adaptive drug formulary recommendations based on outcomes
Natural Language Processing (NLP)	Automation of administrative tasks such as coding and reporting	Drug classification from unstructured clinical notes
Machine Learning	Forecasting patient admissions, optimizing ED operations	Personalized drug selection, drug demand forecasting
Bayesian Networks	Risk assessment and resource allocation optimization	Cost-effectiveness and pharmacoeconomic analysis
Deep Learning (LSTM, CNN)	Dynamic scheduling, predictive maintenance of hospital equipment	Drug utilization analysis and outcome prediction

The applications of AI in hospital administration and formulary design have proven transformative in improving operational efficiency, reducing costs, and enhancing patient care. AI models such as predictive analytics, reinforcement learning, NLP, and deep learning are being integrated into hospital workflows to optimize patient flow, streamline administrative tasks, and improve resource allocation. Similarly, in formulary design, AI assists in personalized medication management, cost-effectiveness analysis, and drug demand forecasting, ensuring that hospitals can provide optimal care while maintaining financial sustainability. As AI continues to evolve, its potential to revolutionize both hospital administration and formulary design will only expand, bringing greater efficiencies and better patient outcomes.

3.6 Challenges in AI Model Deployment

Despite promising results, several challenges impede the widespread adoption of AI in hospital administration and formulary design:

1. **Data Quality and Standardization** – Inconsistent data across systems hampers model training and interoperability.
2. **Bias and Fairness** – AI models may inherit biases present in historical data.
3. **Ethical and Legal Concerns** – Informed consent, data privacy, and algorithmic transparency remain critical issues.
4. **Resistance to Change** – Clinicians may be hesitant to adopt AI recommendations over traditional protocols.

SOLUTIONS AND RECOMMENDATIONS

The integration of Artificial Intelligence (AI) in hospital administration and formulary design presents numerous opportunities to optimize operational efficiencies, improve patient care, and enhance resource management. However, to fully realize these benefits, specific strategies and recommendations must be considered. This section provides a comprehensive set of solutions and recommendations based on the analysis of current AI applications, focusing on improving hospital administration processes and formulary design. The aim is to ensure that AI technologies are used effectively and sustainably within healthcare systems.

4.1 Solutions for Improving Hospital Administration

4.1.1 Enhancing Predictive Analytics for Dynamic Patient Flow Management

One of the most pressing challenges in hospital administration is managing patient flow effectively. Predictive analytics, powered by AI, can provide hospitals with the foresight needed to allocate resources efficiently. However, many hospitals still rely on traditional methods that often fail to anticipate sudden surges in patient numbers, leading to overcrowding and inefficiencies in care delivery.

Solution: Hospitals should adopt AI-driven predictive models to forecast patient admissions, discharge patterns, and emergency department traffic. These models should integrate data from multiple sources, such as historical patient visits, seasonal trends, and public health data (e.g., flu outbreaks). For example, combining predictive models with real-time data from wearable health devices can offer a more dynamic prediction of patient health trends (Lu et al., 2020; Muniasamy et al., 2025a; Muniasamy et al.,2025b). Moreover, hospitals should create decision-support systems that allow administrators to act on these predictions in real-time, ensuring optimal bed management, staffing, and equipment allocation.

Recommendation: Integrate AI predictive models with hospital information systems (HIS) to allow seamless data flow between various departments, enhancing the accuracy and timeliness of predictions. Additionally, hospitals should continually update and refine these models using new patient data to improve their predictive power.

4.1.2 Optimizing Staffing Using Reinforcement Learning

Staffing is a critical component of hospital administration, directly impacting both patient care quality and staff wellbeing. Traditional scheduling systems often fail to account for fluctuations in patient volumes, leading to overstaffing or understaffing. Reinforcement learning (RL), a subset of AI, can help address these challenges by dynamically adjusting staffing schedules based on real-time patient demand.

Solution: Hospitals should implement RL-based staffing models to optimize workforce allocation. RL can be used to balance workloads by ensuring that the right number of healthcare professionals are available at the right time. RL algorithms can take into account variables such as patient volume, departmental needs, staff availability, and shift preferences. This approach helps reduce burnout, improve staff satisfaction, and prevent overstaffing, which is a significant cost driver in healthcare (Wu et al., 2025).

Recommendation: Integrate RL-based scheduling algorithms with hospital electronic health record (EHR) systems to ensure that staffing decisions are based on the most accurate, up-to-date information about patient needs and staff availability. Hospitals should also establish feedback loops where the system can learn from past staffing decisions and continuously improve scheduling accuracy.

4.1.3 Leveraging NLP for Administrative Automation

Hospital administration involves the processing of large volumes of unstructured data, such as clinical notes, discharge summaries, and patient feedback. Natural Language Processing (NLP) can significantly improve the efficiency of administrative processes by automating tasks like medical coding, report generation, and appointment scheduling.

Solution: Hospitals should implement NLP systems to automate routine administrative tasks. NLP can extract relevant information from free-text clinical documents, classify it according to standardized formats, and generate reports without requiring manual intervention. Furthermore, NLP tools can be used to mine patient feedback and clinical notes to identify operational inefficiencies, allowing administrators to address issues such as bottlenecks in care delivery.

Recommendation: Adopt NLP-based automation systems that integrate with existing hospital IT infrastructure, such as EHRs, and enable real-time processing of clinical documents. Regular training and refinement of these systems are necessary to improve their accuracy in interpreting complex medical language.

4.2 Solutions for Enhancing Formulary Design

4.2.1 Implementing AI for Personalized Drug Formulary Management

AI can be instrumental in creating personalized drug formularies that take into account the specific characteristics of individual patients, such as their medical history, genetic profile, and response to previous treatments. By personalizing formulary recommendations, hospitals can improve patient outcomes, reduce adverse drug reactions, and optimize medication costs.

Solution: Hospitals should implement AI-based systems that integrate EHR data and genomics to recommend drugs tailored to individual patients. Such systems can analyze vast datasets to identify the most effective drugs for a given patient profile, improving the likelihood of positive treatment outcomes. In addition to clinical outcomes, AI models can also consider factors like drug interactions, allergies, and comorbidities when making formulary decisions.

Recommendation: Hospitals should partner with pharmaceutical companies and biotech firms to develop AI models that incorporate the latest clinical trial data, genetic research, and real-world evidence to refine personalized formulary decisions. Integrating AI tools with EHRs will allow seamless access to patient data, enabling clinicians to make better-informed prescribing decisions.

4.2.2 AI-Driven Cost-Effectiveness Analysis for Drug Selection

AI models, particularly those based on machine learning and Bayesian analysis, can provide hospitals with valuable insights into the cost-effectiveness of various medications. By incorporating clinical efficacy, side-effect profiles, and patient outcomes, AI can help healthcare providers identify the most cost-effective drugs for inclusion in their formularies.

Solution: Implement AI systems that combine clinical trial data, real-world patient outcomes, and economic analysis to evaluate the cost-effectiveness of different drug treatments. Machine learning models can predict the long-term benefits and costs associated with drug therapies, assisting hospital administrators in making data-driven formulary decisions that balance cost with clinical benefits.

Recommendation: Hospitals should continuously update their pharmacoeconomic models with new data on drug efficacy and costs to ensure that formularies reflect the most up-to-date evidence. Collaboration with pharmaceutical companies and health economists will be crucial in refining these models.

4.2.3 Integrating AI for Real-Time Medication Inventory Management

AI can optimize drug inventory management by predicting future medication needs and reducing stockouts or overstocking. Machine learning algorithms can analyze trends in drug utilization and forecast future demand, ensuring that hospitals maintain an optimal inventory of medications without tying up excessive resources.

Solution: Hospitals should adopt machine learning models that forecast drug demand based on historical usage data, patient demographics, and seasonal trends. These models can adjust inventory levels in real-time, ensuring that critical medications are always available without overstocking less frequently used drugs.

Recommendation: Implement automated systems that integrate inventory management with patient data to ensure that medication stocks are replenished as needed. Collaboration with pharmaceutical suppliers to develop AI-driven supply chain solutions will also help ensure the timely availability of medications.

The solutions and recommendations provided in this section highlight the transformative potential of AI in hospital administration and formulary design. By adopting predictive analytics, reinforcement learning, and NLP for administrative tasks, hospitals can significantly improve operational efficiency, reduce costs, and enhance patient care. Similarly, AI can revolutionize formulary design by enabling personalized medicine, cost-effectiveness analysis, and real-time inventory management. Moving forward, it is essential for hospitals to integrate AI systems into their existing infrastructure, ensuring seamless data flow and real-time decision-making to optimize both patient care and resource utilization.

FUTURE RESEARCH DIRECTIONS

The integration of Artificial Intelligence (AI) in hospital administration and formulary design has seen considerable advancements, but there remain significant opportunities for further exploration and refinement. As healthcare systems become increasingly complex, AI technologies will play a pivotal role in transforming operational processes, improving patient outcomes, and optimizing resource utilization. This section outlines key areas for future research in AI for hospital administration and formulary design, with a focus on unresolved challenges, emerging technologies, and the evolving needs of the healthcare industry.

5.1 AI-Driven Personalization in Hospital Administration

5.1.1 Enhancing Personalization with Patient-Centric AI Models

While AI has proven effective in streamlining hospital administration, future research should focus on developing more sophisticated, patient-centric models. Personalized patient care and efficient resource management require AI systems that can tailor hospital services and administrative processes to individual patient profiles. This personalization could extend to scheduling, treatment plans, and hospital resources, ensuring that decisions are made based on the unique needs of each patient rather than generic algorithms.

Research Directions:

- **Patient-Profile Based Scheduling:** Future research could focus on developing AI models that consider a comprehensive range of patient factors, such as age, medical history, genetic data, and social determinants of health, when making scheduling and resource allocation decisions. Research could explore how AI can predict future patient needs more accurately by combining historical clinical data with real-time health monitoring data.

- **Adaptive AI Systems:** Another promising area is the development of adaptive AI systems capable of learning from ongoing patient interactions and continuously refining administrative processes based on new patient data. These systems would require a combination of machine learning techniques, including reinforcement learning and deep learning, to dynamically adjust hospital operations.

5.1.2 Integrating AI with Internet of Medical Things (IoMT)

The Internet of Medical Things (IoMT) refers to the network of connected medical devices and applications that can communicate patient data in real-time. As hospitals adopt more IoMT devices, there is an increasing need for AI models capable of processing large volumes of real-time data to make immediate administrative decisions.

Research Directions:

- **Real-Time Data Processing for Hospital Operations:** Future research could focus on AI systems that integrate with IoMT devices to monitor patient health continuously and predict when administrative intervention (e.g., resource allocation, staffing) is required. Research could explore the potential for AI to automate decision-making in real-time, such as optimizing bed usage or predicting emergency care needs.
- **Data Privacy and Security in IoMT Integration:** Another important research direction is the development of robust AI models that can securely process sensitive patient data from IoMT devices. Ensuring that patient data is anonymized and protected from cyber threats will be a significant challenge as IoMT adoption increases in hospitals.

5.2 AI in Formulary Design: Leveraging Real-World Evidence

5.2.1 Real-World Data (RWD) and Artificial Intelligence in Drug Selection

Currently, most AI models for formulary design rely heavily on clinical trial data. However, real-world data (RWD) provides a richer source of information, capturing patient outcomes, side effects, and responses across broader, more diverse patient populations. Future research could explore how AI models can be trained using RWD to improve formulary decisions.

Research Directions:

- **Incorporating RWD into AI Formulary Models:** Researchers can investigate methods for incorporating diverse RWD from electronic health records (EHR), claims data, and patient-reported outcomes (PROs) to refine drug formulary decision-making. This could lead to the development of AI models that predict drug effectiveness in real-world settings and not just controlled clinical trial environments.
- **Longitudinal Studies Using AI and RWD:** Long-term studies could focus on how AI models can analyze longitudinal RWD over extended periods to identify trends and patterns in drug efficacy, patient outcomes, and cost-effectiveness. Such studies could help design more accurate and comprehensive drug formularies based on the actual experiences of patients.

5.2.2 AI Models for Multi-Drug Interactions and Personalized Medicine

One of the critical challenges in formulary design is understanding and managing complex drug interactions. As more patients with multiple chronic conditions seek care, managing multi-drug regimens becomes increasingly challenging. AI offers the potential to model complex drug interactions and personalize drug combinations based on individual patient profiles.

Research Directions:

- **Predicting Drug Interactions Using AI:** Future research could focus on developing advanced AI models that predict potential drug-drug interactions and their impact on patient outcomes. These models would use data from large clinical datasets and molecular modeling to simulate how different drugs interact at the biochemical level.
- **Personalized Multi-Drug Therapy Systems:** A promising area of research is the development of personalized medicine algorithms that recommend optimal multi-drug regimens. These systems would combine AI techniques like natural language processing (NLP) to analyze clinical notes, machine learning to analyze genetic data, and deep learning to predict how different drugs will interact in individual patients.

5.3 Enhancing AI Algorithm Interpretability and Trust

5.3.1 Explainable AI (XAI) in Healthcare Decision-Making

While AI has shown remarkable success in healthcare, a major barrier to its widespread adoption is the "black-box" nature of many algorithms. For healthcare providers to trust and adopt AI systems, it is crucial that these models provide explanations for their decisions, particularly in high-stakes environments like hospital administration and formulary design.

Research Directions:

- **Developing Transparent AI Models:** Research should focus on developing AI models that are not only accurate but also explainable. These models would help administrators and clinicians understand how decisions are made, thus building trust in AI systems. One approach could be integrating explainable AI (XAI) techniques into hospital administration AI models to improve decision transparency.
- **Human-AI Collaboration in Decision-Making:** Future research should explore the potential for hybrid models that combine the computational power of AI with human expertise. By providing decision-makers with AI-generated insights and actionable explanations, these systems could improve collaboration between AI systems and healthcare professionals.

5.3.2 Improving Data Quality and Integration Across Healthcare Systems

AI models are only as good as the data they are trained on, and in healthcare, data is often fragmented and siloed across different departments and systems. For AI to be truly effective, data from multiple sources—such as EHRs, pharmacy databases, and laboratory systems—must be integrated and of high quality.

Research Directions:

- **Data Standardization and Integration:** Future research could focus on the development of data standards that allow seamless integration of diverse datasets across hospitals and healthcare networks. This would ensure that AI models can be trained on comprehensive datasets, leading to more accurate predictions and decisions.
- **Addressing Data Quality Issues:** Research should explore techniques to improve the quality of healthcare data, including methods to handle

missing data, ensure data accuracy, and reduce biases in clinical datasets. Such improvements will be critical for training reliable and equitable AI models.

The future of AI in hospital administration and formulary design is promising, with numerous opportunities for research to enhance the efficiency, accuracy, and personalization of healthcare systems. Key research directions include improving patient-centric AI models, integrating real-world data for better formulary decisions, and developing transparent, interpretable AI algorithms. As healthcare continues to evolve, AI will play a pivotal role in optimizing resources, improving patient care, and ensuring the sustainability of healthcare systems. Future research should focus on overcoming the challenges of data integration, algorithm interpretability, and the personalization of AI systems to ensure that AI can be fully leveraged to meet the needs of healthcare providers and patients alike.

CONCLUSION

The integration of Artificial Intelligence (AI) into hospital administration and formulary design represents a transformative shift in how healthcare systems operate. As healthcare systems worldwide grapple with increasing patient demands, resource constraints, and the need for more personalized care, AI offers a promising solution to streamline hospital operations, optimize resource allocation, and enhance patient outcomes. This chapter has explored the various AI models applied in hospital administration and formulary design, emphasizing their potential benefits, challenges, and future research directions. As we look to the future, the continued evolution of AI in these domains promises to reshape healthcare delivery on a global scale.

6.1 Summary of Key Findings

6.1.1 AI in Hospital Administration

The application of AI in hospital administration has significantly improved the efficiency of operations, reduced costs, and enhanced the overall patient experience. Key AI-driven models, such as predictive analytics, resource optimization algorithms, and scheduling systems, have helped healthcare facilities manage patient flow, optimize bed utilization, and streamline staffing processes. AI's ability to process vast amounts of data from Electronic Health Records (EHRs), patient management systems, and real-time monitoring devices allows for more informed decision-making and proactive management.

One of the standout areas of AI application in hospital administration is predictive modeling, which helps forecast patient admission rates, emergency room wait times, and critical care needs. By anticipating patient demand more accurately, hospitals can better allocate resources, reduce bottlenecks, and avoid unnecessary delays. Additionally, the application of machine learning (ML) techniques for optimizing staffing schedules has led to more efficient use of personnel, ensuring that the right number of staff are available at peak times without incurring unnecessary costs.

6.1.2 AI in Formulary Design

In formulary design, AI has revolutionized the way healthcare providers select medications and manage drug inventories. By using machine learning and data analytics, AI can analyze large datasets, including clinical trial results, patient outcomes, and real-world evidence (RWD), to recommend optimal drug choices for specific patient populations. This data-driven approach not only improves patient care by ensuring the most effective medications are selected but also helps healthcare providers manage drug costs more effectively.

AI's potential to predict drug interactions and adverse reactions in real-time is another key advantage in formulary management. By incorporating genetic and molecular data, AI systems can provide personalized drug recommendations based on individual patient profiles, improving the likelihood of successful treatment outcomes. Furthermore, the ability of AI models to simulate different drug regimens and predict their impact on patient outcomes has proven invaluable in designing drug formularies that are both effective and cost-efficient.

6.1.3 Challenges and Barriers

Despite the significant advancements in AI applications, there are several challenges that must be addressed to fully realize the potential of AI in hospital administration and formulary design. One of the primary challenges is the issue of data quality and integration. Healthcare data is often fragmented and stored in siloed systems, making it difficult for AI models to access comprehensive datasets needed for accurate predictions and recommendations. Standardizing healthcare data formats and improving interoperability between systems is essential for AI's widespread adoption.

Another significant barrier is the "black-box" nature of many AI algorithms, which undermines trust and transparency in AI-generated decisions. To gain acceptance among healthcare professionals, AI models must be explainable, providing clear insights into how decisions are made. This is particularly critical in high-stakes areas such as patient care and drug selection, where the stakes are high, and accountability is paramount.

Additionally, while AI can improve operational efficiency, it is essential that it complements rather than replaces human expertise. Future research should focus on developing hybrid AI systems that combine the strengths of AI algorithms with human judgment, ensuring that healthcare professionals remain at the center of decision-making processes.

6.2 Implications for Healthcare Systems

The implications of AI in hospital administration and formulary design are far-reaching. Hospitals that embrace AI technologies stand to benefit from improved operational efficiency, reduced costs, and enhanced patient care. AI models that predict patient demand, optimize hospital resources, and improve staff allocation will enable healthcare providers to deliver better services with fewer resources, addressing the growing demand for healthcare in a sustainable manner.

For formulary design, the ability of AI to analyze large datasets, predict patient responses to drugs, and identify potential drug interactions will result in more personalized treatment regimens. This will not only improve patient outcomes but also reduce healthcare costs by ensuring that patients receive the most appropriate medications without the risks associated with adverse drug reactions.

The growing reliance on AI in healthcare also raises important ethical considerations, such as patient privacy, data security, and the potential for algorithmic bias. To ensure that AI technologies are used responsibly, healthcare systems must implement robust data governance frameworks, prioritize transparency in AI decision-making, and continuously monitor and evaluate the performance of AI systems to detect and mitigate any biases that may arise.

6.3 Future Prospects and Research Directions

As outlined in the chapter, there are numerous avenues for future research in AI applications in hospital administration and formulary design. One key area for future exploration is the integration of real-world evidence (RWD) into AI models. While clinical trial data remains the gold standard in drug efficacy, RWD offers a richer, more diverse set of patient outcomes that can be used to refine drug formularies and personalize treatment plans. Future AI models should aim to incorporate

RWD alongside clinical trial data, providing a more accurate picture of how drugs perform in real-world settings.

Another exciting research direction is the development of more advanced and interpretable AI models. Explainable AI (XAI) will be crucial for gaining the trust of healthcare professionals and ensuring that AI-generated decisions are understandable and actionable. AI systems should provide clear, understandable explanations for their recommendations, allowing clinicians to make more informed decisions and fostering a collaborative approach to healthcare delivery.

Additionally, the integration of AI with emerging technologies such as the Internet of Medical Things (IoMT) and blockchain presents significant opportunities for enhancing hospital administration and formulary design. Real-time data from IoMT devices, combined with AI's analytical capabilities, can improve patient monitoring, reduce hospital readmissions, and help manage resource allocation more effectively. Blockchain, on the other hand, can ensure the security and integrity of healthcare data, enabling safer AI-driven decision-making processes.

6.4 Closing Thoughts

The integration of AI into hospital administration and formulary design holds immense promise for improving healthcare efficiency, reducing costs, and enhancing patient outcomes. AI models have already demonstrated their potential to optimize hospital operations, personalize drug selection, and streamline formulary management processes. However, to fully realize the benefits of AI in healthcare, ongoing research is needed to address challenges related to data quality, algorithm transparency, and the integration of real-world data.

As AI technologies continue to evolve, healthcare systems must embrace a collaborative approach that combines the strengths of AI algorithms with human expertise. By doing so, we can create a future healthcare landscape that is not only more efficient and cost-effective but also more personalized and patient-centric.

The future of AI in hospital administration and formulary design is bright, with numerous opportunities for research and innovation. By continuing to push the boundaries of what AI can achieve in these domains, healthcare systems worldwide will be better equipped to meet the evolving needs of patients and healthcare providers.

REFERENCES

Adhiya, J., Barghi, B., & Azadeh-Fard, N. (2024). Predicting the risk of hospital readmissions using a machine learning approach: A case study on patients undergoing skin procedures. *Frontiers in Artificial Intelligence*, *6*, 1213378. DOI: 10.3389/frai.2023.1213378 PMID: 38249790

Almeman, A. (2024, May 8). The digital transformation in pharmacy: Embracing online platforms and the cosmeceutical paradigm shift. *Journal of Health, Population and Nutrition*, *43*(1), 60. DOI: 10.1186/s41043-024-00550-2 PMID: 38720390

Amann, J., Blasimme, A., Vayena, E., Frey, D., & Madai, V. I. (2020). Explainability for artificial intelligence in healthcare: A multidisciplinary perspective. *BMC Medical Informatics and Decision Making*, *20*(1), 310. DOI: 10.1186/s12911-020-01332-6 PMID: 33256715

Badwan, B. A., Liaropoulos, G., Kyrodimos, E., Skaltsas, D., Tsirigos, A., & Gorgoulis, V. G. (2023). Machine learning approaches to predict drug efficacy and toxicity in oncology. *Cell Reports Methods*, *3*(2), 100413. DOI: 10.1016/j.crmeth.2023.100413 PMID: 36936080

Baio, G. (2014). Bayesian models for cost-effectiveness analysis in the presence of structural zero costs. *Statistics in Medicine*, *33*(11), 1900–1913. DOI: 10.1002/sim.6074 PMID: 24343868

Beis, S., & Anandan, J. (1999). Formulary management in an integrated health care system. *Pharmacy Practice Management Quarterly*, *18*, 43–49. PMID: 10339067

Chenais, G., Lagarde, E., & Gil-Jardiné, C. (2023, May 23). Artificial Intelligence in Emergency Medicine: Viewpoint of Current Applications and Foreseeable Opportunities and Challenges. *Journal of Medical Internet Research*, *25*, e40031. DOI: 10.2196/40031 PMID: 36972306

Churpek, M. M., Yuen, T. C., & Edelson, D. P. (2013). Predicting clinical deterioration in the hospital: The impact of outcome selection. *Resuscitation*, *84*(5), 564–568. DOI: 10.1016/j.resuscitation.2012.09.024 PMID: 23022075

Davenport, T., & Kalakota, R. (2019). The potential for artificial intelligence in healthcare. *Future Healthcare Journal*, *6*(2), 94–98. DOI: 10.7861/futurehosp.6-2-94 PMID: 31363513

Denck, J., Ozkirimli, E., & Wang, K. (2023, September). Machine-learning-based adverse drug event prediction from observational health data: A review. *Drug Discovery Today*, *28*(9), 103715. DOI: 10.1016/j.drudis.2023.103715 PMID: 37467879

Duma, D., & Aringhieri, R. (2023). Real-time resource allocation in the emergency department: A case study. *Omega, 117*, 102844. DOI: 10.1016/j.omega.2023.102844

Fourkiotis, K. P., & Tsadiras, A. (2024). Applying Machine Learning and Statistical Forecasting Methods for Enhancing Pharmaceutical Sales Predictions. *Forecasting*, *6*(1), 170–186. DOI: 10.3390/forecast6010010

Gettman, D. (2023). Integration of Genomics and Artificial Intelligence in Pharmacy Practice: The Era of Predictive, Personalized Care. DOI: 10.13140/RG.2.2.31795.34086

Goyal, P., & Malviya, R. (2023, October 4). Challenges and opportunities of big data analytics in healthcare. [Retraction in: Health Care Sci. 2025 Mar 25;4] [2] [:161. doi: 10.1002/hcs2.70006]. *Health Care Science*, *2*(5), 328–338. DOI: 10.1002/hcs2.66 PMID: 38938583

Green, L. V. (2002–2003). How many hospital beds? *Inquiry : a Journal of Medical Care Organization, Provision and Financing*, *39*(4), 400–412. DOI: 10.5034/inquiryjrnl_39.4.400 PMID: 12638714

He, J., Baxter, S. L., Xu, J., Xu, J., Zhou, X., & Zhang, K. (2019). The practical implementation of artificial intelligence technologies in medicine. *Nature Medicine*, *25*(1), 30–36. DOI: 10.1038/s41591-018-0307-0 PMID: 30617336

Heindel, G. A., & McIntyre, C. M. (2018). Contemporary challenges and novel strategies for health-system formulary management. *American Journal of Health-System Pharmacy*, *75*(8), 556–560. DOI: 10.2146/ajhp170351 PMID: 29626005

IDC (International Data Corporation). (2024). *Worldwide Global DataSphere Forecast*. Retrieved from https://www.idc.com

Iyengar, K., Upadhyaya, G. K., Vaishya, R., & Jain, V. (2020). COVID-19 and applications of smartphone technology in the current pandemic. *Diabetes & Metabolic Syndrome*, *14*(5), 733–737. DOI: 10.1016/j.dsx.2020.05.033 PMID: 32497963

Kaul, A., Enslin, S., & Gross, T. (2020). Health AI: The state of play. *Deloitte Insights*. https://www2.deloitte.com

Komorowski, M., Celi, L. A., Badawi, O., Gordon, A. C., & Faisal, A. A. (2018). The Artificial Intelligence Clinician learns optimal treatment strategies for sepsis in intensive care. *Nature Medicine*, *24*(11), 1716–1720. DOI: 10.1038/s41591-018-0213-5 PMID: 30349085

Lu, L., Zhang, J., Xie, Y., Gao, F., Xu, S., Wu, X., & Ye, Z. (2020). Wearable health devices in health care: Narrative systematic review. *JMIR mHealth and uHealth, 8*(11), e18907. DOI: 10.2196/18907 PMID: 33164904

Miotto, R., Wang, F., Wang, S., Jiang, X., & Dudley, J. T. (2018). Deep learning for healthcare: Review, opportunities and challenges. *Briefings in Bioinformatics, 19*(6), 1236–1246. DOI: 10.1093/bib/bbx044 PMID: 28481991

Mittelstadt, Brent & Allo, Patrick & Taddeo, Mariarosaria & Wachter, Sandra & Floridi, Luciano. (2016). The Ethics of Algorithms: Mapping the Debate. Big Data & Society.

Morley, J., Machado, C. C., Burr, C., Cowls, J., Joshi, I., Taddeo, M., & Floridi, L. (2020). The ethics of AI in health care: A mapping review. *Social Science & Medicine, 260*, 113172. DOI: 10.1016/j.socscimed.2020.113172 PMID: 32702587

Muniasamy, A. (2025b). Revolutionizing health monitoring: Integrating transformer models with multi-head attention for precise human activity recognition using wearable devices. *Technology and Health Care, 31*(1), 395–409. DOI: 10.3233/THC-241064 PMID: 39269866

Muniasamy, A., & Asiri, F. (2025a). Advanced human activity recognition on wearables with multi-scale sparse attention. *Multimedia Tools and Applications.* Advance online publication. DOI: 10.1007/s11042-024-20475-6

Muralitharan, S., Nelson, W., Di, S., McGillion, M., Devereaux, P. J., Barr, N. G., & Petch, J. (2021). Machine learning-based early warning systems for clinical deterioration: Systematic scoping review. *Journal of Medical Internet Research, 23*(2), e25187. DOI: 10.2196/25187 PMID: 33538696

Ngiam, K. Y., & Khor, I. W. (2019). Big data and machine learning algorithms for health-care delivery. *The Lancet. Oncology, 20*(5), e262–e273. DOI: 10.1016/S1470-2045(19)30149-4 PMID: 31044724

Payal, Manju & Ananth Kumar, T. & Kumar K, Suresh. (2022). Integrating Natural language processing (NLP) and Machine learning Techniques for Healthcare Industries. .DOI: 10. 3030. 10.15680/IJIRCCE.2022.1005023l

Peixoto, D., Barbosa, A., Peixoto, H., Lopes, J., Guimarães, T., & Santos, M. (2022). Predictive analytics for hospital inpatient flow determination. *Procedia Computer Science, 210*, 254–259. DOI: 10.1016/j.procs.2022.10.146

Rajkomar, A., Dean, J., & Kohane, I. (2019). Machine learning in medicine. *The New England Journal of Medicine, 380*(14), 1347–1358. DOI: 10.1056/NEJMra1814259 PMID: 30943338

Ramezani, M., Takian, A., Bakhtiari, A., Rabiee, H. R., Ghazanfari, S., & Mostafavi, H. (2023). The application of artificial intelligence in health policy: A scoping review. *BMC Health Services Research, 23*(1), 1416. DOI: 10.1186/s12913-023-10462-2 PMID: 38102620

Raza, M. A., Aziz, S., Noreen, M., Saeed, A., Anjum, I., Ahmed, M., & Raza, S. M. (2022). Artificial intelligence (AI) in pharmacy: An overview of innovations. *Innovations in Pharmacy, 13*(2), 4839. Advance online publication. DOI: 10.24926/iip.v13i2.4839 PMID: 36654703

Shah, N. H., Milstein, A., & Bagley, S. C. (2019). Making machine learning models clinically useful. *Journal of the American Medical Association, 322*(14), 1351–1352. DOI: 10.1001/jama.2019.10306 PMID: 31393527

Strome, T. L. (2020). *Healthcare Analytics for Quality and Performance Improvement* (2nd ed.). Wiley.

Teng, M., Singla, R., Yau, O., Lamoureux, D., Gupta, A., Hu, Z., Hu, R., Aissiou, A., Eaton, S., Hamm, C., Hu, S., Kelly, D., MacMillan, K. M., Malik, S., Mazzoli, V., Teng, Y. W., Laricheva, M., Jarus, T., & Field, T. S. (2022). Health care students' perspectives on artificial intelligence: Countrywide survey in Canada. *JMIR Medical Education, 8*(1), e33390. DOI: 10.2196/33390 PMID: 35099397

Tiwari, A., Behki, P., Kumar, V., & Mahajan, S. (2023). *MODERN HOSPITAL MANAGEMENT SYSTEM. Russell, S., & Norvig, P. (2021). Artificial Intelligence: A Modern Approach* (4th ed.). Pearson.

Topol, E. (2019). *Deep Medicine: How Artificial Intelligence Can Make Healthcare Human Again*. Basic Books.

UChicago Medicine. (2025). *AI Predictive Tool Enhances Patient Deterioration Detection*. Retrieved from https://www.uchicagomedicine.org

Wu, Q., Han, J., Yan, Y., Kuo, Y.-H., & Shen, Z.-J. M. (2025). Reinforcement learning for healthcare operations management: Methodological framework, recent developments, and future research directions. *Health Care Management Science, 28*(2), 298–333. DOI: 10.1007/s10729-025-09699-6 PMID: 40202690

Wu, S., Roberts, K., Datta, S., Du, J., Ji, Z., Si, Y., Soni, S., Wang, Q., Wei, Q., Xiang, Y., Zhao, B., & Xu, H. (2020). Deep learning in clinical natural language processing: A methodical review. *Journal of the American Medical Informatics Association : JAMIA, 27*(3), 457–470. DOI: 10.1093/jamia/ocz200 PMID: 31794016

ADDITIONAL READING

5. Al Kuwaiti, A., Nazer, K., Al-Reedy, A., Al-Shehri, S., Al-Muhanna, A., Subbarayalu, A. V., Al Muhanna, D., & Al-Muhanna, F. A. (2023). A review of the role of artificial intelligence in healthcare. *Journal of Personalized Medicine, 13*(6), 951. DOI: 10.3390/jpm13060951 PMID: 37373940

1. Alajmani, S., & Elazhary, H. (2019). Hospital Readmission Prediction using Machine Learning Techniques. *International Journal of Advanced Computer Science and Applications, 10*(4). Advance online publication. DOI: 10.14569/IJACSA.2019.0100425

2. Habehh, H., & Gohel, S. (2021). Machine learning in healthcare. *Current Genomics, 22*(4), 291–300. DOI: 10.2174/1389202922666210705124359 PMID: 35273459

4. Okonkwo, F., Akonor, B., & Adukpo, T. (2025). Artificial Intelligence in Healthcare Supply Chain Management: Enhancing Resilience and Efficiency in U.S. Medical Supply Distribution. *EPRA International Journal of Economic and Business Review., 12*, 7.

3. Serrano, D. R., Luciano, F. C., Anaya, B. J., Ongoren, B., Kara, A., Molina, G., Ramirez, B. I., Sánchez-Guirales, S. A., Simon, J. A., Tomietto, G., Rapti, C., Ruiz, H. K., Rawat, S., Kumar, D., & Lalatsa, A. (2024). Artificial intelligence (AI) applications in drug discovery and drug delivery: Revolutionizing personalized medicine. *Pharmaceutics, 16*(10), 1328. DOI: 10.3390/pharmaceutics16101328 PMID: 39458657

KEY TERMS AND DEFINITIONS

Artificial Intelligence (AI): Simulation of human intelligence in machines to perform tasks like decision-making and problem-solving.

Hospital Administration: Management of healthcare facilities, focusing on operations, resource allocation, and patient care delivery.

Formulary Design: The process of selecting and managing a list of approved medications for a healthcare system.

Predictive Analytics: Using statistical algorithms and machine learning to forecast future outcomes based on historical data.

Machine Learning (ML): A subset of AI that allows algorithms to improve performance over time with data, without explicit programming.

Natural Language Processing (NLP): AI technology that enables machines to understand and interpret human language.

Explainable AI (XAI): AI systems that provide understandable explanations for their decisions and actions.

Real-World Data (RWD): Data collected from routine clinical practice, offering insights beyond controlled clinical trials.

Drug Formulary: A list of approved medications used to guide prescribing decisions in healthcare settings.

Resource Allocation: The distribution of available resources in healthcare to optimize patient care and operational efficiency.

Patient Flow: The movement of patients through various stages of care in a healthcare facility, ensuring efficient resource use.

Artificial Neural Networks (ANNs): AI models that mimic the human brain, used for pattern recognition and data classification.

Healthcare Supply Chain Management: Coordination of medical supplies, equipment, and medications to ensure timely availability and efficiency.

Optimization Algorithms: Mathematical methods used to find the best solutions in healthcare processes, like staffing and resource allocation.

Adverse Drug Reactions (ADRs): Harmful effects caused by medications, which AI helps predict and prevent.

Cost-Effectiveness Analysis (CEA): An evaluation method comparing the costs and benefits of different healthcare treatments or drugs.

Personalized Medicine: Tailored medical treatment based on individual patient characteristics such as genetics and lifestyle.

Blockchain in Healthcare: A secure, decentralized digital ledger technology used to store and share healthcare data.

Hybrid AI Systems: AI systems that combine machine learning with human expertise to enhance decision-making.

Clinical Decision Support Systems (CDSS): AI tools that assist healthcare professionals by providing evidence-based recommendations and alerts.

Chapter 9
Electronic Health Records Unleashed:
Strategies for Leveraging Big Data in Healthcare Research

Komal Bhardwaj
https://orcid.org/0000-0002-9378-5542
Maharishi Markandeshwar Institute of Management, Maharishi Markandeshwar University, Mullana, India

Aishwarya Tipara
https://orcid.org/0009-0002-0284-0057
Upgrad, Hyderabad, India

Garima
Maharishi Markandeshwar Institute of Management, Maharishi Markandeshwar University, Mullana, India

ABSTRACT

In the era of advanced healthcare technology, the adoption of Electronic Health Records (EHRs) has led to the accumulation of vast troves of clinical data. While EHRs primarily serve as a central repository for patient care, they are increasingly being utilized for secondary purposes, such as clinical research, disease surveillance, and quality improvement initiatives. This study systematically examines the diverse secondary uses of EHR data and their implications for patient privacy. Employing a mixed-methods approach, the research delves into the perceptions and perspectives of key stakeholders, including healthcare providers, hospital administrators, policy-makers, and patient advocacy groups, through in-depth interviews. Additionally, the study analyses the prevalence and trends of secondary EHR data utilization using quantitative data. Crucially, the study provides a critical evaluation of the existing

DOI: 10.4018/979-8-3373-2043-4.ch009

regulatory frameworks, namely the (GDPR) and (HIPAA).

INTRODUCTION

The healthcare industry has experienced significant digital advancements, particularly with the widespread adoption of Electronic Health Records (EHR). This shift has opened the door to data-driven approaches in healthcare, supporting objectives like improving service delivery, facilitating clinical research, enabling public health monitoring, and optimizing healthcare facility management. Telehealth plays a key role in providing healthcare services to both urban and rural populations, while smartphone apps help individuals manage their personal health. The application of big data is crucial in achieving these goals and delivering high-quality services.

One promising approach is individualized predictive analytics, which relies on patient similarities. When a new patient requires care, similar cases from historical data are identified, insights are drawn, and personalized predictions are made. For example, this method has been used in recommending medications, identifying risk factors, predicting cardiac arrest based on telemonitoring, and delivering personalized healthcare.

Healthcare conditions and systems often depend on a range of factors, including genetics, environmental influences, gender, medical history, and lifestyle choices. Personalized healthcare cannot rely solely on clinical trials. Researchers are using advanced algorithms to analyse large clinical datasets and identify disease patterns—referred to as "black-box medicine"—which could greatly enhance personalized healthcare.

Enhanced EHR systems hold potential for more effective use of big data in healthcare. In the future, EHR systems may provide "genomic clinical decision support" to enable personalized and timely care. Clinical decision support tools will help interpret genetic variations and their implications for specific diseases or treatments, facilitating informed decisions based on a patient's genetic profile, such as whole-genome sequencing.

Precision medicine focuses on individual characteristics, taking into account environmental, genetic, social, and psychological factors. It is resource-driven, patient-centred, and data-heavy, with an emphasis on data from whole-genome sequencing and big data analytics as key enablers for precision healthcare.

Clinical Data Production and the Shift Towards Electronic Health Records (EHRS)

Clinical data is continuously generated through various diagnostic activities in hospitals, clinics, and laboratories. This data originates from clinical trials, medical imaging, doctor prescriptions, and wearable sensors connected via wireless body area networks [Figure 1]. Globally, the volume of clinical data is increasing rapidly.

EHRs represent a significant advancement in healthcare, offering potential improvements in patient care, communication, and a reduction in medical errors. Despite these benefits, the adoption of EHR systems has been slow, particularly in primary care and hospital settings in the United States (DesRoches et al., 2008). Research indicates that EHR system users report higher satisfaction, improved decision-making, better communication, and fewer medication errors (DesRoches et al., 2008). The widespread adoption of EHRs accelerated following the implementation of the 2009 Health Information Technology for Economic and Clinical Health (HITECH) Act, which provided financial incentives to encourage healthcare facilities to adopt these systems (Centers for Medicare & Medicaid Services, n.d.).

Figure 1. Clinical data repository exchange

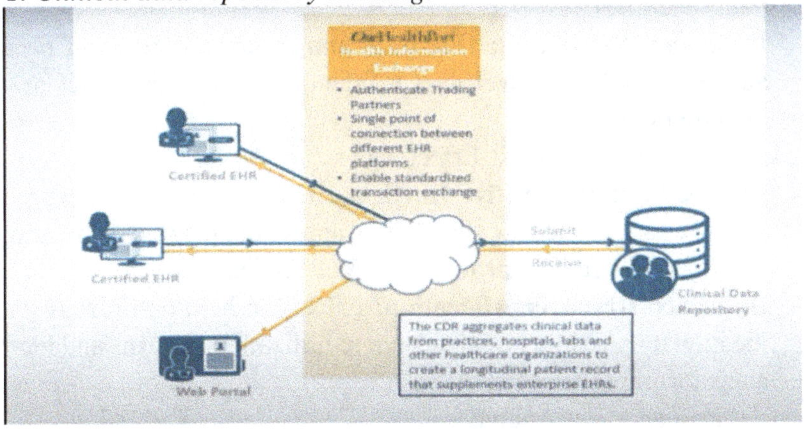

Compared to Traditional Paper-Based Systems, EHRs Offer Several Significant Advantages

1. Improved Data Management and Access:

- **Centralized Repository:** EHRs serve as a central repository for patient data, making it easier to access and manage information across different healthcare settings.
- **Structured Data:** EHRs use standardized data formats, ensuring consistency and improving data quality.
- **Enhanced Search Capabilities:** Advanced search functionalities within EHRs allow for efficient retrieval of specific patient information.

2. Enhanced Decision Support:
    - **Decision Support Systems (DSS):** EHRs can integrate DSS to provide clinicians with real-time information and recommendations based on patient data, leading to more informed decision-making.
    - **Clinical Guidelines and Protocols:** EHRs can be configured to follow evidence-based guidelines and protocols, ensuring adherence to best practices.
3. Improved Patient Safety and Quality of Care:
    - **Reduced Errors:** EHRs can help reduce medical errors by providing alerts for drug interactions, allergies, and other potential safety issues.
    - **Improved Care Coordination:** EHRs facilitate better communication and coordination among healthcare providers, leading to improved patient outcomes.
    - **Enhanced Population Health Management:** EHRs can be used to analyse population-level data to identify trends and target preventive interventions.
4. Increased Efficiency and Cost-Effectiveness:
    - **Reduced Administrative Burden:** EHRs can automate many administrative tasks, such as scheduling appointments and generating bills, freeing up healthcare providers to focus on patient care.
    - **Improved Resource Allocation:** EHRs can help optimize resource allocation by providing data on patient utilization patterns and identifying areas for improvement.
5. Enhanced Research and Analytics:
    - **Data Mining and Analysis:** EHRs can be used for data mining and analysis to identify trends, patterns, and insights that can inform research and improve healthcare practices.
    - **Population Health Research:** EHRs can support population-based research studies to better understand the health needs of communities.

New Challenges for the Protections

To address privacy concerns, various regulations are in place worldwide, such as the General Data Protection Regulation (GDPR) in Europe, the Health Insurance Portability and Accountability Act (HIPAA) in the United States and My Health Record (MHR) in Australia. These regulations aim to safeguard personal data, but the rapid evolution of Data Analytics (DA) and Artificial Intelligence (AI) presents new challenges for these protections.

1. **Examining Secondary Uses:** The chapter explores various applications of EHR data beyond direct patient care and discusses their potential privacy implications.
2. **Identifying Challenges:** The article emphasizes the importance of protecting the security and privacy of Electronic Health Records (EHRs) when they are used for purposes other than the original intended use.
3. **Analysing Regulatory Frameworks:** The chapter provides a detailed analysis of GDPR and HIPAA and their challenges in ensuring data privacy in the context of expanding EHR data usage.
4. **Addressing Ethical Implications:** The chapter discusses the ethical challenges raised by the use of personal data in AI applications and calls for collaborative efforts among medical, legal, and technical experts to address these issues.

The chapter's unique contribution lies in its systematic analysis of the use of sensitive EHR data and the resulting privacy and ethical challenges, given the limited existing literature due to the interdisciplinary nature of this research area.

BACKGROUND

Advancements in Healthcare Technology and the Role of AI in HER

Over the past decade, advancements in technology have significantly transformed healthcare, emphasizing remote care, digital health, and reliance on high-tech solutions (Jazieh & Kozlakidis, 2020). Artificial intelligence (AI) analytic software can draw insights from large datasets, fundamentally changing how care is personalized and delivered to patients (Voets et al., 2022; Nichol et al., 2021; Helm et al., 2020) In this era of rapid growth in health data and computing capabilities, AI is increasingly being utilized across various healthcare domains, including medical diagnosis (Mori et al., 2020), patient monitoring (Golas et al., 2018) treatment (Mervin et al., 2018) and drug discovery (Williams et al., 2015) Intelligent software has demonstrated superior performance compared to traditional methods in terms of accuracy and effectiveness (Chew & Achananuparp, 2022) As a result, AI has the potential to enhance patient outcomes and achieve cost savings for healthcare providers and payers (Irvin et al., 2020; Voermans et al., 2019; Delgadillo, 2022; Hill et al., 2020). For instance, risk stratification algorithms have been effective in reducing misdiagnoses and unnecessary treatments, thus saving costs for providers and payers (Boutilier et al., 2021). Additionally, AI has been developed to tackle costly administrative inefficiencies by streamlining workflows and eliminating non-patient-care tasks (Sharan et al., 2016) . The healthcare industry's shift from a fee-for-service model to value-based care further drives the adoption of technology (Turner et al., 2021; Wolff et al., 2020) . With the Centers for Medicare & Medicaid Services (CMS) implementing various value-based purchasing and bundling programs along with incentive payments, hospitals are motivated to enhance the quality and efficiency of their services (Centers for Medicare and Medicaid Services, 2021) .

Despite the abundance of reports showcasing AI's successes in laboratory settings, evidence supporting its real-world value remains limited due to slow adoption in clinical practice (Voets et al., 2022) . Challenges such as unclear returns on investment hinder the adoption of AI, making it difficult for healthcare providers to justify implementation costs (Wedel & Hagist, 2020). Consequently, the health economic impact of AI has become a critical factor in decision-making (Simoens, 2009) . Health economic evaluations (HEEs) are essential for helping stakeholders optimize resource allocation by assessing the cost-effectiveness of innovative technologies (Tricco, 2018; Xie et al., 2020). Notably, the perceived value of AI applications can vary among different stakeholders, including patients, care providers, researchers, and policymakers (Rossi et al., 2022). However, much of the existing literature evaluating AI algorithms (Voets et al., 2022; Chew & Achananuparp, 2022) tends to be broad and general. This study aims to fill that gap by reviewing contemporary research that compares the financial and efficiency impacts of AI applications with standard care (SoC) or other care types across various levels, including individual, healthcare system, payer, and society.

The integration of Electronic Health Records (EHRs) and Artificial Intelligence (AI) is no longer just about digitizing paper records. Modern AI-based systems are transforming static patient data into dynamic, actionable insights, a crucial development as healthcare providers now manage 50 times more data per patient than they did just five years ago, making traditional EHR software development approaches insufficient for modern healthcare demands. Moreover we can say the current landscape of AI in EHR focuses on three key areas:

1. Automation of Routine Tasks: Modern EHR systems leverage AI to handle time-consuming administrative work.

2. Enhanced Clinical Decision Support: AI-powered EHRs now analyse patient data in real-time, offering evidence-based recommendations during patient encounters.
3. Improved Interoperability: The latest AI implementations tackle healthcare's persistent interoperability challenges head-on. By standardising data formats and enabling smart data sharing, artificial intelligence in EHR is breaking down traditional information silos. Healthcare organisations report significant improvements in cross-system data accessibility after implementing AI-enhanced EHR solutions.

Importantly, these AI-powered EHR systems are evolving to augment current capabilities through strategic integration points, rather than replacing existing EHR infrastructure. This approach allows healthcare providers to enhance their existing EHR investments while gradually adopting more sophisticated AI capabilities.

As we witness this transformation, it becomes evident that the future of healthcare technology lies at the intersection of robust EHR software development and intelligent AI integration. Organizations that recognise and act on this reality today are positioning themselves for success in tomorrow's healthcare landscape.

Furthermore, we aim to explore the challenges and future opportunities presented by state-of-the-art technologies. To our knowledge, this article is one of the few reviews that comprehensively examines the impact of healthcare AI from multiple stakeholder perspectives. The findings from this study will provide valuable insights for future research in this promising field and support informed decision-making regarding the adoption and implementation of AI.

Economics of Artificial Intelligence Models

Artificial intelligence (AI) has been shown to reduce healthcare costs compared to conventional methods. Research indicates that cost savings associated with AI in treatment are more significant than those in diagnosis. AI accelerates both diagnosis and treatment processes, achieving high accuracy in a shorter time frame than traditional approaches. By minimizing bias and subjectivity, AI enhances diagnostic accuracy, thereby reducing the likelihood of erroneous examinations. This technology can also make patients feel more comfortable when consulting with healthcare providers. AI efficiently analyses vast amounts of data to identify which treatments are most likely to yield positive outcomes. Implementing AI in healthcare not only lowers costs but also enables organizations to maximize their return on investment (ROI). Figure 2 illustrates an AI-based model compared to conventional diagnosis and treatment approaches.

Figure 2. AI-based model compared to conventional diagnosis and treatment approaches

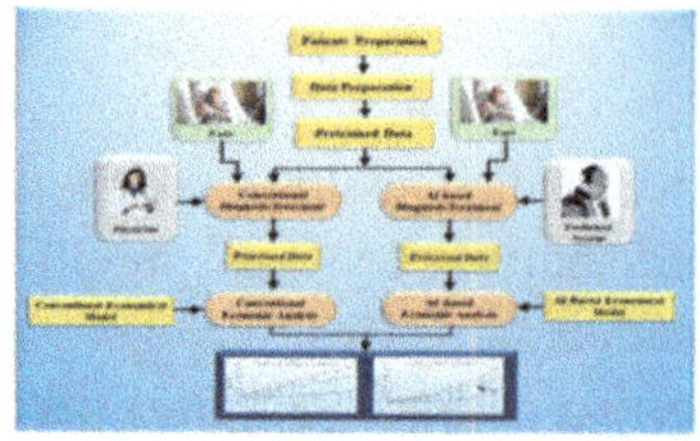

The AI economics model for diagnosis and treatment presents a promising approach to improving healthcare efficiency and reducing costs. The analysis is based on an initial cohort of 20 hospitals and 20 patients per hospital, with an assumed annual growth rate of 10%. A key advantage of the AI-based system is the reduced time required for diagnosis compared to standard methods, leading to significant cost savings over a 10-year period.

The model highlights several key benefits of incorporating AI technologies into healthcare. First, it demonstrates improved efficiency and accuracy in the diagnostic process, leveraging the capabilities of AI-powered tools. This translates to reduced overall healthcare costs, as the AI-based approach streamlines the workflow and minimizes unnecessary expenditures. Additionally, the model suggests enhanced patient outcomes and satisfaction, as the AI-assisted diagnosis and treatment recommendations lead to more personalized and effective care.

Overall, the AI economics model provides a compelling case for the integration of AI in the healthcare sector. By optimizing the diagnosis and treatment process, the model promises to deliver cost savings, improved patient outcomes, and enhanced overall system efficiency.

Utilization of EHR Data

- **Secondary Utilization of EHR Data**

The use of Electronic Health Record (EHR) data for secondary purposes has seen a significant rise, extending beyond its initial role in direct patient care. This growth is driven by the recognition of EHR data's potential to enhance healthcare delivery, support research, and improve public health outcomes. Key trends include:

1. **Applications in Research**: There is a notable increase in the use of EHR data for clinical research. According to Cowie et al. (2017), secondary applications of EHRs, particularly for research, have surged due to the extensive and varied datasets EHRs offer, enabling studies with larger and more diverse populations.
2. **Public Health Surveillance**: EHR data is increasingly used for monitoring and surveillance in public health. During the COVID-19 pandemic, EHR data played a critical role in tracking the virus's spread, identifying vulnerable populations, and assessing treatment effectiveness.
3. **Quality Improvement Initiatives**: Healthcare organizations leverage EHR data to evaluate and enhance care quality by tracking patient outcomes, pinpointing areas for improvement, and applying evidence-based practices.
4. **Predictive Analytics**: The use of EHR data for predictive analytics is growing, helping identify patients at risk for specific conditions or forecast treatment outcomes.
5. **Pharmacovigilance**: Secondary use of EHR data aids in monitoring drug safety and effectiveness in real-world scenarios, complementing traditional clinical trials.
6. **Personalized Medicine**: EHR data is increasingly employed to customize treatments for individual patients based on genetic makeup, lifestyle, and environmental factors.

These trends underscore the diverse applications of secondary EHR data, highlighting its significance in advancing healthcare and medical research.

- **Challenges in secondary use of EHR data**

While the secondary use of EHR data offers numerous applications, it also presents several challenges:

1. **Data Quality**: EHR data often contains inconsistencies, missing information, or errors that affect the reliability of secondary analyses.
2. **Interoperability**: The lack of standardization across different EHR systems hinders data integration and sharing.
3. **Privacy and Security**: Ensuring patient privacy while allowing beneficial secondary use of data remains a significant challenge.
4. **Consent and Ethics**: There is ongoing debate about the need for patient consent for the secondary use of their health data.
5. **Bias**: EHR data may not be representative of the entire population, potentially leading to biased conclusions in research.

Addressing these challenges is crucial for maximizing the benefits of secondary EHR data use while protecting patient rights and ensuring data integrity.

- **Privacy Concerns and Data Breaches**

The adoption of EHRs and big data analytics in healthcare has heightened concerns about patient privacy and the risk of data breaches. As the adoption of Electronic Health Records (EHRs) and big data analytics in healthcare has increased, so have concerns about patient privacy and the risk of data breaches. This section explores the key privacy issues and the impact of data breaches in the healthcare sector.

- **Privacy Concerns:**

1. Unauthorized Access: The digitization of health records increases the risk of unauthorized access to sensitive patient information .
2. Data Mining: The ability to analyse large datasets raises concerns about the potential misuse of patient data for purposes not initially intended .
3. Patient Consent: There's ongoing debate about the extent to which patients should be informed and provide consent for various uses of their health data .
4. Re-identification Risk: Even with de-identified data, there's a risk of re-identifying individuals through data linkage or unique combinations of characteristics.
5. Third-Party Access: Sharing of EHR data with third parties, such as researchers or commercial entities, raises questions about data ownership and control .

- **Data Breaches:**

1. Increasing Frequency: The healthcare sector has seen a significant increase in data breaches over the past decade .
2. Financial Impact: Data breaches in healthcare are among the most costly across all industries, with significant financial implications for affected organizations.
3. Patient Trust: Breaches can erode patient trust in healthcare providers and systems, potentially affecting care-seeking behaviour's.
4. Types of Breaches: Common types include hacking/IT incidents, unauthorized access/disclosure, and loss/theft of devices containing patient data .
5. Regulatory Consequences: Data breaches can result in severe penalties under regulations such as HIPAA in the U.S. and GDPR in Europe.

Addressing these privacy concerns and mitigating the risk of data breaches is crucial for maintaining patient trust and ensuring the ethical use of EHR and big data in healthcare. This requires ongoing efforts in improving cybersecurity measures, enhancing data governance practices, and educating healthcare professionals about data privacy and security. Figure 3 illustrates the life cycle model in secondary use of EHR data.

Figure 3. Life cycle model in secondary use of EHR data

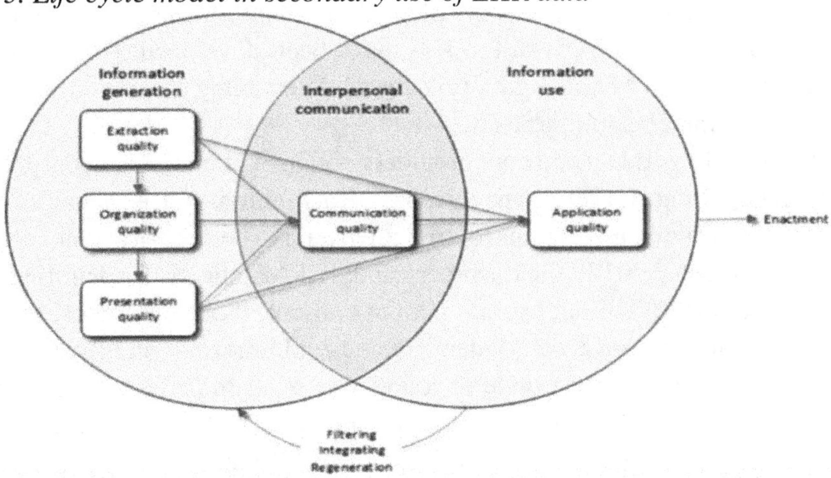

As EHRs become more prevalent, privacy concerns regarding data security and unauthorized access have intensified. EHRs, unlike paper-based systems, are vulnerable to data breaches, raising questions about patient consent and the ethical use of sensitive health information. Research indicates that data breaches in healthcare can erode patient trust, potentially impacting care-seeking behaviours. Moreover, the expansion of EHRs into secondary uses increases the need for robust consent management systems, which would enable patients to control their data use effectively. The ethical implications of using EHR data without patient consent are a significant concern, particularly as healthcare systems adopt AI-driven tools that may extract sensitive information from patient records. Even with de-identified data, risks of re-identification—where anonymized data is re-linked to specific individuals—persist, especially as datasets are combined with external sources. Addressing these ethical considerations requires advanced data governance models that prioritize transparency and patient autonomy.

REGULATORY FRAMEWORKS: GDPR AND HIPAA

As the use of Electronic Health Records (EHRs) and big data in healthcare has grown, so has the need for robust regulatory frameworks to protect patient privacy and ensure data security. Two of the most significant regulations in this area are the General Data Protection Regulation (GDPR) in the European Union and the Health Insurance Portability and Accountability Act (HIPAA) in the United States. To address these privacy issues, regulatory frameworks such as the General Data Protection Regulation (GDPR) in the EU and the Health Insurance Portability and Accountability Act (HIPAA) in the U.S. have been developed. Both GDPR and HIPAA aim to protect patient data privacy while enabling its responsible use for research and public health purposes.

GDPR mandates that healthcare providers obtain explicit patient consent before using their health data for secondary purposes. It also enforces strict penalties for data breaches, encouraging institutions to strengthen their cybersecurity protocols (Voigt & Vondem Bussche, 2017). On the other hand, HIPAA allows de-identified data to be used for research without explicit patient consent, though it imposes stringent requirements on the protection of identifiable health information (Tovino,2016).

While these frameworks provide a foundation for data privacy, emerging technologies like AI challenge their scope. Researchers suggest that GDPR and HIPAA need to adapt to address data governance in the context of AI applications, as machine learning models can inadvertently exploit data patterns that may lead to patient re-identification or biases.

THE ROLE OF ELECTRONIC HEALTH RECORDS IN ENHANCING NURSING DOCUMENTATION AND PATIENT CARE

Electronic Health Records (EHRs) serve as a crucial tool in modern healthcare, significantly improving communication among healthcare providers by establishing a centralized repository for patient information. This centralization enables professionals from various disciplines and locations to access the same patient data, thereby fostering coordinated and comprehensive care. Furthermore, EHRs enhance communication through features such as secure messaging and electronic referrals, which promote collaboration among healthcare providers. By offering a holistic view of a patient's medical history—including past medical conditions, medications, allergies, and test results—EHRs facilitate improved care coordination and continuity. For instance, alerts and reminders for preventive care and screenings are integral components of EHR systems, ensuring timely implementation of necessary health interventions. An example of this is the alert system that notifies healthcare providers when a patient is due for a screening or vaccination, thereby promoting adherence to preventive care protocols.

The adoption of EHRs by nursing staff is paramount to the successful implementation of these systems. Research indicates that Electronic Nursing Records (ENRs) can substantially enhance the quality and safety of patient care. For example, a study conducted in Tunisia demonstrated that the implementation of ENRs improved the traceability of vital signs and infusion administration, both of which are critical for ensuring patient safety (Ginting, Dewi, & Lestari, 2024). The transition to electronic documentation also streamlines nursing processes by reducing the time required for data entry and minimizing errors associated with manual documentation. Nurses have reported increased productivity and greater ease in accessing patient data, which in turn facilitates accurate nursing diagnoses.

Moreover, electronic documentation allows for the integration of standardized nursing terminology, which enhances communication and interoperability with other healthcare systems. This standardization is vital for improving the quality of nursing care and supporting research initiatives (Taneva et al., 2024). Evidence suggests that EHR systems lead to improvements in the accuracy and completeness of nursing documentation, which is essential for patient safety. For instance, the use of ENRs has been linked to significant enhancements in the tracking of vital signs and infusion administration, thereby elevating the overall quality of care provided to patients.

However, several barriers impede the widespread adoption of electronic documentation. Key challenges include inadequate infrastructure, such as unreliable internet connectivity and insufficient access to devices (Danso et al., 2024). Furthermore, regular training and supervision are necessary to ensure that nurses are proficient in utilizing these systems. The transition from paper-based to electronic systems can be met with resistance from nursing staff, particularly if they are not adequately involved in the change process or if the systems are perceived as cumbersome. Additionally, issues related to system integration and interoperability can hinder the full utilization of EHRs, thereby limiting their potential to enhance the quality of care.

There exists a notable gap between the adoption of health technology and its effective use, underscoring the necessity of this study. Despite the widespread implementation of EHRs, the outcomes for nursing staff remain mixed. It is imperative to review empirical evidence evaluating the effectiveness of EHRs in improving nursing documentation, as failure to utilize these systems effectively can adversely affect the quality of nursing care, patient safety, and staff workload.

Although EHRs are widely regarded as a means to enhance documentation and patient safety, inconsistencies in the quality of nursing documentation continue to pose significant challenges. Factors such as poor system usability, limited training, and insufficient nurse involvement in system design often obstruct optimal utilization of EHRs in clinical environments. This literature review aims to evaluate the effectiveness of EHR utilization by nurses and to identify key strategies that support the improvement of nursing documentation quality through technology-based solutions.

The findings of this review are expected to provide a comprehensive understanding of how EHRs are implemented in nursing practice, highlighting both advantages and disadvantages, as well as their impacts on clinical practice and organizational dynamics. The practical implications of these findings are highly relevant to hospital administration and nursing policy. It is essential for hospitals to view EHRs as strategic instruments rather than merely administrative resources. Studies emphasize the importance of involving nurses in the iterative development and evaluation of EHR tools to enhance usability and reduce the documentation burden. Engaging nurses in the design process can address usability issues such as data redundancy and poor workflow navigation, which are significant contributors to documentation burden. Active participation of nurses in all phases of EHR development, from design to evaluation, is critical for successful adoption. When nurses are involved, they exhibit greater acceptance of change and develop the necessary digital competencies.

Ongoing training is essential for nurses to effectively utilize EHR systems. Training programs should be tailored to address specific challenges and enhance digital literacy among nurses, whose proficiency levels can vary widely (Cachata et al., 2024). Periodic training sessions can help nurses adapt to system updates and new functionalities, ensuring they can leverage the full potential of EHR systems to improve patient care.

In conclusion, this literature review demonstrates that the use of Electronic Health Records (EHRs) in nursing practice contributes positively to documentation efficiency, information accessibility, and care coordination, particularly when the systems are well-designed and supported by user training and involvement. While some studies report increased effectiveness and time savings in documentation, others indicate that without adequate organisational support, EHR implementations may lead to increased administrative burdens, heightened mental stress, and disruption of clinical workflows.

SOLUTIONS AND RECOMMENDATIONS

- **Challenges in Leveraging EHR Data for Secondary Purposes**

    1. **Data Quality and Standardisation**: EHR data often suffers from issues related to quality and consistency. Variability in how data is entered, coded, and structured can lead to inaccuracies. Methods and dimensions of electronic health record data quality assessment: enabling reuse for clinical research.

2. **Interoperability Issues**: Different EHR systems may not communicate effectively with each other due to lack of standardisation in data formats. The inability to share and integrate data across systems can hinder comprehensive analysis.
3. **Data Security Concerns:** The sensitivity of health data raises significant security concerns. Cyberattacks on healthcare organizations have increased, with data breaches exposing patient information.
4. **Resource Limitations**: Many healthcare organisations, especially smaller practices, may lack the necessary resources to analyse EHR data effectively. Limited access to skilled data analysts and advanced analytics tools can hinder the ability to derive meaningful insights from EHR data (Bateman, et. al (2015).
5. **Regulatory Compliance**: Navigating complex regulations like HIPAA can limit how EHR data is used for research or public health initiatives.

- **Balancing EHR Data Utilization and Patient Privacy.**

1. **Informed Consent**: Healthcare providers often seek informed consent from patients before using their data for secondary purposes. This practice helps ensure transparency and builds trust.
2. **De-identification**: To protect patient identities, many organizations anonymize data before analysis. The National Institute of Standards and Technology (NIST) provides guidelines for de-identification that help reduce the risk of re-identification.
3. **Data Governance Policies**: This indicates that implementing strong data governance policies is crucial for ensuring that data is accessed and used appropriately and responsibly within an organization.
4. **Ethical Considerations**: Providers must weigh the potential public health benefits against privacy risks. Ethical frameworks, such as those proposed by the American Medical Association (AMA), emphasize the need for balancing individual rights with societal benefits
5. **Collaboration with Oversight Bodies**: Engaging with Institutional Review Boards (IRBs) or ethics committees can guide responsible data use and ensure compliance with ethical standards.

- **GDPR and HIPAA Regulations**

1. **HIPAA (Health Insurance Portability and Accountability Act)**: HIPAA sets standards for the protection of patient health information in the U.S. It mandates safeguards to ensure the privacy and security of EHR data.

2. **GDPR(General Data Protection Regulation)**: GDPR governs data protection and privacy in the EU, emphasizing data subject rights and requiring explicit consent for data processing.
3. **Impact on HER Data Use**: Both regulations require robust data protection measures influencing data management practices in healthcare.

- **Impact of Machine Learning and Data Analytics on EHR Data Security and Privacy**

1. **Enhanced Security Measures**: Machine learning algorithms can enhance security by identifying patterns indicative of security breaches. For example, anomaly detection systems can alert organizations to potential threats in real-time, as discussed by Ahmed et al. (2019).
2. **Data Breach Risks**: However, advanced analytics can also expose vulnerabilities. If machine learning models are not properly secured, they can become targets for cyberattacks.
3. **Privacy Risks with Predictive Analytics**: Using predictive analytics can inadvertently lead to the re-identification of anonymised data.
4. **Bias and Ethical Concerns**: Machine learning algorithms can perpetuate biases present in training data, leading to inequitable healthcare outcomes.
5. **Regulatory Compliance**: Organisations must ensure that their use of machine learning and analytics complies with regulations like HIPAA and GDPR.

FUTURE RESEARCH DIRECTIONS

- **How can the interoperability and privacy issues of EHR be resolved?**

1. Introduction to Blockchain-Based Solutions

Blockchain technology is a potential tool. Blockchain is a decentralised database that uses encrypted data blocks linked in a chain. This technology ensures that all parties involved can verify data access through consensus algorithms, making it difficult to tamper with information without detection.

1) Advantages of Blockchain
   1. Decentralisation: Data is distributed across the network, avoiding a single point of failure.

2. Transparency: All nodes have access to the same data, enhancing accountability.
3. Privacy and Security: Data is encrypted using hash functions, protecting

2) Application in EHR

Blockchain can address interoperability and privacy issues in Electronic Health Records (EHR). Several frameworks have been developed:

1. Medrek: Uses smart contracts on Ethereum to manage patient-provider relationships and data permissions, enhancing interoperability without storing raw medical records.
2. Ancile: Implements private transactions and proxy re-encryption for access control, ensuring patients can manage their data permissions securely.
3. OmniPHR: A peer-to-peer network that integrates EHRs, allowing patients to see their health records from different providers seamlessly.
4. Healthcare Blockchain System: Focuses on remote patient monitoring while maintaining security and privacy through a private blockchain.
5. Med Share: Monitors data access and usage through smart contracts to protect patient privacy.

3) Challenges of Blockchain in EHR

Despite its potential, blockchain faces several challenges:

1. Inefficiency: High computational demands slow down transaction processing compared to centralised systems.
2. Equity Issues: Incentive models may favour well-resourced healthcare providers, leading to disparities in access.
3. High Energy Consumption: Mining operations require substantial energy, raising environmental concerns and contributing to greenhouse gas emissions.
4. Trust Issues: The lack of regulation and understanding of blockchain may lead to distrust among patients and healthcare providers regarding data privacy.

- **How patients and providers can access a blockchain-based Electronic Health Record (EHR)system.**

1) Web Portal:
    1. Patients can access the blockchain-based EHR through a dedicated web portal.
    2. The web portal allows patients to securely enter their medical history, current medications, and other relevant information.
    3. Patients can use the web portal to communicate with their healthcare providers and access their appointment schedules.
    4. The web portal leverages the decentralised and secure nature of the blockchain to ensure the privacy and integrity of patient data.
2) Mobile App:
    1. Patients can download a mobile app to access their blockchain-based EHR on their smartphones or tablets.
    2. The app provides patients with the ability to view their medical data, test results, and other relevant information.
    3. Patients can use the app to communicate with their healthcare providers and manage their appointments.
    4. The mobile app integrates with the blockchain-based EHR system, providing patients with a convenient and secure way to access their health information.
3) Provider Access:
    1. Healthcare providers can access the blockchain-based EHR system through a dedicated web portal or a specialized application.
    2. Providers can use the system to view and update patient records, order tests, and communicate with patients.
    3. The blockchain-based EHR ensures that all changes to patient data are recorded and can be traced, providing a secure and transparent system for healthcare providers.
    4. Providers can leverage the interoperability features of the blockchain-based EHR to seamlessly share patient information with other healthcare organizations, improving coordination of care.

By leveraging the decentralized and secure nature of blockchain technology, these blockchain-based EHR systems aim to empower patients with greater control over their health data while also providing healthcare providers with a more efficient and transparent way to manage patient records and care coordination.

While blockchain-based Electronic Health Record (EHR) systems offer several advantages, there are also some potential disadvantages to consider:

1. Adoption Challenges:

- Transitioning from traditional EHR systems to a blockchain-based approach can be a complex and resource-intensive process for healthcare organizations.
- Widespread adoption may be hindered by the need for significant infrastructure changes and the learning curve associated with new technologies.

2. Scalability Concerns:
   - Blockchain networks can face scalability issues, particularly when dealing with the large volumes of data generated in healthcare settings.
   - The decentralized nature of blockchain may introduce latency and performance challenges as the network grows.
3. Interoperability Barriers:
   - While blockchain-based EHRs aim to improve interoperability, integrating with existing legacy systems and ensuring seamless data exchange can be a significant challenge.
   - Achieving true interoperability across different blockchain networks and healthcare providers may require additional standardization and coordination efforts.
4. Regulatory Compliance:
   - Healthcare organizations must ensure that blockchain-based EHR systems comply with various regulatory requirements, such as HIPAA, in terms of data privacy, security, and governance.
   - Navigating the evolving regulatory landscape can add complexity and uncertainty to the adoption process.
5. Cost Considerations:
   - Implementing and maintaining a blockchain-based EHR system may require significant upfront investments in infrastructure, training, and ongoing maintenance.
   - The potential cost savings from improved efficiency and reduced administrative overhead may not be immediately realized, especially for smaller healthcare providers.
6. Resistance to Change:
   - Healthcare professionals and patients may be hesitant to adopt a new technology, especially if they are comfortable with the existing EHR systems.
   - Overcoming the fear of the unknown and building trust in the blockchain-based approach can be a challenge.

CONCLUSION

In conclusion, as the secondary use of Electronic Health Records (EHRs) continues to expand across clinical research, public health surveillance, and quality improvement, ensuring robust privacy protections and ethical governance becomes imperative. This chapter has underscored the value of EHR data while revealing significant challenges related to patient consent, data security, and regulatory adequacy. Through a mixed-methods approach involving stakeholder perspectives and data analysis, the findings highlight gaps in current frameworks like GDPR and HIPAA, particularly in addressing evolving data-sharing practices. Furthermore, the ethical considerations of using sensitive health data in AI-driven systems demand interdisciplinary collaboration to develop context-aware policies and transparent technological solutions. Moving forward, safeguarding patient trust will require not only legal compliance but also ethical foresight and innovation in privacy-preserving technologies to strike a balance between data utility and individual rights.

REFERENCES

Ahmed, M., & Barkat Ullah, A. S. (2017, August). False data injection attacks in healthcare. In *australasian conference on data mining* (pp. 192-202). Singapore: Springer Singapore.

Bateman, A. W., Gunderson, J., & Mulder, R. (2015). Treatment of personality disorder. *Lancet, 385*(9969), 735–743. DOI: 10.1016/S0140-6736(14)61394-5 PMID: 25706219

Boutilier, J. J., Chan, T. C., Ranjan, M., & Deo, S. (2021). Risk stratification for early detection of diabetes and hypertension in resource-limited settings: Machine learning analysis. *Journal of Medical Internet Research, 23*(1), e20123. DOI: 10.2196/20123 PMID: 33475518

Cachata, D., Costa, M., Magalhães, T., & Gaspar, F. (2024). The Integration of Information Technology in the Management and Organization of Nursing Care in a Hospital Environment: A Scoping Review. *International Journal of Environmental Research and Public Health, 21*(8), 968. DOI: 10.3390/ijerph21080968 PMID: 39200579

Centers for Medicare and Medicaid Services. (2021). *The Hospital Value-Based Purchasing (VBP)*. Program.

Chew, H. S. J., & Achananuparp, P. (2022). Perceptions and needs of artificial intelligence in health care to increase adoption: Scoping review. *Journal of Medical Internet Research, 24*(1), e32939. DOI: 10.2196/32939 PMID: 35029538

Cowie, M. R., Blomster, J. I., Curtis, L. H., Duclaux, S., Ford, I., Fritz, F., Goldman, S., Janmohamed, S., Kreuzer, J., Leenay, M., Michel, A., Ong, S., Pell, J. P., Southworth, M. R., Stough, W. G., Thoenes, M., Zannad, F., & Zalewski, A. (2017). Electronic health records to facilitate clinical research. *Clinical Research in Cardiology; Official Journal of the German Cardiac Society, 106*(1), 1–9. DOI: 10.1007/s00392-016-1025-6 PMID: 27557678

Danso, K. O., Asagba, P. O., Yarhere, I. E., Adumattah, P., & Amoaful, S. (2024). Implementing and Adopting EHR Systems in Developing Countries. *Ghana Journal of Nursing and Midwifery, 1*(4), 30–62. DOI: 10.69600/gjnmid.2024.v01.i04.30-62

Delgadillo, J., Ali, S., Fleck, K., Agnew, C., Southgate, A., Parkhouse, L., Cohen, Z. D., DeRubeis, R. J., & Barkham, M. (2022). Stratified care vs stepped care for depression: A cluster randomized clinical trial. *JAMA Psychiatry, 79*(2), 101–108. DOI: 10.1001/jamapsychiatry.2021.3539 PMID: 34878526

DesRoches, C. M., Campbell, E. G., Rao, S. R., Donelan, K., Ferris, T. G., Jha, A., Kaushal, R., Levy, D. E., Rosenbaum, S., Shields, A. E., & Blumenthal, D. (2008). Electronic health records in ambulatory care—A national survey of physicians. *The New England Journal of Medicine*, *359*(1), 50–60. DOI: 10.1056/NEJMsa0802005 PMID: 18565855

Douma, M. C., Rejeb, M. B., Zardoub, N., Braham, A., Chouchene, H., Bouallegue, O., & Latiri, H. S. (2024). Impact of Implementing Electronic Nursing Records on Quality and Safety Indicators in Care. *The Libyan Journal of Medicine*, *19*(1), 2421625. DOI: 10.1080/19932820.2024.2421625 PMID: 39570988

Ginting, D. S., Dewi, W. N., & Lestari, W. (2024). Nurses' experiences using electronic medical record (EMR): A systematic review. *Malahayati International Journal of Nursing and Health Science*, *7*(8), 976–983. DOI: 10.33024/minh.v7i8.625

Golas, S. B., Shibahara, T., Agboola, S., Otaki, H., Sato, J., Nakae, T., Hisamitsu, T., Kojima, G., Felsted, J., Kakarmath, S., Kvedar, J., & Jethwani, K. (2018). A machine learning model to predict the risk of 30-day readmissions in patients with heart failure: A retrospective analysis of electronic medical records data. *BMC Medical Informatics and Decision Making*, *18*(1), 1–17. DOI: 10.1186/s12911-018-0620-z PMID: 29929496

Helm, J. M., Swiergosz, A. M., Haeberle, H. S., Karnuta, J. M., Schaffer, J. L., Krebs, V. E., & Ramkumar, P. N. (2020). Machine learning and artificial intelligence: Definitions, applications, and future directions. *Current Reviews in Musculoskeletal Medicine*, *13*(1), 69–76. DOI: 10.1007/s12178-020-09600-8 PMID: 31983042

Hill, N. R., Sandler, B., Mokgokong, R., Lister, S., Ward, T., Boyce, R., Farooqui, U., & Gordon, J. (2020). Cost-effectiveness of targeted screening for the identification of patients with atrial fibrillation: Evaluation of a machine learning risk prediction algorithm. *Journal of Medical Economics*, *23*(4), 386–393. DOI: 10.1080/13696998.2019.1706543 PMID: 31855091

Irvin, J. A., Kondrich, A. A., Ko, M., Rajpurkar, P., Haghgoo, B., Landon, B. E., Phillips, R. L., Petterson, S., Ng, A. Y., & Basu, S. (2020). Incorporating machine learning and social determinants of health indicators into prospective risk adjustment for health plan payments. *BMC Public Health*, *20*(1), 1–10. DOI: 10.1186/s12889-020-08735-0 PMID: 32357871

Jazieh, A. R., & Kozlakidis, Z. (2020). Healthcare transformation in the post-coronavirus pandemic era. *Frontiers in Medicine*, *7*, 429. DOI: 10.3389/fmed.2020.00429 PMID: 32850915

Mervin, M. C., Moyle, W., Jones, C., Murfield, J., Draper, B., Beattie, E., Shum, D. H. K., O'Dwyer, S., & Thalib, L. (2018). The cost-effectiveness of using PARO, a therapeutic robotic seal, to reduce agitation and medication use in dementia: Findings from a cluster–randomized controlled trial. *Journal of the American Medical Directors Association, 19*(7), 619–622. DOI: 10.1016/j.jamda.2017.10.008 PMID: 29325922

Mori, Y., Kudo, S. E., East, J. E., Rastogi, A., Bretthauer, M., Misawa, M., Sekiguchi, M., Matsuda, T., Saito, Y., Ikematsu, H., Hotta, K., Ohtsuka, K., Kudo, T., & Mori, K. (2020). Cost savings in colonoscopy with artificial intelligence-aided polyp diagnosis: An add-on analysis of a clinical trial (with video). *Gastrointestinal Endoscopy, 92*(4), 905–911. DOI: 10.1016/j.gie.2020.03.3759 PMID: 32240683

Nichol, A. A., Batten, J. N., Halley, M. C., Axelrod, J. K., Sankar, P. L., & Cho, M. K. (2021). A typology of existing machine learning–based predictive analytic tools focused on reducing costs and improving quality in health care: Systematic search and content analysis. *Journal of Medical Internet Research, 23*(6), e26391. DOI: 10.2196/26391 PMID: 34156338

Rossi, J. G., Rojas-Perilla, N., Krois, J., & Schwendicke, F. (2022). Cost-effectiveness of artificial intelligence as a decision-support system applied to the detection and grading of melanoma, dental caries, and diabetic retinopathy. *JAMA Network Open, 5*(3), e220269–e220269. DOI: 10.1001/jamanetworkopen.2022.0269 PMID: 35289862

Sharan, A. D., Schroeder, G. D., West, M. E., & Vaccaro, A. R. (2016). Understanding business models in health care. *Clinical Spine Surgery, 29*(4), 158–160. DOI: 10.1097/BSD.0000000000000380 PMID: 27018909

Simoens, S. (2009). Health economic assessment: A methodological primer. *International Journal of Environmental Research and Public Health, 6*(12), 2950–2966. DOI: 10.3390/ijerph6122950 PMID: 20049237

Tricco, A. C. (1967). PRISMA extension for scoping reviews (PRISMA-ScR): Checklist and explanation. *Angewandte Chemie International Edition in English, 6*(11), 951.

Turner, H. C., Archer, R. A., Downey, L. E., Isaranuwatchai, W., Chalkidou, K., Jit, M., & Teerawattananon, Y. (2021). An introduction to the main types of economic evaluations used for informing priority setting and resource allocation in healthcare: Key features, uses, and limitations. *Frontiers in Public Health, 9*, 722927. DOI: 10.3389/fpubh.2021.722927 PMID: 34513790

Voermans, A. M., Mewes, J. C., Broyles, M. R., & Steuten, L. M. (2019). Cost-effectiveness analysis of a procalcitonin-guided decision algorithm for antibiotic stewardship using real-world US hospital data. *OMICS: A Journal of Integrative Biology*, *23*(10), 508–515. DOI: 10.1089/omi.2019.0113 PMID: 31509068

Voets, M. M., Veltman, J., Slump, C. H., Siesling, S., & Koffijberg, H. (2022). Systematic review of health economic evaluations focused on artificial intelligence in healthcare: The tortoise and the cheetah. *Value in Health*, *25*(3), 340–349. DOI: 10.1016/j.jval.2021.11.1362 PMID: 35227444

Voigt, P., & Von dem Bussche, A. (2017). The eu general data protection regulation (gdpr). *A practical guide, 1st ed., Cham: Springer International Publishing, 10*(3152676), 10-5555.

Von Wedel, P., & Hagist, C. (2020). Economic value of data and analytics for health care providers: Hermeneutic systematic literature review. *Journal of Medical Internet Research*, *22*(11), e23315. DOI: 10.2196/23315 PMID: 33206056

Williams, K., Bilsland, E., Sparkes, A., Aubrey, W., Young, M., Soldatova, L. N., De Grave, K., Ramon, J., de Clare, M., Sirawaraporn, W., Oliver, S. G., & King, R. D. (2015). Cheaper faster drug development validated by the repositioning of drugs against neglected tropical diseases. *Journal of the Royal Society, Interface*, *12*(104), 20141289. DOI: 10.1098/rsif.2014.1289 PMID: 25652463

Wolff, J., Pauling, J., Keck, A., & Baumbach, J. (2020). The economic impact of artificial intelligence in health care: Systematic review. *Journal of Medical Internet Research*, *22*(2), e16866. DOI: 10.2196/16866 PMID: 32130134

World Health Organization. (2016). *Global Report on Diabetes*. World Health Organization.

Xie, Y., Nguyen, Q. D., Hamzah, H., Lim, G., Bellemo, V., Gunasekeran, D. V., Yip, M. Y. T., Qi Lee, X., Hsu, W., Li Lee, M., Tan, C. S., Tym Wong, H., Lamoureux, E. L., Tan, G. S. W., Wong, T. Y., Finkelstein, E. A., & Ting, D. S. (2020). Artificial intelligence for teleophthalmology-based diabetic retinopathy screening in a national programme: An economic analysis modelling study. *The Lancet. Digital Health*, *2*(5), e240–e249. DOI: 10.1016/S2589-7500(20)30060-1 PMID: 33328056

ADDITIONAL READING

Haque, S. N., Roy, S. S., & Kaiser, M. S. (2023). Privacy-preserving federated learning for healthcare data using blockchain. *Healthcare Analytics*, *3*, 100135. DOI: 10.1016/j.health.2023.100135

Haripriya, R., Khare, N., & Pandey, M. (2025). Privacy-preserving federated learning for collaborative medical data mining in multi-institutional settings. *Scientific Reports*, *15*(1), 12482. DOI: 10.1038/s41598-025-97565-4 PMID: 40217112

KUMAR. PRANJAL & Chauhan, Siddhartha. (2021). Big Data Analytics & Artificial Intelligence in Healthcare. DOI: 10.21203/rs.3.rs-150303/v1

Mandl, K. D., & Kohane, I. S. (2023). A 21st-century health IT system—Creating a real-world learning health system. *The New England Journal of Medicine*, *388*(11), 1010–1018.

S., Sangeetha. (2023). Privacy-Preserving Federated Learning for Healthcare Data. .DOI: 10.4018/979-8-3693-0593-5.ch008

KEY TERMS AND DEFINITIONS

Electronic Health Records (EHRs): Digitized versions of patients' medical histories maintained by healthcare providers, including data on diagnoses, medications, treatment plans, and test results. EHRs are essential for modern patient care and increasingly used for secondary research and analytics.

Secondary Use of Data: The practice of using health data collected for primary clinical care in additional contexts such as research, public health surveillance, or healthcare policy development, often raising privacy and ethical considerations.

HIPAA (Health Insurance Portability and Accountability Act): A U.S. federal law enacted in 1996 that establishes standards to protect patients' medical records and personal health information, particularly in the context of electronic data transmission.

GDPR (General Data Protection Regulation): A comprehensive data protection regulation enacted by the European Union that governs how personal data, including health information, is collected, processed, and shared, emphasizing user consent and data minimization.

Data De-identification: The process of removing or masking personal identifiers from datasets to protect individual privacy, especially before data is used for secondary purposes like research or AI training.

Chapter 10

Attention-Driven Sparse Graph Convolutional Networks for Early Detection of Liver Disorders From Medical Data

Shahnazeer C.K.
https://orcid.org/0009-0002-3380-2109
Pondicherry University, Karaikal, India

Sureshkumar G.
https://orcid.org/0000-0002-3823-9776
Pondicherry University, Karaikal, India

ABSTRACT

Liver diseases are increasing, necessitating better predictive models for early detection and effective treatments. This research paper presents an Attention-Driven Sparse Graph Convolutional Network (SGCNN) model based on medical data for early liver disease prediction. The model uses graph-based representations to depict connections between features and the attention mechanism, allowing for the flexible selection of specific connections. This sparsity and attention-based model reduces computation costs while maintaining high accuracy, making it suitable for real-time applications. The framework includes data preprocessing, graph construction, and classification tasks. The results show that the proposed method outperforms conventional learning models in efficiency and precision. The article highlights the

DOI: 10.4018/979-8-3373-2043-4.ch010

potential of attention-driven sparse graph convolutional networks as a valuable tool for early detection in healthcare.

INTRODUCTION

Liver diseases exist as a major global health problem, which is the reason for a high morbidity and mortality rates. These maladies are usually hidden in their beginning stages and because of this, identification can be the only way to have an effective treatment and to manage it. The field of medicine has been totally transformed by the use of machine learning and deep learning techniques which allow disease prediction and early diagnosis. Likewise, graph-based learning solutions have been highly recognized dwelling on their capability of modeling tricky relationships in medical data. In contrast to the standard measure, the graph-based technique is able to catch both the feature-level and the structural dependencies which in turn are indispensable for the analysis of health data. Researchers have done some work to look into the application of graph convolutional networks (GCNs) in disease prediction due to their efficiency in graph-structured data handling. Point out an example when GCNs have been used to predict cancer subtypes, which has to do with the fact that multiple omics data details have been added, therefore their accuracy has been improved (Hu et al., 2024). The team was able to achieve success through the use of the graph-based approach for heart disease risk prediction by integrating the patient's demographic and clinical information and, therefore, improving personalized medicine practices(Y. Li et al., 2020). Besides, the researchers have exploited the graph learning techniques to make it possible to detect diabetes by utilizing the patient data which in turn paved the way for the formation of a reliable prediction framework (Baskar et al., 2020).

To make GNC predictive ability stronger, attention mechanisms integrating into these models like dynamic weighting of important features and relationships have been instrumentalized. It has been proven by studies that attentiveness significantly enhances the performance of disease classification tasks, e.g., the early diagnosis of Alzheimer's, via the prioritizing of the critical brain regions in the neuroimaging data (Huang et al., 2025). The attention models have also been used in respiratory disease prediction, and are suitable for the target of issues in clinical practice (Zhang et al., 2024).

The use of sparsity techniques in graph representations has also brought about the alleviation of computational complexity as well as the maintenance of accuracy. Sparse graph convolutional networks have been successfully deployed in diagnosing lung diseases, thus leading to the development of real-time diagnoses with a computational power of a minimal amount (Kexin Ding et al., 2022). Sparsity incorporation of complex datasets has also shown its worth in processing large medical datasets for chronic liver diseases (Sangeetha et al., 2023). A sparse graph-based infrastructure is oftentimes also employed for forecasting liver fibrosis development, revealing their adaptability to liver-related disease research (Kowsalya Selvaraj & Saraswathi Subbian, 2023).

The latest developments in graph-based models show the scalability of these models for multi-illness prediction schemes. To illustrate, a study was conducted involving multiple chronic diseases and the multi-modal graph-based approach in which the flexibility of graph-based learning was revealed (Wang et al., 2021). Hybrid models, meanwhile, combining graph learning and deep neural networks not only have shown impressive accuracy in liver disease diagnosis but also have the advantages of both graph representations and feature extraction capabilities (Sangeetha S, 2016) . The fusion of graph-based learning, attention mechanisms, and sparsity opens a bright avenue for the accelerated prediction of diseases. This investigation is designed to deliver additional capabilities needed to deal with the lower computational needs and the accuracy of the prediction in the situation of liver disease detection.

The current paper does an effective job at introducing the SGCNN model. However, a more thorough literature review that is more comprehensive will make the work more appealing. A literature review where the most recent deep learning models used in liver disease detection are (etc.) and probably the best belonging to GNNs, RNNs, and Transformer architectures would be appropriate and enlightening. Furthermore, examining graph-based learning's success rate in similar clinical prediction activities might highlight the weaknesses of the current model and how it overcomes those.

The current research work only to a small extent discusses the development of liver disease predictors, while in addition, it is necessary to concentrate much more on the issue of the global health burden that these diseases represent, such as the statistical trends, the challenges of diagnostic methods, and the gaps in treatment. This would not only be the motivation for the proposed framework but also make the matter clearer and more concrete. Henceforth, article is well-targeted to researchers and professionals in the domains of AI in healthcare, medical informatics, and predictive analytics. The technical depth combined with real-world applicability makes it suitable for a book chapter audience seeking innovative, AI-driven healthcare solutions.

BACKGROUND

The literature survey collectively enlists numerous real-life applications of machine learning, predominantly graph-based models and attention mechanisms, in early diagnosis and prognosis of different diseases, with the outcomes of the resources to healthcare being significant. An increase in the use of machine learning methods in applications to predict diseases, namely, in healthcare, has been evident with several studies trying to use it to augment diagnostic accuracy in different ways. CNNs were the technology artifact used by a research team for diagnosing liver diseases through detecting medical images, a step that resulted in a huge leap toward diagnostic accuracy (J. Li et al., 2022).

In a related study, a group of experts was able to use recurrent neural networks (RNNs) to display specificities in diagnosing liver cirrhosis early, the implementation of the model revealed a rise in accuracy. The method of neural network architecture used in the study emphasized the sequential patterns that allow the model to be predictive over the traditional ways (W. Liu et al., 2025). Moreover, in a GNNs experiment network of long-range connections was used for the feature space encoding, and then a Variational type of Autoencoder (VAE) was employed to generate the trajectory in the latent space which allowed the network to encapture complex disease dynamic with the graph motion model (D. Liu et al., 2021). A different study focused on the integration of deep learning models with multi-modal medical data, utilizing both clinical records and genomic data for more robust liver disease classification, demonstrating the potential of hybrid approaches in complex healthcare applications (K. Liu et al., 2019).

It is also the case that attention mechanisms have been recognized to be the main driver in terms of the validation of disease classification models. A research paper introduced attention-based models to prioritize relevant clinical features, significantly enhancing the precision of cardiovascular disease prediction models (Chong Yin et al., 2024). Another study conducted a study that included the application of attention-enhanced models for the prediction of chronic kidney disease, where attention mechanisms were used to find the key features of the disease and thus were the most important for the progression of the disease (J. Li et al., 2024). In addition, the concept of the sparse graph-based approach has also been the subject of considerable attention in the latest literature, mainly due to its capacity to cut down the computational complexity while still managing to produce the high-performance result. A study delved into the use of sparse graph convolutional networks (SGCNs) to forecast Alzheimer's disease, implementing sparsity which made it faster for large-scale datasets to be processed while still giving the predictive accuracy outcome that is normally achieved through dense networks, because sparsity in Alzheimer's disease networks is built by the idea of computational efficiency (Yang et al., 2023).

Furthermore, a model that combined both sparse graphs and attention mechanisms was proposed to the lung cancer detection-area while it was able to identify crucial tumor traits and save computational energy at the same time (Liang et al., 2024). Another research was aimed at using sparse graph learning for heart disease prediction, where the model was able to process medical data successfully, resulting in the identification of the hidden links between various risk factors (Zhou et al., 2024). On the other side, multi-task learning along with graph convolutional networks were used to perform multi-disease prediction, where the ability to infer diseases like diabetes, hypertension, and obesity due to the shared information led to the better prediction of such diseases (Hassan et al., 2017).

The rising incidence of liver diseases from steatosis and fibrosis to hepatocellular carcinoma (HCC) highlights the need for powerful predictive models. Traditional diagnostic methods frequently are lacking to detect early-stage disease or stratify Patient according to the risk of progressive disease. In the last decade, artificial intelligence (AI) (i.e., machine learning (ML) and deep learning (DL)) has increasingly demonstrated its dominance in liver disease prediction accuracy. The authors review herein recent critical developments on AI/ML systems for liver disease classification, fibrosis assessment, and hepatocarcinogenesis risk prediction, emphasizing on explainability, feature selection, and performance testing.

Nakatsuka et al. (2025) proposed a deep learning model to predict hepatocellular carcinoma (HCC) with hepatic steatosis by steatosis liver disease (SLD), based on hematoxylin and eosin-stained whole-slide biopsy patterns. This study included 685 patients (46 patients developed HCC within 7 years, 639 patients did not). A keras-based deep CNN was trained on 28000 tiles from these images and achieved a predictive accuracy of 81.0% and area under the curve (AUC) of 0.80. The model also showed high performance in an independent validation cohort (accuracy, 82.3%; area under the curve, 0.84), comparable to that of logistic regression models using fibrosis stage only. One strength of this study was interpretability made possible by saliency maps, which revealed nuclear atypia, high nuclear-cytoplasmic ratios, immune infiltration, and fibrosis patterns. Such subtle pathological indicators indicate that the DL model is capable of encapsulating the more generalizing morphological appearance, thus overcoming the limitations of fibrosis based conventional metrics. Its clinical relevance is considerable – this system may catch the early stages of hepatic carcinogenesis in patients with mild fibrosis that would be treated as low risk individuals in the absence of analysis.

Dabbah et al. (2024) accepted the burden of diagnosis of advanced fibrosis (AF) in patients with metabolic dysfunction-associated steatotic liver disease (MASLD) -the condition previously known as NAFLD. They developed a battery of five machine learning classifiers, including the extreme gradient boosting (XGBoost) classifier with the best performance as reflected by an AUC of 0.91, which was significantly superior to historical scores such as the Fibrosis-4 index (FIB-4: AUC = 0.78) and the NAFLD Fibrosis Score (NFS: AUC = 0.81). Validation on a primary care sample (n=540) emphasized its relevance to screening scenarios in the real-world. Notably, the authors incorporated SHAP(Shapley Additive Explanations) to promote model interpretability by clinicians. HbA1c, GGT, AST and age were identified as the four top predictors, and SHAP analysis enabled reclassification of 73%) of false positives (all with specificity 0.76). Due to the high NPV (99%) of the model patients with negative predictions could be safely ruled out, potentially leading to a significantly lower number of unnecessary referrals or imaging. This method demonstrates the responsible AI use of healthcare by combining high-performance prediction with interpretability.

Noor et al. (2025) proposed a hybrid feature optimization method fusing ranking and projection-based method for the CLD detection, and then the filters and deep neural networks (DNNs) were employed. We focused on our approach and methodology of maximising the feature input by SHAP for the global interpretability of both the most influential clinical and biochemical parameters are input for the model input. The model accuracy, 90.12% was demonstrated to be higher than traditional ML classifiers by experimental results. This work clearly demonstrated the advantage of integrating feature selection with DL architectures, which can enhance model generalization and lower the cost burden. Reliability was guaranteed using SMOTE scheme to cope with class imbalance and robust cross validation. This approach has potential of being used for implementation in decision-support systems for universal CLD detection in all healthcare environments.

Theerthagiri (2024) also developed histogram-based gradient boosting (HGBoost) classifier for liver disease prediction with recursive feature selection for relevance ranking. The system was evaluated on the Indian Liver Patient Dataset (ILPD) and compared with other classifiers such as MLP, AdaBoost, Random Forest, and GBoost. The developed model provided better accuracy (4–9% better) and lower MSE in comparison with other algorithms. An important premise of this work has been attention on computational efficiency and interpretability. The recursive feature selection provided the automatic removal of noisy and irrelevant features and the classification accuracy of HGBoost remained high. The authors propose that HGBoost could be used for population-level liver disease screening, especially in low resource settings.

In another image-based classification domain, the authors proposed a CNN-based model trained with CT scans for the automatic diagnosis of hepatic cirrhosis. The model was impressively accurate in classifying cases with 93.25%, above baselines from CNNs and even radiologist-perceived predictions. Convolutional and pooling layers were stacked to learn abstract features from abdominal CT images by the authors. In addition, the model included dropout layers as a solution for overfitting, and data augmentation for improving robustness.

This study underscores the role of image-based DL in aiding radiological diagnosis particularly in areas with scarce access to hepatologists. In the identical steatotic liver disease and HCC-related clinical scenario, digital pathology has been extended still by employing CNNs in analysis of WSI. Nakatsuka et al. (2025) re-investigated histological HCC predictors beyond standard staging looking at high resolution image tiles of biopsies. This study demonstrates how CNNs, focused exclusively on histopathologic discriminators including hepatocyte morphology and immune infiltration patterns, are able to recognise subtle microanatomic features associated with risk of malignancy. Such integration of computational pathology and deep learning offers new tools for early detection of cancerous conversion that complement pathologists and hepatologists with diagnostic layers without the need of new staining or imaging modalities.

Saeed et al. (2025) with the overview on application of ML and DL for the prediction of HCC on HCV patients. Emphasizing that HCV accounts for 78% of global HCC, the authors criticize the invasiveness of "classic" tools for diagnosis such as liver biopsy and ultrasonography, with the latter being non-sensitive especially at early stage. The research highlights the promising perspective of AI technology in facilitating the HCC prediction based on non-invasive clinical, laboratory, imaging and histological information. ML models including Decision Trees, Support Vector Machines (SVM) and Multi-linear Regression are known for their capacity to discover patterns from complex datasets, and they are adapted to process multimodal medical data. After PRISMA-based screening from 128 articles to 12, the review summarizes the utility of AI in the diagnosis, prognosis and treatment of HCC. Conventional screening modalities (US, CT, MRI, AFP, and serum biomarkers) are reviewed with discussion of AI as a potential adjunct combining these modalities in patient specific risk assessment. ADTree and SVM models are emphasized due to their accuracy, and it is demonstrated that CNN outperforms traditional methodologies in imaging-based prediction. The paper deals with issues such as lack of data and imbalance, recommending ensemble methods and transfer learning. Ending with discussion about the scope of AI, algorithm performance and leading predictive characteristics as future research questions, this review serves as an essential reference source for researchers and clinicians engaging in AI imaging bookmarking and review cave is being edited applications in liver disease diagnosis.

Udompap et al. (2025), present a novel study to analyze whether AI can predict metabolic dysfunction-associated steatotic liver disease (MASLD), an asymptomatic and challenging to detect early condiition, from tones of AI-powered electrocardiograms (AI-ECGs). Using a CNN model, the authors developed and validated their method on a large MASLD cohort of 3468 cases and 25,407 controls collected from the Rochester Epidemiology Project, which was externally validated within the Mayo Clinic Enterprise. The AUC for the AI-ECG model was 0.69 in the development cohort and 0.62 in the validation cohort, equivalent or better than traditional clinical parameters like BMI (AUC 0.71), ALT (0.64) or diabetes status (0.66). The CNN was trained with a matrix format of the 12-lead ECG data (12×5000) and multiple clinical variables were analyzed alone and in combination with ECG data. The combined model of ECG, age, sex, BMI, diabetes, ALT demonstrated the best performance for the AP (AUCs: 0.76 in the discovery cohort and 0.72 in the validation cohort). Subgroup analyses supported the robustness of the model in populations with or without cardiovascular disease (CVD) and metabolic comorbidities. This study highlights the clinical value of ECG as a noninvasive, inexpensive and widely available screening tool for MASLD, particularly in locations outside hepatology services. It is a window for earlier diagnosis, early interventions and better patient outcomes through lifestyle change and risk stratification. In addition, the study provides evidence in support of the future exploration of AI-augmented ECG analysis to expand the sensitivity for the detection of a wider range of metabolic liver diseases, indicating the generalizability and merit of AI-CNN models as an alternative diagnostic tool in modern clinical settings.

Kiran et. al. introduces a CNN-based deep learning model for an enhanced diagnosis of cirrhosis, a life-threatening liver disease characterized by an irreversible scarring. Classical diagnostic methods, including liver biopsy and laboratory tests, are invasive and operator-dependent, supporting the interest for automated imaging-based solutions. For the identification between cirrhotic and non-cirrhotic tissues, the CNN model is trained with liver ultrasound and CT- scan images. Using the image-label pairs, we can train the model in a supervised learning way and add dropout layers and data augmentation to improve the generalization and reduce overfitting. It exhibits favorable performance in terms of the standard metrics: accuracy, precision, recall and F1-score, as compared with conventional diagnostic instruments. The investigation also benefits from transfer learning with pre-trained architectures such as VGG16 and ResNet50, which makes it possible to achieve high accuracy (over 90%) with small amount of data. This approach greatly enhances the efficiency and learning capability of models by utilizing the well-trained image models for feature re-use. Besides the classification performance, the proposed CNN can provide the class activation maps, which can be used to localize the pathological liver regions, which is beneficial on interpretability and clinical trust. Practically, the framework holds great promise for clinical translation as a rapid and reliable tool that radiologists can use to surpass the visual diagnosis, expedite the rate of diagnosis of cirrhosis, and start interventions in a timely fashion. The ability of the model to quickly analyze imaging data can decrease reliance on invasive procedures and subjective judgments, facilitating earlier diagnosis and better outcomes for patients.

By including multi-center data, fibrosis stage prediction to increase granularity, and cross-modality validation for broader clinical applicability, the study encourages future research for generalizability. This work is illustrative of the transformative impact of AI-based radiological analysis in liver disease diagnosis, enabling non-invasive, scalable, and interpretable diagnostic solutions in hepatology.

The AWARE study that aimed to improve non-invasive diagnosis of advanced fibrosis in people with fatty liver disease, which is becoming significantly more prevalent worldwide (NAFLD/MASLD). Given the drawbacks of conventional methods, such as transient elastography and liver biopsy, the authors established a model based on machine learning (ML) and gradient boosting classifiers. This model, developed based on a cohort consisting of 2463 patients from European and North American population, included widely available clinical indicators such as age, BMI, platelet count, AST, ALT, prevalence of type 2 diabetes and LSM. The AWARE notch model performed best with an AUROC of 0.85 compared to common fibrosis scores such as FIB-4 and NFS (AUROC 0.79 and 0.78, respectively). Most importantly, it had a high negative predictive value (NPV) and could rule out advanced fibrosis for 91% of patients, thereby potentially reducing the need for approximately 30% of liver biopsies. A notable strength of AWARE is its interpretability and transparency, which would be appealing to the clinician and more user-friendly than black-box models, while its lightweight nature allows operational, effortless integration within primary care and telehealth. The method attempts to find relevant features for medical decision making, while maintaining usability. Moreover, AI-supported diagnostics in hepatology have a promising perspective, particularly when combined with telemedicine and wearable technology for longitudinal data collection on disease-risk. Authors' plea for future prospective validation of the model in larger cohorts and proposed incorporation of imaging biomarkers to enhance the diagnostic accuracy of ML models. In summary, the AWARE study is a major innovation in applying machine learning to develop a scalable, accurate, and accessible fibrosis prediction method for early intervention and optimal management of chronic liver disease.

A number of common themes cut across the studies. First, the application of deep learning to image modalities — whether CT or histopathology — shows great potential to identify intricate patterns that may go unnoticed by human readers. CNNs are a group of deep networks equipped with the hierarchical feature encoding property and have shown superior results in the risk prediction of HCC as well as the diagnosis of cirrhosis. These models and the interpretability tools, in particular when taken together with additional interpretability tools such as saliency maps or SHAP, mitigate the 'black box' critique that is an obstacle to clinical use. Second, imaging data alone, will not replace laboratory results and epidemiological features, especially for the differentiation between stages of fibrosis and chronic liver disease. Algorithms, such as XGBoost and HGBoost, combined with the "right" feature-selection techniques (e.g., recursive elimination, projection-based ranking) largely improve predictive performance. And interestingly, explainability continues to be key aspect in responsible AI adoption: for example, research that uses SHAP values to explain and improve models. Third, pre-training samples such as state preprocessing and class balance adjustment by SMOTE or redundancy-based sampling are also important for producing sound model predictions. Furthermore, considering multimodal data (e.g., combining 2D shear wave elastography and clinical biomarkers) enables a broad diagnostic overview and enhances model stability and generalizability.

Taken together, these developments indicated the transition from proof-of-concept to infrastructure-ready AI assisted liver disease prediction. The studies that were reviewed demonstrate that algorithm and feature-engineering development lead to actionable diagnostic rules with improved overall diagnostic accuracy, interpretability, and clinical relevance along the spectrum of liver diseases, ranging from early fibrosis to HCC. The literature covered in this review underscores the key role of AI, especially ML and DL, in the development of liver disease diagnosis and prognosis. Saeed et al. studies prediction of HCC among HCV patients with ML/DL models on multimodal sources of data. Udompap et al. presents the AI-augmented ECG to screen for MASLD and provides a connection between cardiometabolic traits and liver disease. Kiran et.al. introduces a CNN deep learning approach for non-invasively diagnosing cirrhosis based on ultrasound/CT images, deviating from conventional means. Gradient boosting is implemented in the AWARE study to obtain highly accurate and clinically interpretable predictions of the stages of fibrosis in patients with NAFLD.

PROPOSED SYSTEM

The proposed system is in line with the methodical technique, which predicts liver diseases from medical data. Initially, the main issue is data preprocessing, where the medical data that is raw gets cleaned and normalized to guarantee quality and consistency. Then, the system creates a graph representation of the data, where one node is a medical feature or patient record, and the edges detail their interconnections. CNN framework, a graph processing technique, is used to analyze this graph, which benefits from capturing the complex relationships among the diseases and genes. A mechanism of attention is used for the system to emphasize the dire features; for instance, it will be like prioritizing the most related connections in the graph, as seen in Figure 1. The method is to sparsity methods that reduce the computational complexity by excluding less relevant nodes and edges; thus, the model efficiency and scalability are not violated. Eventually, the model is trained using labeled data, and its performance is evaluated through precision, accuracy, and other relevant metrics. The outcome will be a predictive model that is efficient and accurate in identifying liver diseases at an early stage. This makes it a smart tool for healthcare applications.

Figure 1. Proposed system flow diagram

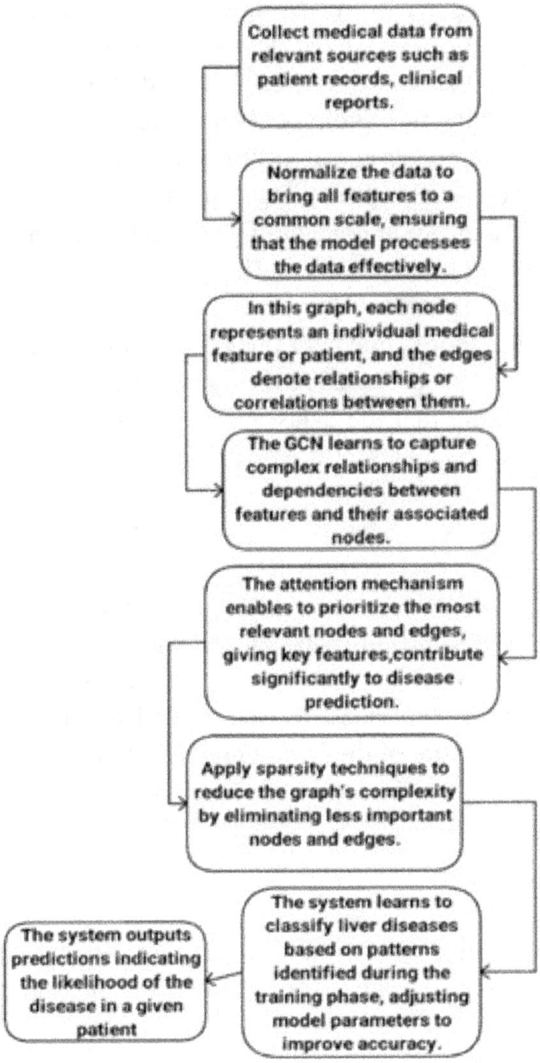

By going into detail about the clinical characteristics that were obtained during the preprocessing of the data, and the reasons for choosing graph-based modeling over other representation techniques, the article can present a stronger argument. By also revealing the indicators like demographic, behavioral, and biochemical that served as the nodes of the graph during the construction process, a full scope will be achieved, and interpretability will be facilitated. While the paper maintains a logical sequence, the transitions between data preprocessing, graph construction, and classification could be made smoother with clearer subsection headings and brief introductions to each major processing step. A schematic diagram of the end-to-end pipeline would also improve the flow and reader understanding.

Firstly, the proposed system for liver disease prediction kick-offs with a formalized approach to data collection and processing. The entire step-by-step process is conducted through math models and algorithms, which is the core part of the transformation of raw data materials into actionable predictions. The detailed explanation of each step involved in the system, including relevant equations integrated into the process, is graphically presented below and is also given somewhere in the text. The procedure rests on the premise that raw medical data ought to be first collected. The latter includes patient records, medical images, laboratory test results, and other clinical parameters that may be stored in various formats. Preprocessing techniques are then applied to ensure that the dataset is appropriate for model training. The techniques handle missing values, outliers, and normalization the dataset as in (1).

$$X=\{x1,x2,...,xN\} \quad (1)$$

The (1) is composed of N feature vectors with one vector translating to one patient's entire set of clinical features as demonstrated in the chart. As a solution to the mislaying of missing value attributes, the system admin rehashes a new value μ_i once for each feature across the whole data base and place it instead of a void of data. If x_{ij} symbolizes the jth feature of the ith patient, the imputation process reads as (2).

$$x_{ij} = \begin{cases} x_{ij}, \text{ if } x_{ij} \text{ is available} \\ \mu_j, \text{ if } x_{ij} \text{ is missing} \end{cases} \quad (2)$$

Then the data undergoes removal of outliers. An outlier is looked upon as an outlier if a feature's value x_{ij} is away from the defined measure set by the mean μ_j and a standard deviation threshold σ_j in (3).

$$|x_{ij}-\mu_j| > 3\cdot\sigma_j \quad (3)$$

Outliers are removed or replaced with boundary values that have enough consistency from the rest of the data. Normalization then takes the following step to make sure that all features are on the same scale which is very important for further processing steps. The normalization formula for each feature xi is given by (4).

$$x_i'=x_i-\mu_i/\sigma_i \tag{4}$$

where μ_i is the mean and σ_i is the standard deviation of the characteristic xi, respectively. Here, all of the features are standardized into having a mean of zero and the variance of the unit, and thus, they fit in well during model training. Once the data is preprocessed, it is converted to a graph structure for the next steps of processing. Medical data along with patient records and clinical features is now a graph (5).

$$G=(V,E) \tag{5}$$

where V is represented by the set of nodes (each representing a feature of the patient record), and E is the set of edges (each representing a relationship between the features of the patient records). Adhesion matrix A shows the connections between the adjacent nodes in the graph that are first created. The matrix (6).

$$A_{ij} = \begin{cases} 1, \textit{ if nodes i and j are connected} \\ \qquad \textit{otherwise} \end{cases} \tag{6}$$

The adjacency matrix of the graph provides a measure of the similarity, which is often based on the correlations or the distances between the features in the dataset. After that, a Graph Convolutional Network (GCN) is utilized on the data to capture feature dependencies and to learn node representations. A GCN is a way to convolve the features of a graph utilizing repeated graph convolution operations. In each layer l, the convolution operation is represented as (7).

$$H(l+1)=\sigma(AH(l)W(l)) \tag{7}$$

where H(l) is the feature layer matrix at level l, W(l) is the weight matrix at level l, and f is the activation function (for ex., ReLU). When the convolution operation is used along with the graph, the order of the nodes in the graph will then be interpreted using the outcomes of the operation. By implementing the introduction of the model with attention, we focus on the most informative nodes during convolution. The attention coefficient α_{ij} for the relationship between nodes i and j is calculated as (8).

α_{ij}=exp(LeakyReLU(aT[Wh_i||Wh_j]))/(∑k∈N(i)exp(LeakyReLU(aT[Wh_i||Wh_k]))

(8)

where h_i and h_j are the feature vectors for nodes i and j, respectively, a is a learnable attention vector, N(i) is the set of neighbors of node i, and || denotes concatenation. The next step in the process is the optimization of the graph for computational efficiency by the introduction of sparsity. This is done by selectively pruning less important edges in the graph, reducing the graph's size and complexity. The sparse adjacency matrix As is computed by retaining only the top K largest elements of the adjacency matrix A (9).

A_s=Top-K(A, K) (9)

where Top-K(A, K) selects the top K largest elements from the matrix A. Once the data is represented as a sparse graph, the model leads to the training phase. The model is trained by minimizing a loss function, typically cross-entropy loss for classification tasks. The cross-entropy loss L for a multi-class classification problem is defined as (10).

L=−$\sum_i$∑cy_i,clog(y^i,c),(i=1 to N),(C=1 to C)(10)

where y_i,c is the true label for the ith node and class c, and y^i,c is the predicted probability for the ith node and class c. During training, the model is updated iteratively to minimize the loss function, refining its ability to predict disease states based on input data. The output predictions for each node are derived using a softmax function applied to the raw logits z_i (11).

y^i=Softmax(z_i)=(exp(z_i)/(∑jexp(z_j)) (11)

where z_i represents the raw output for node i. When the model is trained, the performance thereof is evaluated using standard evaluation metrics such as Accuracy (Acc) is offered as (12).

Acc=(1/N)$\sum_i$I(y^i=y_i), (i=1 to N) (12)

where I(·) is the indicator function, which equals 1 if the predicted label y^i matches the true label y_i. Lastly, after evaluating the model, predictions can be made for new, unseen data. The predicted probability of disease for a new patient is calculated using the softmax function applied to the raw output z_{new} as in (13).

$$y\text{^}new=Softmax(z_{new}) \tag{13}$$

Once the model is trained and evaluated, it is ready for Real-time predictions are now being used to help healthcare professionals recognize liver disease at an early stage. This entire process, whether from collecting data to deploying it, can give the surety of the system's resilience and efficacy in the use of graph-based learning and optimization techniques for the prediction of diseases.

SOLUTIONS AND RECOMMENDATIONS

The research model tends to under-emphasize the limitations of the proposed approach, particularly in regard to scalability for large-scale hospital deployments and potential sensitivity to noisy or missing clinical data. Adding a critical evaluation of these areas can enhance credibility and practical impact.

The results show that monitoring of medical parameters like Blood Bilirubin Levels (BBL), Liver Enzyme Levels (LEL), Albumin Levels (AL), and Platelet Count (PC) is of key importance to overall health and detecting potential medical conditions. When BBL values surpass the limit, liver dysfunction is the likely cause and could be the result of complications like jaundice or biliary obstruction. The same applies to LEL, where a higher-than-normal value indicates liver damage and inflammation that can be linked to acute disorders such as hepatitis or cirrhosis, which in turn, need prompt medical help. AL, in most cases, within the normal range, signifies that the liver is healthy, while those below the threshold might indicate malnutrition or the presence of liver disease-caused problems like poor healing. The low PC count seems to be an important aspect also as low platelet counts are detected in thrombocytopenia, which serves as the basis for excessive bleeding and bruising, especially in individuals with pre-existing conditions like liver cirrhosis. Hence, these outcomes solely support the view that these parameters should be kept within their specific limits at all times. Changes in any of them will act as strong messages for diseases that are primitively hidden and thus will call for a range of therapies that involve more continuous monitoring and medical interventions.

The proposed system should greatly consider integrating a broader comparative assessment of the study across multiple real-world datasets in order to push the research's impact as far as possible. The introduction of ablation studies provides a way to measure the effect of sparsity and attention components separately. It is also important to clearly explain the strategies that were used for hyperparameter tuning.

The data is collected from all the patients who had their blood, liver, albumin, and Platelets checked and their values are made relative to their threshold to provide a clear understanding of their behavior.

In Figure 2 (Blood Bilirubin Levels), the BBL average is about 1.0 mg/dL, but there are many instances where the threshold of 1.2 mg/dL is exceeded. Approximately 15 % of the data points reveal values that exceed the threshold, a clear sign of liver failure. Too high BBLs can eventually bring about jaundice, liver failure, and other associated diseases. BBLs lasting an extended period usually call for urgent care, because they frequently come about with liver damage or biliary blockage.

Figure 2. Comparison of BBL of Proposed framework

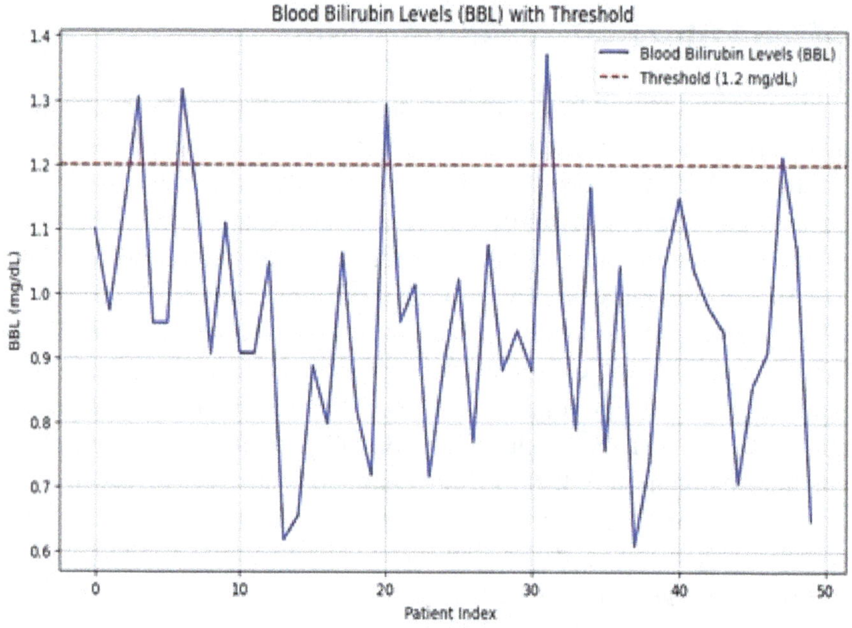

As regards to Figure 3 (Liver Enzyme Levels), on the other hand, the average LEL is 35 U/L, with more than 40 U/L being the referring value of 10% of the data points. The tone set by the readings implies that the person could be sick with inflammation of their liver or with a liver injury. However, the maximum levels are 55 U/L, which is a strong evidence of liver injury and should be closely monitored. The underlying conditions are hepatitis or cirrhosis that warrant medical care if values continue to be above the threshold.

Figure 3. Analysis of enzymes in the liver

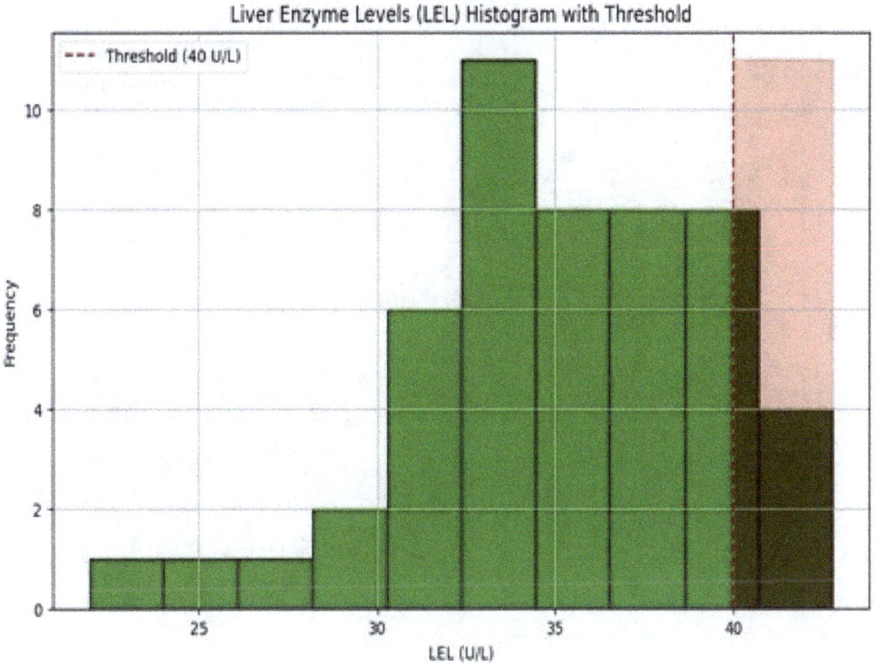

In Figure 4 (Albumin Levels), Indoor greetings fleece most AL values which are located on a higher level of 3.5 g/dL than the threshold, with a 5% overlapping percentage of the data points that belong to this area. People with low AL can have a value of 2.8 g/dL which indicates probable malnutrition or liver disease. The consequences of such low values are water retention, ascites, and longer healing time of wounds, the need for intervention to stop the underlying causes is strongly reflected.

Figure 4. Albumin levels in liver comparison

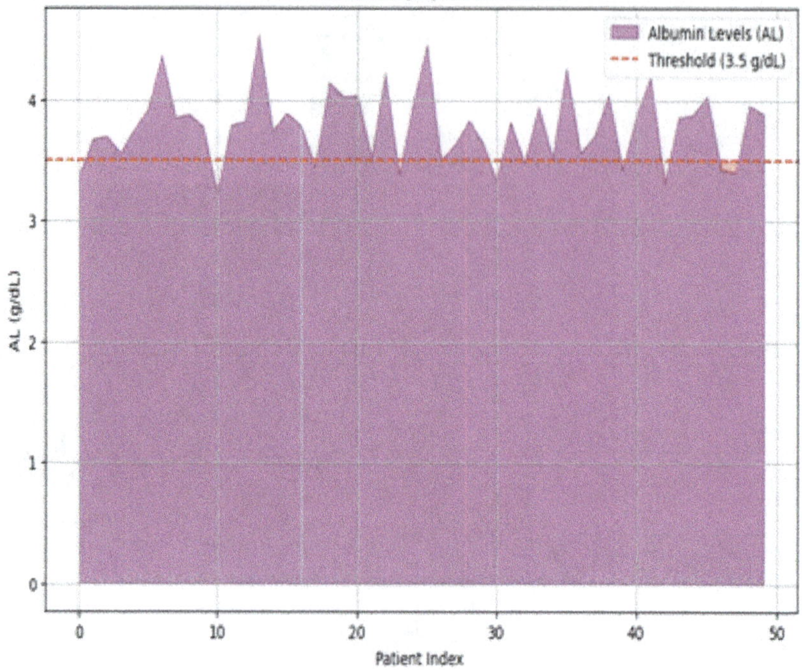

In Figure 5 (Platelet Count), where the average PC for instance is around $160 \times 10^3/\mu L$, there are approximately 12% of the values go lower than the $150 \times 10^3/\mu L$ threshold. The lowest recorded value which was $120 \times 10^3/\mu L$ is a situation that may signal the fact that a person may have a problem of thrombocytopenia. This condition increases the risk of bleeding and bruising, and its impact is particularly critical in patients with conditions like liver cirrhosis, where platelet count abnormalities can lead to life-threatening complications. These observations are consistent with the evidence that the role of keeping each parameter at its threshold for proper health management is significant. If these signs show up exceeding the defined limits, they become a matter of high concern and may lead to health problems that need immediate medical help in order to stop more severe complications.

Figure 5. Platelet Count rates by the proposed framework

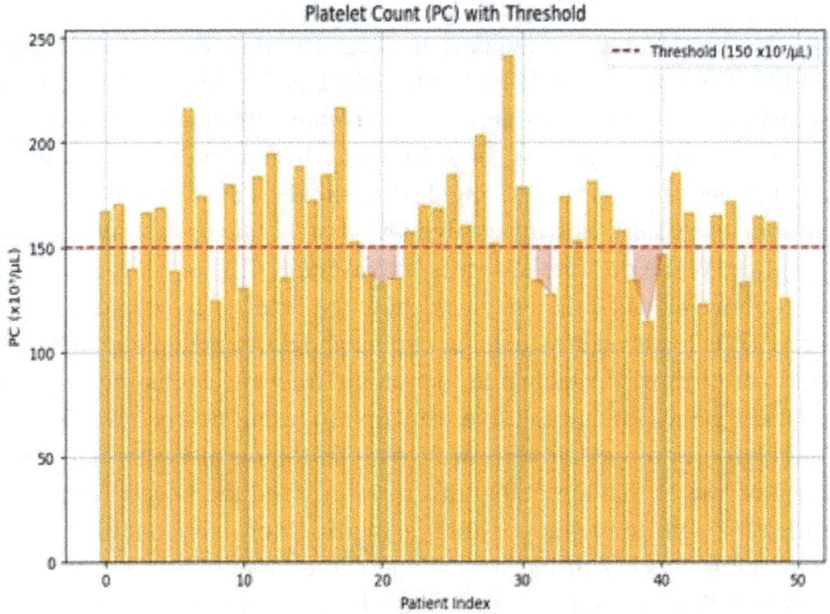

Hence, the research model lies on the right track with the book's theme since it outlines the top up-to-date AI trends in healthcare, more specifically real-time predictive models and the personalized disease prognostic model. It wisely addresses the inefficiency in computational power and the problem of interpretation with traditional models by coming up with the GNN approach that is both structured and scalable. Nevertheless, referring to the modern healthcare digital transformation landscape as a base for the new model's theme can be more informative.

FUTURE RESEARCH DIRECTIONS

One of the major strengths of the article is its integration of sparsity and attention mechanisms in a graph structure, which contributes to both accuracy and computational efficiency. These innovations are well-suited for deployment in edge-healthcare devices and real-time diagnostic settings. Leveraging this strength, future work can explore multi-disease prediction frameworks using similar architecture.

A key weakness of the article is the lack of clarity on the model's behavior under class imbalance, which is common in medical datasets. Furthermore, performance variability across diverse patient demographics was not addressed. Including stratified testing or cross-validation based on subgroups would help address this limitation.

CONCLUSION

In conclusion, the study of the core medical criteria—Blood Bilirubin Levels (BBL), Liver Enzyme Levels (LEL), Albumin Levels (AL), and Platelet Count (PC)—illustrates the great importance of each parameter being within its respective threshold limit. The average BBL of 1.0 mg/dL, 15% with data points which are approximately higher than the 1.2 mg/dL threshold, is a reason to be alert when high bilirubin levels start showing as high levels suggest liver dysfunction that may cause jaundice. While on liver enzymes, the average LEL of 35 U/L, out of 10% half that is above 40 U/L, the enzymes show the level of liver injury or inflammation 55 U/L is the level at which the patient should consult a doctor as it might be hepatitis or cirrhosis. Meanwhile, the albumin levels, excluding a few values that are unacceptably low for the liver function to occur, nearly have the majority over the 3.5 g/dL baseline and thus are mostly in the normal liver function range the low 5% of values that are below this threshold and the lowest value of 2.8 g/dL recorded, though, show the possible malnutrition or liver condition which can delay the healing process of the wound and cause more dangerous health issues such as wound decompensation. Lastly, the platelet count, with an average of 160 $\times 10^3/\mu L$ and 12% of data points which are lower than 150 $\times 10^3/\mu L$, indicates that low platelet count could lead to thrombocytopenia which in turn increases the risk of bleeding and bruising. The bottom line counting of 120 $\times 10^3/\mu L$ implies some potentially serious medical conditions, especially in patients with liver cirrhosis.

REFERENCES

Baskar, K., Venkatesan, G. K. D. P., & Sangeetha, S. (2020). A Survey of Workload Management Difficulties in the Public Cloud. *In Intelligent Computing in Engineering: Select Proceedings of RICE 2019* (pp. 491–499). DOI: 10.1007/978-981-15-2780-7_54

Chong Yin, Siqi Liu, Fei Lyu, Jiahao Lu, Sune Darkner, Vincent Wai-Sun Wong, & Pong C. Yuen. (2024). XFibrosis: Explicit Vessel-Fiber Modeling for Fibrosis Staging from Liver Pathology Images. *Computer Vision and Pattern Recognition*, 11282–11291.

Hassan, T. M., Elmogy, M., & Sallam, E.-S. (2017). Diagnosis of Focal Liver Diseases Based on Deep Learning Technique for Ultrasound Images. *Arabian Journal for Science and Engineering*, *42*(8), 3127–3140. DOI: 10.1007/s13369-016-2387-9

Hu, X., Sun, L., Zheng, R., Xia, X., Liu, M., Chen, W., Zhang, X., & Wang, C. (2024). Application of graph theory in liver research: A review. *Portal Hypertension & Cirrhosis*, *3*(4), 234–248. DOI: 10.1002/poh2.97

Huang, Y., Pu, Q., Lan, W., Huang, C., & Zhong, C. (2025). SMDPG: Identifying Metabolite-Disease Associations via Optimized Negative Sampling and Sparse Graph Convolutional Network. *IEEE Transactions on Computational Biology and Bioinformatics*, 1–12. DOI: 10.1109/TCBBIO.2025.3532256

Kexin Ding, Mu Zhou, Zichen Wang, Qiao Liu, Corey W. Arnold, Shaoting Zhang, & Dimitri N. Metaxas. (2022). Graph Convolutional Networks for Multi-modality Medical Imaging: Methods, Architectures, and Clinical Applications. *Electrical Engineering and Systems Science -Image and Video Processing, 3.*

Selvaraj, K., & Subbian, S. (2023). Inter-Scale Amalgam Cluster Dense Graph Convolutional Network for Hepatocellular Carcinoma Detection. *International Journal of Intelligent Engineering and Systems*, *16*(6), 356–365.

Li, J., Fu, T., Song, H., Fan, J., Xiao, D., Lin, Y., Gu, Y., & Yang, J. (2024). Embedding-Alignment Fusion-Based Graph Convolution Network With Mixed Learning Strategy for 4D Medical Image Reconstruction. *IEEE Journal of Biomedical and Health Informatics*, *28*(5), 2916–2929. DOI: 10.1109/JBHI.2024.3365203

Li, J., Kong, M., Wang, D., Yang, Z., & Hao, X. (2022). Prediction of lncRNA–Disease Associations via Closest Node Weight Graphs of the Spatial Neighborhood Based on the Edge Attention Graph Convolutional Network. *Frontiers in Genetics*, *12*. Advance online publication. DOI: 10.3389/fgene.2021.808962

Li, Y., Zhao, Y., Zhang, F., Liao, M., Yu, L., Chen, B., & Wang, Y. (2020). Liver segmentation from abdominal CT volumes based on level set and sparse shape composition. *Computer Methods and Programs in Biomedicine*, *195*, 105533. DOI: 10.1016/j.cmpb.2020.105533

Liang, Z., Zhang, S., Wei, A., Liu, Z., Wang, Y., Hu, H., Chen, W., & Qi, L. (2024). CylinGCN: Cylindrical structures segmentation in 3D biomedical optical imaging by a contour-based graph convolutional network. *Computerized Medical Imaging and Graphics*, *111*, 102316. DOI: 10.1016/j.compmedimag.2023.102316

Liu, D., Luo, Y., Zheng, J., Xu, H., Zhang, J., & Deng, L. (2021). GCNSDA: Predicting snoRNA-disease associations via graph convolutional network. *2021 IEEE International Conference on Bioinformatics and Biomedicine (BIBM)*, 183–188. https://doi.org/DOI: 10.1109/BIBM52615.2021.9669505

Liu, K., Sun, X., Jia, L., Ma, J., Xing, H., Wu, J., Gao, H., Sun, Y., Boulnois, F., & Fan, J. (2019). Chemi-Net: A Molecular Graph Convolutional Network for Accurate Drug Property Prediction. *International Journal of Molecular Sciences*, *20*(14), 3389. DOI: 10.3390/ijms20143389

Liu, W., Lu, P., & Zhou, J. (2025). Enhancing Disease-metabolite Associations Prediction with Weighted Graph Convolutional Networks Based on Community-driven Link Completion. *IEEE Transactions on Computational Biology and Bioinformatics*, 1–13. DOI: 10.1109/TCBBIO.2025.3532644

Sangeetha, S. (2016). A study on problems and challenges faced by micro small and medium enterprises: A special reference to manufacturing sector in Coimbatore district. *International Journal of Academic Research and Development*, *1*(9), 29–33.

Sangeetha, S., Suganya, P., Shanthini, S., Murthy, G. N. K., & Sathya, R. (2023). Crime Rate Prediction and Prevention: Unleashing the Power of Deep Learning. *Proceedings of the 4th International Conference on Smart Electronics and Communication, ICOSEC 2023*. https://doi.org/DOI: 10.1109/ICOSEC58147.2023.10276012

Wang, T., Shao, W., Huang, Z., Tang, H., Zhang, J., Ding, Z., & Huang, K. (2021). MOGONET integrates multi-omics data using graph convolutional networks allowing patient classification and biomarker identification. *Nature Communications*, *12*(1), 3445. DOI: 10.1038/s41467-021-23774-w

Yang, B., Yang, Y., Wang, M., & Su, X. (2023). MRGCN: Cancer subtyping with multi-reconstruction graph convolutional network using full and partial multi-omics dataset. *Bioinformatics (Oxford, England)*, *39*(6). Advance online publication. DOI: 10.1093/bioinformatics/btad353

Zhang, C., Zhang, Z., Zhang, F., Zeng, B., Liu, X., & Wang, L. (2024). A computational model for potential microbe–disease association detection based on improved graph convolutional networks and multi-channel autoencoders. *Frontiers in Microbiology, 15*. Advance online publication. DOI: 10.3389/fmicb.2024.1435408

Zhou, L., Wang, N., Zhu, Z., Gao, H., Zhou, Y., & Fang, M. (2024). Identification of subtypes in digestive system tumors based on multi-omics data and graph convolutional network. *International Journal of Machine Learning and Cybernetics, 15*(9), 3567–3577. https://doi.org/10.1007/s13042-024-02109-3

Nakatsuka, T., Tateishi, R., Sato, M., Hashizume, N., & Kamada, A.. (2025). Deep learning and digital pathology powers prediction of HCC development in steatotic liver disease. *Hepatology (Baltimore, Md.), 81*(3), 976–989. DOI: 10.1097/HEP.0000000000000904

Dabbah, S., Mishani, I., Davidov, Y., & Ben Ari, Z. (2025). Implementation of Machine Learning Algorithms to Screen for Advanced Liver Fibrosis in Metabolic Dysfunction-Associated Steatotic Liver Disease: An In-Depth Explanatory Analysis. *Digestion, 106*(3), 189–202. DOI: 10.1159/000542241

Noor, S., AlQahtani, S. A., & Khan, S. (2025). Chronic liver disease detection using ranking and projection-based feature optimization with deep learning. *AIMS Bioengineering, 12*(1), 50–68. DOI: 10.3934/bioeng.2025003

Theerthagiri, P. (2025), Liver disease classification using histogram-based gradient boosting classification tree with feature selection algorithm, *Biomedical Signal Processing and Control,* Volume 100, Part C,107102, ISSN 1746-8094, https://doi.org/10.1016/j.bspc.2024.107102

Saeed, F., Shiwlani, A., Umar, M., Jahangir, Z., Tahir, A., & Shiwlani, S. (2025). Hepatocellular Carcinoma Prediction in HCV Patients using Machine Learning and Deep Learning Techniques. *Jurnal Ilmiah Computer Science, 3*(2), 120–134. https://doi.org/10.58602/jics.v3i2.48

Udompap, P., Liu, K., Attia, I. Z., Canning, R. E., Benson, J. T., Therneau, T. M., Noseworthy, P. A., Friedman, P. A., Rattan, P., Ahn, J. C., Simonetto, D. A., Shah, V. H., Kamath, P. S., & Allen, A. M. (2025). Performance of AI-Enabled Electrocardiogram in the Prediction of Metabolic Dysfunction-Associated Steatotic Liver Disease. *Clinical Gastroenterology and Hepatology, 23*(4), 574–582.e3. DOI: 10.1016/j.cgh.2024.08.009

Kiran, A., Neerugatti, V., & Kumar, D. S. J. Somasekar, Santhosh Boddupalli, B. Sai Praneetha (2024), Revolutionizing cirrhosis liver disorder diagnosis: A deep learning approach with convolutional neural networks,V. Sharmila et al. (Eds), Challenges in Information, Communication and Computing Technology,449-454, Taylor & Francis Group

ADDITIONAL READING

Savaş, S. (2025). Explainable Artificial Intelligence for Diagnosis and Staging of Liver Cirrhosis Using Stacked Ensemble and Multi-Task Learning. *Diagnostics (Basel)*, *15*(9), 1177. https://doi.org/10.3390/diagnostics15091177

Edwin Raja, S., Sutha, J., Elamparithi, P., Jaya Deepthi, K., & Lalitha, S. D. (2025). Liver tumor prediction using attention-guided convolutional neural networks and genomic feature analysis. *MethodsX*, *14*, 103276. https://doi.org/10.1016/j.mex.2025.103276

KEY TERMS AND DEFINITIONS

Graph Convolutional Networks (GCNs): Neural networks that work with graph data to help predict diseases by capturing relationships between medical features.

Attention Mechanisms: A method in AI that helps models focus on the most important parts of data for better predictions.

Sparse Graph Representations: A simplified graph with fewer connections that keeps important information while using less computing power.

Multi-modal Graph-Based Learning: A technique that combines different types of medical data in a graph to improve disease prediction.

Liver Diseases: Serious health problems affecting the liver, often hard to detect early and needing accurate diagnosis.

Chapter 11
Artificial Intelligence Enabled Dynamic Drug Overdose Response System

Sachin Sharma
https://orcid.org/0000-0002-7821-3685
Amity University, Mohali, India

Kumar Mayank
https://orcid.org/0009-0009-6056-4880
Graphic Era University, Dehradun, India

Prachi Pandey
Graphic Era University, Dehradun, India

ABSTRACT

The present-day medical industry is battling an ever-increasing number of drug overdose cases, which has led to a global public health emergency and necessitated the development of alternative measures. This chapter presents the Dynamic Drug Overdose Response System (DDORS), an innovative program that makes use of artificial intelligence (AI) to rethink strategies for preventing and responding to drug overdoses. The system integrates real-time data analysis with machine learning algorithms, as well as a user-friendly healthcare application developed using Flutter all of which together form. This chapter also describes how an AI-based diabetes prediction & classification system was designed to demonstrate the wide-ranging applicability of diagnostic tools in healthcare settings where artificial intelligence is concerned. Such an inclusion affirms our belief in the need for a holistic approach

DOI: 10.4018/979-8-3373-2043-4.ch011

towards addressing different types of healthcare challenges, from acute crises to chronic conditions like diabetes.

INTRODUCTION

With the increase in drug overdose cases, there is a pressing need for new public health strategies. DDORS proposes combining AI with real-time data analytics and mobile technology to establish a responsive system that can predict, prevent and respond to drug overdoses. By using past records in addition to sophisticated machine learning algorithms, DDORS hopes to decrease the number of OD incidents as well as enhance emergency intervention time. For wide-reaching compatibility and ease of use across different platforms, the framework used in building this system is Flutter. This means that it can be accessed by people from various backgrounds who may be restricted by geography or other technological limitations. Through the mobile app healthcare workers are able to communicate fast among themselves and with first responders and community members. In order to illustrate more possibilities of artificial intelligence in health care provision, a diabetes prediction and classification system developed alongside DDORS is discussed in this article. Similar techniques are applied here where patterns are identified within patient records through AI leading to early detection and personalized treatment plans. The additional inclusion of this system shows how far-reaching AI can be when it comes to addressing different healthcare needs using advanced technology. There are a few common sorts of screenings utilized to analyze diabetes or evaluate a person's chance of creating it:

- Fasting Plasma Glucose (FPG) Test: This test measures your blood sugar level after an overnight quick. A fasting plasma glucose level of 126 milligrams per deciliter (mg/dL) or higher demonstrates diabetes.
- Oral Glucose Tolerance Test (OGTT): This includes drinking a sugary arrangement and after that measuring blood sugar levels two hours afterward. A blood sugar level of 200 mg/dL or higher after two hours shows diabetes.
- Random Plasma Glucose Test: This test includes measuring blood sugar levels at any time, notwithstanding of after you final ate. A random blood sugar level of 200 mg/dL or higher, together with side effects of diabetes, demonstrates diabetes.
- Hemoglobin A1c (HbA1c) Test: This test measures your normal blood sugar level over the past 2-3 months. An HbA1c level of 6.5% or higher shows diabetes.

- Risk Assessment Questionnaires: These are utilized to evaluate a person's chance components for creating diabetes. They regularly inquire almost family history, age, weight, physical movement level, and other components.
- Glycated Albumin Test (GA): This test measures the rate of glycated egg whites within the blood, giving an sign of blood sugar levels over the past 2-3 weeks.
- Continuous Glucose Monitoring (CGM): CGM includes wearing a little sensor beneath the skin to degree blood sugar levels all through the day and night. It can give point by point data around glucose designs and patterns.

The strategies and clues utilized in distinguishing the nearness of drugs within the body shift concurring to the sort of sedate; be that as it may, there are a few common pointers and approaches:

The general signs and symptoms for identifying drug overdose are the following:

- Mental Functions: Disarray, Furiousness beyond limit or irritation beyond limit, Sleepiness or coma, Inconscience or dullness to external stimuli
- Breathing Problems: Rhythmical shallow breaths, Difficulty breathing, Absence of breathing
- Heart Problems: Fast or irregular pulse rate, Slow pulse rate, Low blood pressure levels, Nervous System Abnormalities: Epileptic fit(s), Muscle jerks or convulsions
- Other Physical Indications: Throwing up and feeling like vomiting, Having blue skin colouration due to low oxygen supply (cyanosis), Large open / very small closed circular muscles in centre of iris (pupils), Too much perspiration / cold damp skin with appearance somewhat like wax (clammy skin), Ache around navel area (abdominal pain)
- Different Drugs Show Different Signs: Opioids: Smaller than normal pupils; slow respiration; bluish discoloration caused by lack of O2 (cyanosis); unawareness. Stimulants e.g., cocaine, methamphetamine etc.: Restlessness; increased activity level; faster heartbeat rates than normal; chest pains felt as tight squeezing sensations lasting seconds/minutes long enough for someone else to notice them as well – followed by sudden muscle contractions throughout most parts/layers comprising each affected joint/space on one side only which may include either upper limbs alone but not lower extremities; arms and legs flailing uncontrollably at times (seizures).
- Depressants e.g., benzodiazepines, barbiturates etc.: Very strong desire to sleep more than usual amounts of time taken up by such activity alone or together with other similar ones until further notice; breathing slowly; loss of coordination.

- Alcohol: Disorientation, coma, throwing up, slow breathing, unawareness.

Together, DDORS and the diabetes prediction and classification system represent the future of AI-enabled healthcare. By harnessing the power of AI, real-time data, and user-friendly applications, these systems offer hope for more effective responses to public health crises and improved patient outcomes. Our research underscores the critical role technology plays in addressing global healthcare challenges and lays the foundation for a future where AI is an integral part of medical practice. The escalating emergency of medicate overdoses requests inventive and immediate arrangements. Traditional reaction instruments, whereas vital, frequently face impediments in speed, asset allotment, and prescient capabilities. Typically where Artificial Intelligence (AI)-enabled dynamic medicate overdose reaction frameworks rise as a transformative approach, advertising the potential to revolutionize how we combat this open health crisis. These sophisticated frameworks use the control of AI, machine learning, and real-time information to create a proactive, versatile, and exceedingly proficient system for anticipating and reacting to overdoses. At its center, an AI-enabled energetic overdose reaction framework points to move from receptive intercessions to prescient avoidance and quick, optimized crisis reaction.

By coordination assorted information streams—including emergency medical services (EMS) calls, hospital admissions, social media patterns, illicit drug showcase insights, and indeed wastewater analysis—AI algorithms can identify rising hotspots, predict overdose surges, and pinpoint high-risk people or communities. This predictive capability permits for the vital pre-positioning of assets, such as naloxone distribution, mobile outreach groups, and community-based bolster administrations, accurately where and when they are most required. Beyond expectation, these frameworks empower crisis responders with real-time situational mindfulness. Wearable sensors, keen celerity frameworks, and coordinates communication stages can give pivotal data around a person's condition, the nearness of specific substances, and the foremost viable intervention procedures (Rawat et al., 2025). AI can direct dispatchers in prioritizing calls, recommend optimal courses for to begin with responders, and indeed help paramedics with real-time symptomatic bolster and treatment conventions. Besides, the "dynamic" aspect of these frameworks implies they continually learn and adjust. As new data becomes accessible, the AI models refine their forecasts and reaction recommendations, guaranteeing the framework remains exceedingly viable in an ever-evolving emergency. Eventually, by harnessing AI, we will move towards a future where overdose responses are not just quicker, but more brilliant, more focused on, and eventually, more life-saving. The heightening sedate overdose emergency, especially driven by opioids, has developed as a basic open wellbeing challenge universally, claiming endless lives and straining healthcare frameworks.

Within the United States alone, over 107,000 overdose passings were detailed in 2023, with opioids bookkeeping for more than 80,000 of these fatalities. This emergency, fueled by the expanding predominance of synthetic opioids like fentanyl, underscores the critical require for imaginative, data-driven arrangements to moderate its destroying affect. Traditional approaches to overdose avoidance and reaction, such as manual surveillance, prescription drug monitoring programs, and crisis medical intercessions, have struggled to keep pace with the scale and complexity of the scourge. These strategies frequently depend on labor-intensive forms, delayed information reporting, and divided frameworks, coming about in missed openings for opportune mediations. The coming of Artificial Intelligence (AI) offers a transformative opportunity to address these inadequacies by empowering energetic, real-time, and exact reactions to sedate overdoses. An AI-enabled Dynamic Drug Overdose Response System (DDORS) leverages progressed computational strategies, such as machine learning (ML), natural language processing (NLP), and predictive modeling, to improve observation, discovery, anticipation, and treatment of medicate overdoses. By coordination tremendous datasets from electronic health records (EHRs), medical analyst reports, wearable gadgets, and social determinants of wellbeing, such a framework can recognize at-risk people, predict overdose patterns, optimize asset assignment, and encourage quick mediations, eventually sparing lives and diminishing the societal burden of compulsion.

This chapter investigates the conceptual system, mechanical components, applications, challenges, and future potential of an AI-enabled DDORS, emphasizing its role in revolutionizing the reaction to the overdose emergency. The establishment of an AI-enabled DDORS lies in its capacity to prepare and analyze large-scale, heterogeneous information sources in genuine time. Unlike conventional surveillance frameworks, which frequently endure from delays in information collection and detailing, AI-driven frameworks can total and decipher information from different streams, counting EHRs, prescription drug monitoring programs (PDMPs), emergency medical services (EMS) information, and indeed unstructured content from medical examiners' reports (Sharma et al., 2025). Machine learning algorithms, a cornerstone of AI, empower the framework to recognize designs and patterns in overdose incidents by analyzing factors such as medicine histories, statistic profiles, and geospatial information. For occasion, predictive modeling can survey hazard factors—such as earlier substance utilize, mental wellbeing analyze, or financial conditions—to hail people at tall hazard of overdose. Ponders, such as those by Goodman-Meza et al., have illustrated the adequacy of NLP in classifying substances included in overdose passings by mining unstructured medical records, achieving tall precision in recognizing patterns and supporting hypothesis era. These capabilities permit open wellbeing authorities to move past receptive measures, empowering proactive methodologies like focused on naloxone conveyance or custom fitted open wellbeing campaigns. By coordination real-time information from wearable gadgets, such as heart rate screens or glucose sensors, an AI-enabled DDORS can assist improve its predictive control, recognizing physiological changes characteristic of an impending overdose and activating immediate cautions to to begin with responders or healthcare providers.

The application of AI in overdose reaction expands beyond surveillance to personalized mediation and treatment optimization (Devliyal et al., 2024). Machine learning models, such as those based on Bayesian non-parametrics or profound learning, can foresee individualized treatment reactions by analyzing patient-specific information, counting genetic inclinations, restorative histories, and social determinants. For case, AI can optimize dosing regimens for medicines like buprenorphine or methadone, utilized in medication-assisted treatment (Mat) for opioid use disorder (OUD), by continuously learning from persistent results. This energetic alteration guarantees most extreme efficacy whereas minimizing adverse impacts, tending to the confinements of inactive treatment conventions. Besides, AI-driven apparatuses like CURATE.AI have appeared guarantee in fitting combination treatments for OUD, adjusting measurements based on real-time understanding reactions. Such personalized approaches are basic intending to the heterogeneity of addiction, where components like polydrug utilize or co-occurring mental wellbeing disorders complicate treatment. By joining social and natural data—such as lodging precariousness or community-level overdose rates—AI can moreover advise holistic intercessions, interfacing at-risk people with social administrations or recovery programs. This multifaceted approach adjusts with the broader objective of lessening overdose fatalities whereas advancing long-term recovery. A key component of an AI-enabled DDORS is its capacity for early discovery and quick reaction.

Tools like eToxPred, which anticipate the toxicity of chemical compounds, can distinguish developing synthetic drugs with tall overdose potential early in their circulation, empowering preemptive activity. Additionally, NLP-driven frameworks can analyze social media, EMS reports, or hospital confirmation information to identify surges in overdose episodes, giving real-time alarms to open wellbeing specialists. For instance, UCLA analysts have created calculations that prepare restorative examiners' passing certificates to recognize overdose causes with unprecedented speed, reducing the lag time in surveillance information from months to weeks. This fast discovery is basic for deploying assets like naloxone, an opioid overdose inversion sedate, to high-risk ranges. AI can optimize the dispersion of naloxone by foreseeing where overdoses are likely to happen, guaranteeing that first responders and community organizations are enough prepared. Moreover, mobile health (mHealth) applications, fueled by AI, can enable people to survey their own chance for OUD in private, overcoming boundaries like shame or need of access to healthcare. These apps can give assets, interface clients to suppliers, and indeed coordinated with wearable gadgets to screen crucial signs, activating crisis reactions when essential.

Despite its transformative potential, executing an AI-enabled DDORS faces a few challenges. Information quality and integration stay noteworthy obstacles, as healthcare frameworks regularly work in silos, with conflicting information groups and restricted interoperability. Incomplete or one-sided datasets, such as those skewed by underreporting in underserved communities, can compromise the exactness of AI expectations. Moral concerns too emerge, especially with respect to quiet security and the potential abuse of delicate wellbeing information. Guaranteeing compliance with controls like HIPAA whereas keeping up vigorous information security is vital. Additionally, the "black box" nature of a few AI models, especially profound learning, raises concerns approximately interpretability, as clinicians and policymakers may falter to believe expectations without clear clarifications. To address this, reasonable AI strategies, such as highlight significance examination, are being developed to improve transparency. Moreover, incongruities in access to innovation and healthcare foundation seem exacerbate disparities, limiting the system's reach in rustic or low-income ranges. Overcoming these challenges requires a multidisciplinary approach, combining skill from information science, open health, and social work to guarantee impartial and dependable usage. The societal and economic suggestions of an AI-enabled DDORS are significant.

Advances in multiomics information investigation, which combines genomics, proteomics, and metabolomics, may improve the system's capacity to foresee person reactions to compulsion treatments. Wearable gadgets and Internet of Things (IoT) advances will encourage empower real-time checking, making a closed-loop framework where information collection, investigation, and intervention happen consistently. Partnerships between the scholarly community, industry, and government are fundamental to scale these frameworks, guaranteeing they are available over different populaces. Open-source stages, like those utilized in COVID-19 investigate, seem encourage information sharing and quicken advancement. Additionally, tending to the social determinants of addiction—such as destitution, injury, and stigma—through AI-driven experiences will be vital for long-term victory. By combining mechanical ability with a human-centered approach, an AI-enabled DDORS has the potential to convert the overdose response landscape, advertising hope within the fight against one of the most pressing public health emergencies of our time.

BACKGROUND

Opioid dependency is convoluted, with a lot of various genetic and environmental factors influencing. Opioid overdose as the deadliest outcome is one of the leading causes of accidental deaths in America. Our research studied how opioid overdose changes the brain by determining variations in particular neuronal DNA markers. Comparatively, we observed widespread alterations in these markers among cases that had died from opioids compared to controls. We were able to predict accurately if samples came from overdose cases or controls through use of machine learning based on these markers. Several other studies showed that genes affected differently between individuals who overdosed on opioids and other drugs. Additionally, five genes related greatly to these alterations were linked not only to opioid addiction but also traits such as fear, sexual behavior, and educational level. This unravels the neurobiological bases of dependence on opioids and underscores the role played by genetic and environmental forces in feeding into this crisis over these drug substances (Ward et al., 2019). Schell et al. (2021) explores the research paper focus on importance of knowing what causes opioid overdose death in a neighborhood so that prevention activities can be directed appropriately.

For example, in Rhode Island, data on opioid overdose deaths and other community features were matched with the American Community Survey. Socioeconomic factors like education level, income earned, and occupation held were found to predict these deaths as anticipated using machine learning techniques. Nevertheless, we discovered predictors not previously identified including residency tenure, ethnicity of residents and loneliness as seen from the isolation indices. In such ways, we can identify areas at high risk through predictive models for resources distribution aimed at combating opioid epidemic more effectively within the ever-changing trends. Bozorgi et al. (2021) explores Unintentional death in the US caused by drug overdose is a leading reason for the decline of life expectancy. The increased rates of overdose, particularly opioids, are a major public health concern due to increasing number of nonfatal overdoses and hospitalizations. However, it should be noted that non-fatal incidents are often more prevalent than fatal ones with their severe health implications. Several recurrent overdoses can result into chronic physical and cognitive impairments while risky behaviors with drugs also put people at risk of contracting like hepatitis and HIV. Some measures to address the overdose epidemic include

Medication-Assisted Treatment (MAT), Narcan distribution, support programs as well as prescription drug monitoring programs. There are however still very few interventions that can help prevent these deaths from happening. Knowing neighborhood-level predictors of drug overdose is vital for community-based intervention; however, only few studies have been conducted in this area. Traditional statistical approaches have some limitations, but machine learning allows one to search for patterns in complex datasets more flexibly. The main objective of this study is to fill this gap through innovative machine learning and geospatial techniques aimed at predicting drug overdose risks at the neighborhood level. Feng et al. (2019) discuss Drug induced liver injury (DILI), that is a common adverse effect that often results in delays in drug development or removal from the market. Early prediction of DILI is difficult but important to ensure drug safety. This research paper describes the construction of a deep learning model using gene expression data to predict DILI. The model was optimized by selecting different genes and tuning parameters. A support vector machine (SVM) was also developed for comparison purposes. The best deep learning model achieved 97.1% accuracy, surpassing the SVM model's accuracy (88.9%). Validation and animal experiments confirmed the accuracy of this deep learning model. This could be useful in generating substantial data needed for effective decision-making during drug discovery and clinical use, thus ensuring better practices of drug safety evaluation procedures.

Islam et al. (2018) depicts Pharmaceutical industry and medical diagnosis are highly affected by Adverse Drug Reactions (ADRs). Basically, the extensive preclinical testing undertaken doesn't guarantee totally complete safety. Thus, statistical, data mining and machine learning methods using Electronic Health Records (EHRs) have been increasingly employed for detection and prediction of ADRs.To this concern, a hybrid model is put forward that combines both data mining and machine learning for identification of ADRs as well as their intensity. Proportionality Reporting Ratio (PRR) and Chi-Square test are necessary for establishing drug-symptom associations. These findings feed into machine learning algorithms Random Forest or Support Vector Machine (SVM), together with demographic details about patients which predict outcomes of ADRs. The model has achieved an accurate rate of 91% when predicting 'death' as an outcome of ADRs.

IMPORTANCE OF DRUG OVERDOSE RESPONSE SYSTEM

The basic significance of a robust Drug Overdose Response System (DORS) for patients cannot be exaggerated, particularly within the confront of raising overdose epidemics all inclusive. Such frameworks are not only receptive measures; they speak to a multifaceted approach to moderating harm, saving lives, and giving crucial pathways to recuperation for people hooking with substance utilize clutters. From prompt crisis mediation to long-term back, a well-designed DORS acts as a crucial security net, ensuring helpless populaces and lightening the immense strain put on healthcare frameworks and communities. At its center, the essential work of a DORS is quick and viable crisis mediation. This starts with quick access to life-saving medicines, most eminently naloxone. Naloxone, an opioid enemy, can invert the impacts of an opioid overdose inside minutes, reestablishing breathing and awareness. The broad accessibility of naloxone, coupled with preparing for to begin with responders (paramedics, police, firefighters) and progressively, laypersons (family members, friends, community outreach workers), is essential to a fruitful DORS. Each minute counts amid an overdose; brain harm can occur rapidly due to oxygen hardship. A framework that encourages prompt recognition of an overdose and prompt organization of naloxone significantly increments the chances of survival and decreases the probability of long-term neurological complications for the quiet (Kapruwan et al., 2025a).

Without such a framework, endless people would surrender to preventable passings, taking off families and communities shattered. Past quick inversion, a comprehensive DORS expands to the facilitated endeavors of emergency medical services (EMS). This incorporates quick celerity, talented paramedics prepared to supply progressed life bolster, and effective transport to fitting therapeutic offices. Patients who have gotten naloxone still require medical appraisal and regularly advance care, as the impacts of naloxone can wear off, driving to re-narcosis, or there may be co-ingestions or basic medical conditions that require tending to (Devgan et al., 2025). The seamless move from pre-hospital mediation to hospital-based care is vital for stabilizing the understanding, overseeing any complications, and ensuring a thorough medical evaluation. This coordinated reaction avoids secondary complications and offers the understanding a basic window for advance intervention. Besides, a imperative viewpoint of a DORS is the arrangement of post-overdose care and linkage to progressing treatment. An overdose occasion, whereas unnerving, can too be a essential minute for a persistent, serving as a "teachable moment" or a emergency point where they may be more open to assist.

A genuinely successful DORS recognizes this opportunity and coordinating pathways to compulsion treatment and harm lessening administrations (Gupta & Sharma, 2024). This could include peer support specialists meeting patients in crisis divisions, giving quick sympathy and association, or coordinate referrals to inpatient or outpatient treatment programs, medication-assisted treatment (Mat) clinics, and counseling services. The objective is to move past only sparing a life within the minute to advertising a tangible way towards sustained recovery and well-being. Without these linkages, patients are at a essentially higher hazard of encountering repeated overdoses, sustaining a perilous cycle. Information collection and surveillance are moreover vital components of a strong DORS. Real-time information on overdose episodes, demographics of affected people, substances included, and areas of events are basic for understanding the scope of the issue, recognizing rising patterns (e.g., the spread of fentanyl or other strong engineered opioids), and allocating resources successfully. This information advises open wellbeing mediations, permits for the focused on distribution of naloxone, helps recognize high-risk zones for expanded outreach, and guides approach choices. For occasion, an startling cluster of overdoses in a specific neighborhood may trigger a quick open wellbeing reaction, counting focused on naloxone dissemination, community alarms, and expanded outreach administrations. This proactive utilize of information changes the DORS from a simply responsive component into a capable device for public health prevention and moderation.

Besides, a DORS cultivates a culture of hurt reduction inside communities. By advancing naloxone openness, educating overdose acknowledgment, and decreasing the shame related with sedate utilize and overdose, these frameworks engage people to act and back their peers. This community-based approach democratizes overdose reaction, making it less dependent exclusively on professional crisis services and more ingrained within the fabric of way of life. Decriminalization endeavors and Good Samaritan laws, regularly integrated with DORS, assist empower people to call for offer assistance during an overdose without fear of legal repercussions, hence expanding the probability of convenient mediation. This move in open recognition, from judgment to kindness and support, is basic for reaching people who might something else maintain a strategic distance from looking for offer assistance. The financial and social benefits of a DORS are too substantial. Whereas the immediate costs of emergency reaction and treatment might appear high, they are dwarfed by the long-term costs related with untreated substance utilize disarranges, counting chronic wellbeing issues, imprisonment, misfortune of efficiency, and untimely passing. By avoiding overdose fatalities and encouraging access to treatment, a DORS diminishes healthcare consumptions, increments workforce interest, and strengthens the social texture of communities. Saving a life isn't fair an ethical basic; it is an venture in human capital and societal well-being.

At last, the significance of a DORS is intensified for particular powerless populations. Homeless people, those recently released from incarceration, people with co-occurring mental wellbeing disarranges, and individuals who infuse drugs are frequently at a excessively higher chance of overdose. A DORS that's socially competent and particularly tailored to reach these populaces, through road outreach, syringe benefit programs, and coordinates care models, is foremost. These frameworks guarantee that the foremost marginalized people, who may face significant barriers to conventional healthcare, still have get to to life-saving mediations and pathways to recuperation. A comprehensive Drug Overdose Response System is far more than fair an emergency benefit; it could be a basic public health framework that touches each arrange of an overdose occasion and past. From the immediate reversal of a possibly deadly overdose to directing patients towards supported recuperation and illuminating broad open health strategies, a DORS shields lives, mitigates enduring, and offers trust to people and communities grappling with the destroying affect of substance utilize clutters. Its significance for patients lies in its capacity to convert a minute of emergency into an opportunity for life-saving intervention, compassionate care, and eventually, a chance at a more advantageous future.

Prospposed System

Creating a system that predicts and classifies diabetes is a significant development in healthcare because it can help with early detection, individualized treatment, and cost reduction. However, this also comes with several challenges especially on data precision ethics and technicalities. The benefits of a Diabetes Forecasting and Categorization Mechanism:

- Timely Detection and Intervention: It can pick out those people who are prone to contracting diabetes thus providing an opportunity for early prevention against the illness.
- Personalized Medicine: The approach diagnoses different types of diabetes hence enabling personalized treatment plans that lead to better management of the condition.
- Less Expensive Healthcare: Long term hospitalization costs could be reduced through early recognition as well as correct categorization because this will lower complications.
- Better Patient Outcomes: When treatment decisions are made earlier on and they are more accurate due to improved classification, then patients will have improved outcomes in terms of their health and also quality of life.
- More Effective Planning For Health Services: By forecasting how likely it is for members within a given population to develop diabetes, care providers may allocate resources better or even manage patient care effectively.
- Research and Development: This system provides researchers with predictive models which can be used in identifying risk factors associated with diabetes such as genetic markers among others so that new prevention strategies and treatments could be developed.

The challenges of a Diabetes Prediction and Classification System:

- Data Quality and Accuracy: The efficiency of the program is determined by how good the data it uses is. When collecting data, errors could be made or sometimes there may be disparities leading to wrong forecasts.
- Ethical and Privacy Concerns: Privacy laws must be adhered to strictly when handling confidential health information. In addition, ethical guide-

lines should not be violated as they can cause discrimination against patients through misuse of these records.

- Technical Complexity: Technological know-how is necessary for developers because they need large computational resources alongside sophisticated machine learning models so that their predictive models become more accurate.
- Bias and Fairness: Certain groups might receive unfair predictions from this system due to some unintended biases embedded during training; therefore eliminating bias while ensuring fairness remains paramount.
- Integration with Existing Healthcare Systems: Compatibility issues arising from resistance towards change make it difficult for this system integration into an existing healthcare infrastructure which utilizes electronic health records (EHR).
- Regulatory Compliance: For compliance purposes, healthcare regulations must be followed together with data protection laws. For example, in America systems are expected to meet the HIPAA standards while those within Europe ought to adhere to GDPR requirements.
- Patient Involvement and Instruction: Patient involvement and instruction are imperative for this organization to succeed. People must comprehend predictions and categories so they can decide what to do next about their own health.
- Development of Prototype for Healthcare preventing the overdose of drugs by providing diabetes prediction and classification system, Healthcare App using Flutter. [Figure 1]

Figure 1. Development process of prototype.

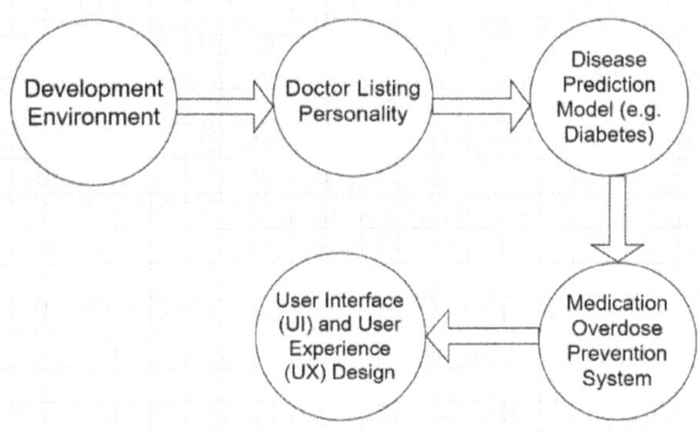

The approach for utilizing machine learning techniques to diagnosis the diabetes using prediction as well as classification system. Figure 2 explores the proposed framework.

Figure 2 Proposed Framework.

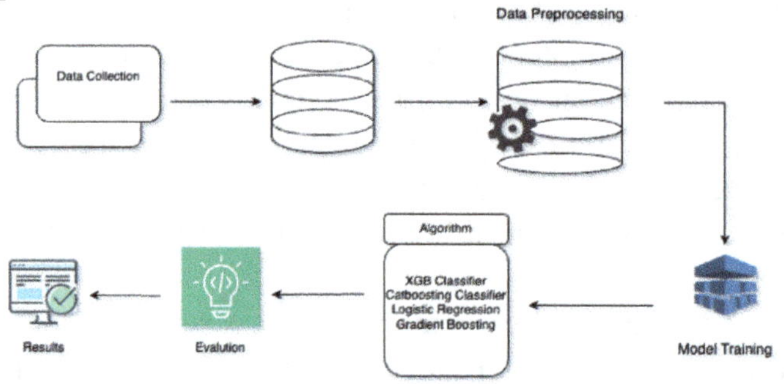

Dataset: For Diabetes Prediction System. Our dataset has a size of 10,000 rows. The dataset contains these following parameters: Age, Hypertension, Heart–disease, Smoking history, BMI, HbA1c levels, Blood glucose levels, and Gender.

For Diabetes Classification System: Our dataset has a size of 800 rows. The dataset contains these following parameters: Pregnancies, Glucose, Blood Pressure, Skin Thickness, Insulin, BMI, Diabetes Pedigree Function, Age

Preprocessing: For Diabetes Prediction System. Check Duplicates: Identifying duplicate entries in a dataset to ensure data integrity and avoid redundancy. In Python's Pandas, this can be achieved using df.duplicated() to find duplicates and df.drop_duplicates() to remove them.

Recategorizing (Feature: Smoking Status): Recategorizing involves modifying categorical data, like combining, splitting, or renaming categories. If your dataset has a "Smoking Status" feature, you might recategorize it to simplify or standardize the categories.

Transformers: These are tools used to preprocess data, making it suitable for analysis or modeling. Common transformers include:

- Standard Scaler: Standardizes features by removing the mean and scaling to unit variance. Often used in machine learning workflows to normalize data.
- One-Hot Encoder: Converts categorical data into numerical format, creating binary columns for each category.

For Diabetes Classification System:

- Check Null Figures: Identifying missing or null values in a dataset. This is part of data preprocessing since missing values can impact analysis and modeling. Techniques to handle null values include removal, imputation, or replacement with a specific value.
- KNN Imputer: A method to fill in missing values based on the nearest neighbors' approach. This is part of data preprocessing because it addresses missing data.
- Power Transformer (Yeo-Johnson Method): A transformation technique used to stabilize variance and make data more normally distributed. This is part of preprocessing to prepare data for modeling.
- SMOTEEN: A data augmentation technique used to address class imbalance by combining SMOTE (Synthetic Minority Over-sampling Technique) with EN (Edited Nearest Neighbors). This is part of preprocessing when dealing with imbalanced datasets.

Machine Learning Techniques Used: For Diabetes Prediction System. For prediction system, Xgboost Algorithm is being used. XGBoost (Extreme Gradient Boosting) is a powerful and efficient machine learning algorithm for supervised learning tasks, especially classification and regression. XGBoost is an optimized implementation of the gradient boosting framework, designed to be fast, efficient, and highly flexible.

For Diabetes Classification System: For classification system, following algorithms are used i.e. XGBClassifier, CatBoosting Classifier, Logistic Regression, Gradient Boosting, Support Vector Classifier, AdaBoost Classifier, Random Forest, K-Neighbors Classifier, and Decision Tree.

SOLUTIONS AND RECOMMENDATIONS

Figure 3 depicts the screenshots of prototype. Figure 4 explores the accuracy Graph. Table 1 discusses the result of diabetes prediction system. Table 2 explores the accuracy results of diabetes prediction system. Table 3 depicts the accuracy results of hyperparameter tuning. Table 4 explores the comparative analysis.

Figure 3. Screenshots of prototype.

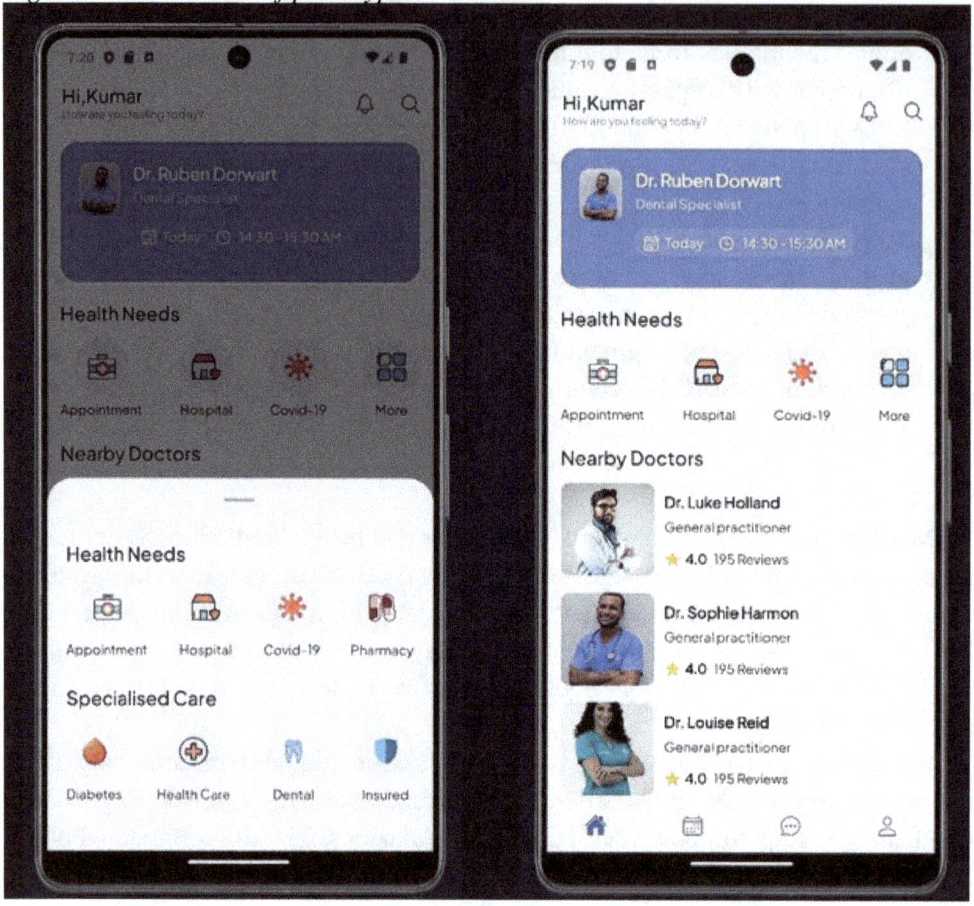

Table 1. Result of diabetes prediction system.

Model	**Xgboost**
Mean Accuracy	93.6%
Test Accuracy	97.19%

Table 2. Accuracy results of diabetes prediction system.

Model Name	**Accuracy (in percentage)**
XGB Classifier	95.7985
CatBoosting Classifier	95.7983
Logistic Regression	94.1176
Gradient Boostin	93.2773
Support Vector Classifier	92.437
AdaBoost Classifier	92.437
Random Forest	91.1596
K-Neighbors Classifier	91.1576
Decision Tree	90.7563

Figure 4. Accuracy Graph.

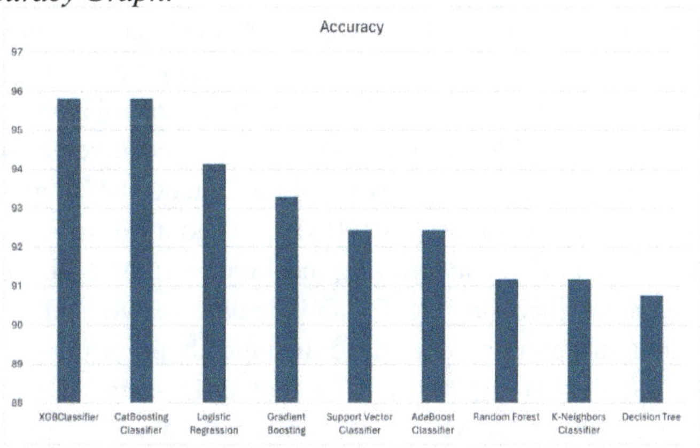

Evaluating the tuned models on the resampled dataset, this code assesses their performance after hyperparameter tuning.

Table 3. Accuracy results of hyperparameter tuning.

Model's Name	**Accuracy (in %)**
CatBoosting Classifier	96.63
XGBclassifier	95.79
Gradient Boosting	95.79

Table 4. Comparative analysis

References	Algorithm Used	Accuracy(in Percentage)
Xue et al. (2020)	SVM (Simple Vector Machine)	96%
Birjais et al. (2019)	Gradient Boosting	86%
Le et al. (2020)	K-NN	96%
Dinh et al. (2019)	SVM	78.7%
Saravananathan and Velmurugan (2016)	J48	62.8%
Proposed System	CatBoosting Classifier	96.63

ADVANTAGES

The opioid emergency, nearby other drug overdose challenges, has developed as a basic public health issue, with over 106,500 medicate overdose deaths detailed within the United States between June 2022 and June 2023, of which more than 80,000 were ascribed to opioids. The complexity of this emergency, fueled by the rise of synthetic opioids like fentanyl, requests inventive arrangements that rise above conventional approaches. Artificial Intelligence (AI)-enabled Dynamic Drug Overdose Response Systems (DDORS) speak to a transformative approach to tending to this epidemic. By integrating machine learning (ML), deep learning (DL), natural language processing (NLP), and big data analytics, these frameworks offer real-time, data-driven interventions to distinguish, prevent, and react to medicate overdoses (Devliyal et al., 2024). This chapter investigates the multifaceted advantages of AI-enabled DDORS and their future viewpoints, highlighting their potential to revolutionize overdose avoidance, treatment, and recovery whereas addressing challenges such as information quality, ethical concerns, and framework integration. AI-enabled DDORS use predictive modeling and real-time information investigation to improve reconnaissance and early location of sedate overdoses. By analyzing differing datasets—such as electronic health records (EHRs), prescription drug monitoring programs (PDMPs), and social media data—AI algorithms can recognize designs and trends related with overdose dangers. For occurrence, machine learning models can foresee people at high risk of opioid overdose by analyzing medicine histories, statistic profiles, and clinical information. Considers have illustrated that transient profound learning models connected to EHRs can foresee opioid overdose dangers with tall precision, empowering convenient intercessions. Moreover, AI-driven reconnaissance frameworks, such as the Electronic Surveillance Framework for the Early Notification of Community-Based Epidemics (Essence), can track overdose episodes in genuine time, giving open health authorities with significant bits of knowledge to deploy assets effectively. This capability is basic in tending to the quick spread of synthetic opioids, which frequently sidestep conventional observing frameworks due to their strength and variability. One of the foremost significant focal points of AI-enabled DDORS is their capacity to deliver personalized chance evaluations and interventions. Machine learning algorithms can coordinated multiomics information, hereditary data, and patient-specific variables to make individualized risk profiles. For illustration, AI can recognize patients inclined to opioid use disorder (OUD) by analyzing genetic inclinations and behavioral designs, permitting for custom fitted anticipation techniques. Moreover, dynamic frameworks like CURATE.AI can alter treatment regimens in genuine time based on understanding reactions, optimizing measurements to maximize viability whereas minimizing adverse impacts. This personalized approach is especially valuable in overseeing complex conditions like OUD, where person reactions to treatment vary widely (Bhatt & Sharma, 2025). By decreasing the dependence on one-size-fits-all interventions, AI-enabled DDORS progress persistent results and diminish the probability of relapse or overdose. AI-enabled DDORS upgrade the effectiveness of crisis reactions to drug overdoses by optimizing asset assignment and reaction times. Machine learning models can analyze geospatial information, emergency call logs, and hospital admission records to predict overdose hotspots, empowering paramedics and to begin with responders to prioritize high-risk areas (Rawat et al., 2025b). For occasion, ponders have appeared that ensemble learning models can anticipate opioid overdose dangers at a neighborhood level, permitting for targeted arrangement of naloxone and other life-saving mediations. Also, AI can streamline paramedic reaction documentation by utilizing NLP to extricate basic data from unstructured information, such as post-mortem examination accounts or emergency medical benefit reports, making strides surveillance and reaction coordination. This capability is significant in tending to the time-sensitive nature of overdose occurrences, where fast intercession can cruel the distinction between life and passing. AI-enabled DDORS bolster long-term recuperation by optimizing treatment plans and reducing relapse rates. Machine learning calculations can foresee the victory of substance utilize disorder treatment programs by analyzing patient information, such as treatment adherence and social determinants of wellbeing. For example, AI models have been utilized to anticipate early dropout dangers in recuperation programs, empowering clinicians to actualize focused on mediations to improve retention. Furthermore, AI-driven frameworks can coordinated real-world prove from clinical trials and quiet results to refine treatment protocols, guaranteeing they are evidence-based and versatile to rising patterns. By encouraging data-driven decision-making, these frameworks improve the viability of medication-assisted treatments (Mat), such as buprenorphine-naloxone, and progress long-term recuperation results. AI-enabled DDORS can decrease shame related with medicate overdoses by automating chance evaluations and intercessions, minimizing the require for subjective human judgment. For occasion, AI-driven mobile apps can give watchful, user-centered bolster for people in recovery, advertising assets like peer support networks and real-time counseling. These frameworks can too progress get to to care by recognizing underserved populations through statistic and financial information analysis, guaranteeing that assets like naloxone dispersion and treatment programs reach those most in require. By joining AI with telehealth stages, DDORS can amplify care to provincial and marginalized communities, addressing disparities in access to addiction treatment and overdose avoidance services. The integration of AI into DDORS can essentially decrease the financial burden of the overdose emergency. Traditional overdose response procedures, such as manual observation and trial-and-error treatment approaches, are resource-intensive and frequently inefficient. AI-driven frameworks streamline these forms by automating information examination, reducing the require for labor-intensive checking, and optimizing asset assignment.

AI-enabled DDORS can support the improvement of evidence-based approaches and administrative systems to address the overdose emergency. By analyzing large-scale datasets, AI can recognize holes in current arrangements, such as insufficient access to Mat or deficiently naloxone dissemination. For illustration, the U.S. Food and Drug Administration (FDA) has recognized the part of AI in drug development and security, with activities just like the CDER AI Council investigating its applications in pharmacovigilance. AI-driven experiences can educate administrative methodologies, such as the FDA's Project Optimus, which points to optimize dosing in oncology but may be adjusted for compulsion treatment. By giving policymakers with data-driven suggestions, DDORS can drive systemic changes to combat the overdose plague successfully. In spite of their advantages, AI-enabled DDORS confront a few challenges that must be tended to to maximize their affect. Information quality and reliability are basic concerns, as AI models depend on precise and comprehensive datasets. Inclinations in EHRs, such as those emerging from billing-focused information collection, can lead to inaccurate forecasts and exacerbate health disparities. Also, the need of interpretability in a few AI models, especially profound learning calculations, postures challenges for clinical selection, as healthcare suppliers require straightforward decision-making forms. Ethical concerns, such as persistent security and the potential for AI to propagate shame, must too be addressed through robust data governance and user-centric plan. At long last, the integration of AI into existing healthcare frameworks requires critical venture in foundation, preparing, and regulatory systems, which may limit adaptability in resource-constrained settings. An Artificial Intelligence Enabled Dynamic Drug Overdose Response System offers various points of interest that can essentially upgrade crisis therapeutic care and combat the opioid emergency. Here are a few key preferences:

- Quick Reaction Times: AI calculations can analyze real-time information from different sources, such as crisis calls, social media, and healthcare records, to recognize areas with a tall likelihood of sedate overdose occurrences. By rapidly pinpointing these ranges, crisis administrations can be dispatched instantly, possibly sparing lives.
- Prescient Analytics: AI-enabled frameworks can utilize chronicled information and prescient modeling to figure potential overdose hotspots and patterns. This proactive approach permits healthcare suppliers and policymakers to apportion assets more productively, actualize focused on intercessions, and execute preventive measures in high-risk zones.
- Personalized Mediation: AI calculations can analyze person hazard components, such as past overdose history, substance utilize designs, and statistic data, to tailor intercession techniques. This personalized approach guarantees that people at higher chance get the suitable level of bolster and help.
- Optimized Asset Allotment: By analyzing information on overdose occurrences, crisis room affirmations, and healthcare utilization designs, AI-enabled frameworks can offer assistance healthcare frameworks optimize asset assignment. This incorporates guaranteeing a satisfactory supply of naloxone (opioid overdose inversion medicine), staffing crisis divisions suitably, and planning care over distinctive healthcare suppliers.
- Improved Coordination and Communication: AI-enabled frameworks can encourage consistent communication and coordination among different partners included in overdose reaction, counting crisis administrations, healthcare suppliers, law authorization offices, and community organizations. This integration of data makes a difference streamline the reaction handle, minimize delays, and guarantee a more viable and facilitated approach to overdose administration.
- Nonstop Observing and Criticism Circle: AI calculations can persistently screen information streams and give criticism to move forward the precision and adequacy of the framework over time. This iterative handle empowers the framework to adjust to changing circumstances, developing patterns, and unused challenges in overdose avoidance and reaction.
- Versatility and Openness: AI-enabled overdose reaction frameworks can be scaled up to cover bigger geographic zones and populaces, making them open to communities of all sizes. This adaptability guarantees that indeed rustic or underserved zones can advantage from progressed overdose discovery and mediation capabilities.

Case Study

The United States, unfortunately, serves as a critical case think about within the urgent require for and advancing execution of Sedate Overdose Response Systems (DORS) due to its extreme and delayed opioid epidemic. Whereas challenges hold on, different states, cities, and organizations have developed innovative and impactful DORS models. Here are a number of prominent cases illustrating different features of a comprehensive DORS:

- **Naloxone Distribution and Community-Based Harm Reduction (e.g., North Carolina Harm Reduction Coalition):** North Carolina has been heavily impacted by the opioid crisis. The North Carolina Harm Reduction Coalition (NCHRC) is a driving illustration of a grassroots organization that has altogether contributed to DORS through widespread naloxone dispersion and overdose anticipation instruction. NCHRC's show illustrates the significant affect of community-based naloxone distribution in decreasing overdose fatalities and its critical return on investment. It highlights the significance of empowering people who are most likely to witness an overdose to be first responders.
    - Community-Led Naloxone Distribution: NCHRC operates through an extensive network of volunteers and outreach workers, prioritizing the distribution of naloxone kits to high-risk populations, including people who inject drugs, individuals in medication-assisted treatment, and formerly incarcerated persons. This "take-home naloxone" model engages laypersons to respond to overdoses immediately.
    - Overdose Education: Alongside naloxone distribution, NCHRC provides comprehensive training on overdose recognition, how to administer naloxone, and what to do after an overdose. This instruction helps to destigmatize overdose reaction and construct community capacity.
    - Legal Protections (Good Samaritan Laws): North Carolina has Good Samaritan laws (like NCGS §90-12.7) that protect individuals who seek help for an overdose from prosecution for minor drug-related charges. This vital legal assurance energizes bystanders to call 911, expanding the likelihood of professional medical intervention.
    - Cost-Effectiveness: Studies on NCHRC's program have shown significant societal benefits. For case, by December 2016, an evaluated 352 overdose passings were avoided in North Carolina due to naloxone dispersion, with an average of $2,742 of advantage for each dollar spent on the program.

- Advocacy and Policy Influence: NCHRC actively engages in advocacy to promote harm reduction policies, including increased access to naloxone and syringe service programs, which are integral to a broader DORS.

- **Public Safety-Led Post-Overdose Outreach Programs (e.g., Quick Response Teams - West Virginia, Franklin County, Ohio):** In many communities, law enforcement and EMS are often the first on the scene of an overdose. Recognizing this, a few zones have created collaborative "Speedy Reaction Groups" (QRTs) that bridge open security with open wellbeing. QRTs represent a move from absolutely reformatory approaches to medicate utilize towards a more open health-oriented demonstrate inside open security. They illustrate the adequacy of combining crisis reaction with quick linkage to care, recognizing the basic window of opportunity after an overdose.
    - Multi-Disciplinary Teams: QRTs typically consist of a paramedic, a law enforcement officer, and a recovery specialist or peer support worker. These groups react to overdose occasions, regularly inside 24-72 hours of the introductory incident.
    - Warm Hand-offs to Treatment: The primary goal of QRTs is to engage individuals who have recently experienced a non-fatal overdose and offer immediate support and linkage to treatment. The recovery specialist plays a vital part in building believe and encouraging a "warm hand-off" to continuous care, counting medication-assisted treatment (Mat) or other recovery administrations.
    - Harm Reduction Supplies: QRTs often distribute naloxone kits to the overdose survivor and their family/friends, along with fentanyl test strips and information on safer drug use practices.
    - Data-Driven Response: Some QRTs leverage data from overdose calls (e.g., through platforms like the Overdose Detection Mapping Application Program - ODMAP) to identify hot spots and direct their outreach efforts efficiently. For case, in Arlington District, Virginia, an increment in overdoses identified through ODMAP information activated a spike alarm, leading to focused on public health informing.
    - Reduced Recidivism: By intervening swiftly after a non-fatal overdose, QRTs aim to reduce the likelihood of repeat overdoses and improve engagement with treatment pathways.
- **State and Local Integration (e.g., Rhode Island, California):** Effective DORS requires coordination across various levels of government and community organizations. States like Rhode Island and California have executed strategies to coordinated state and nearby efforts. These state-level activities illustrate how robust information framework and inter-agency collaboration

can lead to more agile and compelling overdose reaction. By sharing data and planning endeavors, states can actualize more focused on and impactful interventions across diverse communities.

- o Surveillance Response Intervention (SRI) Calls (Rhode Island): The Rhode Island Department of Health (RIDOH) holds weekly SRI calls where real-time overdose data from hospitals (e.g., 48-Hour Opioid Overdose Reporting System) is shared with state agencies and local partners. This permits for rapid recognizable proof of overdose clusters and focused on responses. Public health advisories are dispersed if a community surpasses its predetermined overdose limit, actuating versatile outreach groups to hot spots.
- o Data-Driven Dashboards (California): California utilizes dashboards that provide data on opioid prescribing, overdose deaths, emergency room visits, and hospitalizations by region, substance, and demographics. This information illuminates intervention needs and permits for following of the epidemic.
- o Coalitions and Workgroups: Both states emphasize forming coalitions and workgroups that bring together partners from various sectors (public health, law enforcement, treatment providers, community organizations) to design and implement comprehensive overdose prevention efforts.
- o Consistent Messaging and Resource Allocation: State and local integration ensures aligned prevention messaging and coordinated use of resources, reaching those most in need.

- **Overdose Fatality Reviews (OFRs):** While not a real-time response system, OFRs are a critical retrospective component of a comprehensive DORS, particularly in the US. They include multidisciplinary groups looking into the circumstances encompassing overdose passings. OFRs give invaluable experiences into the complex pathways driving to overdose passings, moving past person fault to recognize systemic issues. They are significant for continuous improvement of DORS, guaranteeing that interventions are evidence-informed and address basic vulnerabilities.
    - o Multidisciplinary Review: OFRTs (Overdose Fatality Review Teams) typically include representatives from public health, law enforcement, medical examiners, social services, mental health, and community organizations.
    - o Comprehensive Data Collection: Reviews delve into the decedent's life cycle, including drug use history, co-morbidities, encounters with the criminal justice system, treatment history, and other relevant factors.

- o Identifying Missed Opportunities: The goal is to identify systemic gaps, missed opportunities for intervention, and contributing factors that may have led to the overdose death. This advises approach changes, open health intercessions, and preparing needs.
- o Informational Sharing and Best Practices: Findings from OFRs are used to inform local and state strategies, disseminate best practices, and improve the overall DORS. For illustration, New Jersey expanded its OFRTs to 17 new provinces, permitting nearby health offices to analyze information and evaluate methodologies.

These case thinks about highlight a few basic subjects within the development of effective DORS within the USA:

- o Naloxone is Foundational: Widespread accessibility and training on naloxone remain the cornerstone of immediate overdose response.
- o Collaboration is Key: Successful DORS requires strong partnerships between public health, public safety, healthcare providers, and community organizations.
- o Data-Driven Decision Making: Real-time and retrospective data analysis is essential for understanding the epidemic, identifying trends, and targeting interventions effectively.
- o Harm Reduction Integration: Moving beyond solely focusing on abstinence, DORS models increasingly integrate harm reduction principles to meet people "where they are."
- o Linkage to Care: Connecting overdose survivors with ongoing treatment and recovery support is crucial to prevent re-overdose and promote long-term well-being.
- o Addressing Stigma: Efforts to reduce the stigma associated with drug use and overdose are vital to encourage help-seeking behavior and foster community support.

France offers a captivating case ponder in sedate overdose reaction due to its verifiably different approach to addiction compared to countries just like the US. Whereas France has not experienced an "opioid emergency" of the same size as North America, it has developed a strong DORS characterized by a solid accentuation on public health, hurt lessening, and widespread access to opioid agonist treatment (OAT).

- o Pioneering Buprenorphine: France was an early adopter and a global leader in the widespread prescription of buprenorphine (Subutex, Suboxone) for opioid use disorder (OUD) starting in 1996, in response to the HIV epidemic among people who inject drugs. This was a radical move from the traditional, more prohibitive methadone-only demonstrate.

- o Decentralized Prescription: Unlike the US, where buprenorphine prescribing has historically been heavily regulated, French general practitioners (GPs) can easily prescribe buprenorphine. This altogether lowered barriers to access, making treatment promptly accessible in communities and coordination it into essential care.
- o Methadone Access: While buprenorphine is more widely prescribed, methadone is also available, primarily through specialized addiction centers and hospitals, with some allowance for community pharmacy dispensing.
- o High Treatment Coverage: France boasts one of the highest OAT coverage rates in Europe, with an estimated 87% of people with OUD receiving either buprenorphine or methadone. This high treatment saturation is considered a essential reason for France's comparatively low opioid overdose death rates.
- o Publicly Funded and Free: OAT and harm reduction services are largely publicly funded and free of charge, significantly reducing financial barriers to treatment and care.
- o Syringe Exchange Programs (SEPs): France established SEPs relatively early, recognizing their importance in preventing HIV and Hepatitis C transmission among people who inject drugs. These programs are often coordinates into broader "low-threshold" centers.

Support Centers for the Reduction of Drug-related Harms (CAARUDs): These centers are crucial hubs for France's DORS. They offer a run of administrations beyond just syringe exchange, including:

- o Information and Counseling: Providing personalized advice and information to drug users.
- o Access to Basic Care: Assisting with hygiene, basic emergency care, and referrals to specialized or general treatment systems.
- o Social Mediation: Helping users integrate into their neighborhoods and prevent public disturbances related to drug use.
- o Naloxone Distribution: CAARUDs play a role in distributing naloxone kits.
- o Drug Checking (Limited): Some centers offer drug checking services, allowing users to test their drugs for unknown or dangerous substances, with warnings disseminated through the network.
- o Supervised Consumption Sites (SCS) / Drug Consumption Rooms (DCRs): France has cautiously piloted SCS, such as "La Salle" in Paris. These locales give a secure and clean environment for individuals to expend pre-obtained

drugs beneath the supervision of prepared staff, with quick therapeutic intercession accessible in case of overdose. They too serve as section focuses for treatment and social bolster.

- o National Health Policy: Health policy, including addiction treatment and harm reduction, is largely decided by the central government in Paris. This centralization encourages the improvement and execution of common objectives and national methodologies.
- o Strong NGO Networks: France benefits from strong national networks of medical-social addiction NGOs (like Fédération Addiction) that work in close alliance with the Ministry of Health. This collaboration guarantees that arrangements are educated by on-the-ground substances which administrations are executed viably.
- o Integrated Medical-Social Approach: The French system combines medical treatment with social support, recognizing that addiction is not just a medical issue but also has significant social determinants. This coordinates approach empowers engagement with treatment, harm diminishment practices, and community-based recuperation.
- o Naloxone Access (Evolving): While France's overdose rates have historically been low due to OAT, there has been a growing recognition of the importance of naloxone.
  - ▪ Increased Availability: Naloxone is available in France in different forms, including an intranasal spray and injectable forms. It can be obtained at community pharmacies.
  - ▪ Prescription Requirement (Historical/Evolving): Historically, obtaining take-home naloxone free of charge in pharmacies required a prescription. Whereas there have been endeavors to extend get to, expelling this medicine barrier is an ongoing dialog to advance engage laypersons as to begin with responders.
  - ▪ Training and Distribution: Distribution occurs through various settings, including addiction treatment centers (CSAPA), harm reduction centers (CAARUD), and hospitals.

France keeps up a generally repressive legal system concerning drug utilize, where ownership and utilize of illegal drugs can still lead to legitimate results, coexisting with its strong harm decrease and treatment approaches. This paradox can make obstructions to care, reinforce shame, and prevent the usage of certain imaginative hurt diminishment programs. Whereas opioids have been well-managed, there have been watched increments in passings including other substances, such as cocaine. The DORS ought to stay versatile to advancing sedate markets (Kapruwan et al., 2025). Whereas there's a solid national approach, a few community-based organizations' endeavors, like domestic conveyance of methadone or extended naloxone and syringe trade programs, have been "inconsistent" and need steady government subsidizing. The French Sedate Overdose Reaction Framework serves as a compelling case consider, especially in its proactive, open health-oriented approach. Its chronicled accentuation on far reaching, low-threshold access to opioid agonist treatment, combined with a comprehensive arrange of hurt lessening administrations and centralized arrangement coordination, has demonstrably kept overdose mortality rates essentially lower than in numerous other developed countries. Whereas it hooks with a "paradox" of prohibitionist laws nearby magnanimous open well-being approaches, France's show offers profitable lessons on how contributing in treatment and hurt decrease as center components of a DORS can viably anticipate a far reaching overdose emergency and ensure open wellbeing.

FUTURE RESEARCH DIRECTIONS

Looking into the future, the prospects for an Artificial Intelligence Enabled Dynamic Drug Overdose Response System are promising and multifaceted. Here are a few potential future points of view:

- Improved Predictive Capabilities: AI calculations will proceed to advance, getting to be indeed more advanced in anticipating and distinguishing ranges with a tall probability of sedate overdose occurrences. By analyzing a broader run of information sources, counting social media, healthcare records, and natural variables, these frameworks can give more exact expectations, permitting for proactive intercession and asset allotment.
- Integration with Wearable Technology: As wearable gadgets ended up more progressed and far reaching, they can be coordinates into AI-enabled overdose reaction frameworks. Wearables seem persistently screen crucial signs and identify early signs of overdose, consequently activating alarms to crisis administrations or caregivers. This proactive approach seem essentially decrease reaction times and progress results.
- Telemedicine and Remote Assistance: AI-enabled frameworks seem encourage farther overdose intercessions through telemedicine stages. Utilizing AI-powered chatbots or virtual associates, people encountering an overdose or seeing one seem receive real-time direction on regulating naloxone or performing essential life back procedures until crisis responders arrive.
- Information Sharing and Collaboration: Within the future, AI-enabled overdose response frameworks may encourage information sharing and collaboration among different partners, counting healthcare suppliers, law authoriza-

tion organizations, community organizations, and open wellbeing specialists. By pooling together anonymized information from assorted sources, these frameworks can produce more comprehensive experiences into overdose patterns and hazard variables, empowering more compelling avoidance and mediation procedures.

- Moral and Security Contemplations: As AI innovations gotten to be more coordinates into overdose reaction frameworks, there will be expanded consideration on moral and security concerns. Future advancements must prioritize straightforwardness, responsibility, and client assent to guarantee that these frameworks work morally and regard individuals' rights to privacy and independence.

The future of AI-enabled DDORS lies within the proceeded advancement of predictive modeling procedures. Next-generation machine learning models, such as graph convolutional neural networks (GCNNs) and recurrent neural networks (RNNs), will empower more exact forecasts of overdose dangers by joining complex, time-series information. For case, GCNNs can demonstrate drug-target intuitive and protein systems, recognizing novel helpful targets for enslavement treatment. Similarly, RNNs can analyze longitudinal understanding information to anticipate dynamic overdose dangers, empowering proactive mediations. These advancements will be upheld by the developing accessibility of high-quality, multimodal datasets, such as those combining genomic, proteomic, and social determinants of health information. As these models ended up more modern, they will empower DDORS to expect and relieve overdose dangers with unprecedented precision. AI-enabled DDORS will play a significant part in progressing exactness medication for addiction treatment.

By leveraging single-cell and spatial transcriptomic investigation, AI can distinguish novel biomarkers and helpful targets for OUD and other substance utilize clutters. For occurrence, automated pattern recognition in spatial transcriptomics can connect histological designs with quality expression information, giving experiences into the neurobiological components of addiction. These advancements will empower the improvement of personalized treatment plans tailored to person hereditary and environmental profiles, improving treatment viability and diminishing relapse rates. Furthermore, AI-driven medicate revelation stages, such as DeepMind's AlphaFold, can quicken the improvement of novel anti-addiction drugs by anticipating protein structures and drug interactions with high accuracy. The integration of AI with wearable gadgets and IoT advances will empower the extension of real-time monitoring frameworks for overdose anticipation.

Future DDORS could join biosensors that identify early signs of overdose, such as changes in heart rate or oxygen levels, and automatically regulate naloxone or alarm crisis administrations. These frameworks will be supported by edge computing, permitting for quick data handling at the point of care. In addition, AI-driven versatile apps will provide continuous support for people in recovery, offering personalized coping techniques and real-time connections to peer support networks. These innovations will move the paradigm from receptive to preventive overdose reaction, significantly decreasing mortality rates. AI-enabled DDORS will empower more successful community-based mediations by leveraging enormous information and predictive analytics. For case, AI can analyze social media information and community wellbeing records to recognize developing sedate patterns, such as the spread of unused engineered opioids. These insights can inform focused on open health campaigns, such as instructive programs and drug-checking administrations at celebrations, which enable users to form educated choices.

Moreover, AI can optimize the dispersion of harm reduction assets, such as naloxone and syringe exchange programs, by distinguishing high-risk communities and anticipating asset needs. These community-based procedures will upgrade the reach and affect of overdose avoidance efforts, especially in underserved regions. Long term victory of AI-enabled DDORS will depend on intrigue collaboration and information sharing among analysts, clinicians, policymakers, and innovation designers. Open establishment models, such as those integrating genomic, proteomic, and clinical information, will encourage the advancement of standardized AI devices for overdose reaction. For case, activities like the Wyss Institute's "Code to Cure" newsletter highlight the significance of collaborative environments in progressing AI-driven medicate disclosure and reaction frameworks. By cultivating associations between academia, industry, and government, DDORS can overcome current restrictions, such as information silos and administrative obstructions, and quicken the sending of inventive arrangements. Future AI-enabled DDORS must address moral and administrative challenges to guarantee capable execution. Advances in explainable AI (XAI) will progress the interpretability of machine learning models, empowering clinicians to believe and approve AI-driven suggestions. Also, robust information governance systems, such as those joining blockchain for secure information sharing, will secure persistent security and guarantee compliance with controls like HIPAA.

The FDA's progressing endeavors to create AI-specific administrative systems, such as the 2025 draft direction on AI in sedate improvement, will give a guide for joining DDORS into clinical hone. By prioritizing ethical considerations and administrative compliance, future frameworks will adjust innovation with understanding safety and public trust. Whereas current AI-enabled DDORS are essentially centered on North America, future perspectives incorporate worldwide versatility and adjustment to diverse healthcare frameworks. AI-driven frameworks can be tailored to address region-specific drug challenges, such as the rise of methamphetamine overdoses in Asia or cocaine-related issues in South America. By leveraging worldwide wellbeing information and collaborating with international organizations, DDORS can give adaptable arrangements that account for social, financial, and regulatory contrasts. For illustration, AI can analyze worldwide pharmacovigilance information to recognize rising sedate dangers and educate international arrangement reactions. This worldwide perspective will guarantee that AI-enabled DDORS contribute to a facilitated, worldwide exertion to combat medicate overdoses. The widespread selection of AI-enabled DDORS will require critical upskilling of healthcare workforces to guarantee successful usage. Future preparing programs will need to prepare clinicians with the aptitudes to decipher AI-driven insights and coordinated them into clinical hone. For illustration, medical instruction should incorporate modules on AI education and enslavement treatment to prepare suppliers for developing sedate dangers.

Moreover, AI can support the advancement of decision-support instruments that direct clinicians in genuine time, diminishing the cognitive burden of overseeing complex overdose cases. By contributing in workforce improvement, healthcare frameworks can maximize the benefits of DDORS and guarantee their economical integration into clinical workflows. AI-enabled Dynamic Drug Overdose Response Systems represent a worldview move in tending to the worldwide drug overdose emergency. Their advantages—ranging from improved observation and personalized mediations to cost-effectiveness and integration with rising technologies—position them as a foundation of advanced open health strategies. By leveraging predictive modeling, real-time observing, and data-driven decision-making, these frameworks can spare lives, decrease healthcare costs, and improve get to to care. Looking to end of, the advancements in predictive modeling, exactness pharmaceutical, and worldwide collaboration will encourage improve the affect of DDORS, whereas tending to ethical and administrative challenges will guarantee their responsible implementation. As the opioid emergency and other drug-related challenges proceed to advance, AI-enabled DDORS offer a adaptable, innovative arrangement to relieve their destroying impacts, clearing the way for a more secure and healthier future.

CONCLUSION

This chapter highlights an Artificial Intelligence (AI) Empowered Dynamic Drug Overdose Response System would likely highlight its potential to revolutionize emergency therapeutic care and combat the opioid crisis. The integration of AI into overdose response systems has illustrated the capacity to essentially diminish response times. By leveraging real-time data analytics and prescient calculations, crisis organizations can be dispatched speedily to areas where overdoses are likely to happen, possibly sparing lives. AI-enabled Dynamic Drug Overdose Response

Framework represents a worldview shift in tending to the drug overdose emergency. By saddling the control of machine learning, common language processing, and predictive modeling, it offers a comprehensive, data-driven approach to observation, anticipation, and treatment. From recognizing high-risk people to optimizing naloxone distribution and personalizing treatments, AI-driven frameworks can altogether upgrade the speed and efficacy of interventions. In any case, realizing this potential requires overcoming challenges related to information quality, ethics, and value. With proceeded investment in investigate, framework, and collaboration, AI-enabled DDORS can not as it were decrease overdose fatalities but moreover pave the way for a more strong and responsive public health framework. As the emergency advances, so as well must our devices, and AI stands at the forefront of this basic advancement, advertising a lifeline to communities devastated by addiction.

REFERENCES

Bhatt, S., & Sharma, S. (2025). Generative Artificial Intelligence Based Biomedical Applications for Pharmaceutical Industry. In *2025 International Conference on Computational, Communication and Information Technology (ICCCIT)*, 1–6. https://doi.org/DOI: 10.1109/ICCCIT62592.2025.10927855

Birjais, R., Mourya, A. K., Chauhan, R., & Kaur, H. (2019). Prediction and diagnosis of future diabetes risk: A machine learning approach. *SN Applied Sciences*, *1*(9), 1112. Advance online publication. DOI: 10.1007/s42452-019-1117-9

Bozorgi, P., Porter, D. E., Eberth, J. M., Eidson, J. P., & Karami, A. (2021). The leading neighborhood-level predictors of drug overdose: A mixed machine learning and spatial approach. *Drug and Alcohol Dependence*, *229*, 109143. DOI: 10.1016/j.drugalcdep.2021.109143 PMID: 34794060

Devgan, K., Sharma, S., Jangra, D., & Sharma, S. (2025). Artificial Intelligence-Enabled Apple Disease Monitoring System for environmental protection and resource conservation. In Advances in computational intelligence and robotics book series (pp. 271–300). https://doi.org/DOI: 10.4018/979-8-3373-3246-8.ch011

Devliyal, S., Goyal, H. R., & Sharma, S. (2024). ICDRET: A dynamic cyber risk estimation technique for intelligent Cyber-Physical Systems in PCS. *The Open Bioinformatics Journal*, *18*(1), e18750362380269. Advance online publication. DOI: 10.2174/0118750362380269250502062754

Devliyal, S., Sharma, S., & Goyal, H. R. (2024). EIAIMSPS: Edge inspired artificial intelligence-based multi stakeholders Personalized Security Mechanism in ICPS for PCS. *International Journal of Advanced Computer Science and Applications*, *15*(8). Advance online publication. DOI: 10.14569/IJACSA.2024.01508117

Dinh, A., Miertschin, S., Young, A., & Mohanty, S. D. (2019). A data-driven approach to predicting diabetes and cardiovascular disease with machine learning. *BMC Medical Informatics and Decision Making*, *19*(1), 211. Advance online publication. DOI: 10.1186/s12911-019-0918-5 PMID: 31694707

Feng, C., Chen, H., Yuan, X., Sun, M., Chu, K., Liu, H., & Rui, M. (2019). Gene expression data based deep learning model for accurate prediction of Drug-Induced liver injury in advance. *Journal of Chemical Information and Modeling*, *59*(7), 3240–3250. DOI: 10.1021/acs.jcim.9b00143 PMID: 31188585

Gupta, A., & Sharma, S. (2024). Deep Learning Inspired Biomarker Diagnostic Enabled Heart Health Monitoring System for Cardiac Arrest Detection. In *2024 International Conference on Emerging Technologies and Innovation for Sustainability (EmergIN)*, 13–17. https://doi.org/DOI: 10.1109/EmergIN63207.2024.10960916

Islam, T., Hussain, N., Islam, S., & Chakrabarty, A. (2018). Detecting Adverse Drug Reaction with Data Mining And Predicting its Severity With Machine Learning. In 2018 IEEE Region 10 Humanitarian Technology Conference (R10-HTC), 1–5. https://doi.org/.DOI: 10.1109/R10-HTC.2018.8629806

Kapruwan, A., Sharma, S., & Goyal, H. R. (2025). ESCBR: Expert System Enabled Case-based Reasoning Approach in IDDCS for CIND. *Recent Patents on Engineering*, *19*. Advance online publication. DOI: 10.2174/0118722121336689250116074945

Kapruwan, A., Sharma, S., & Goyal, H. R. (2025a). iDDCS: Cervical intraepithelial neoplasia severity detection during vagina birth using artificial intelligence approach. *Multidisciplinary Science Journal*, *7*(8), 2025192. DOI: 10.31893/multiscience.2025192

Le, T. M., Vo, T. M., Pham, T. N., & Dao, S. V. T. (2020). A novel Wrapper–Based feature selection for early diabetes prediction enhanced with a metaheuristic. *IEEE Access : Practical Innovations, Open Solutions*, *9*, 7869–7884. DOI: 10.1109/ACCESS.2020.3047942

Rawat, D., Sharma, S., & Bhadula, S. (2025). CT Imaging-Based Deep Learning System for Non-Small Cell Lung Cancer Detection and Classification. *International Journal of Advanced Computer Science and Applications*, *16*(5). Advance online publication. DOI: 10.14569/IJACSA.2025.0160561

Rawat, D., Sharma, S., & Bhadula, S. (2025b). Machine Vision Technique with Image Segmentation in Digital Diagnostic System for Lung Cancer Detection. In *2025 International Conference on Pervasive Computational Technologies (ICPCT)*, 35–40. https://doi.org/DOI: 10.1109/ICPCT64145.2025.10939214

Saravananathan, K., & Velmurugan, T. (2016). Analyzing Diabetic Data using Classification Algorithms in Data Mining. *Indian Journal of Science and Technology*, *9*(43). Advance online publication. DOI: 10.17485/ijst/2016/v9i43/93874

Schell, R. C., Allen, B., Goedel, W. C., Hallowell, B. D., Scagos, R., Li, Y., Krieger, M. S., Neill, D. B., Marshall, B. D. L., Cerda, M., & Ahern, J. (2021). Identifying predictors of opioid overdose death at a neighborhood level with machine learning. *American Journal of Epidemiology*, *191*(3), 526–533. DOI: 10.1093/aje/kwab279 PMID: 35020782

Sharma, S., Tyagi, R., & Mohan, S. (2025). Blockchain-Based Security and Privacy in Digital Healthcare Recommender Systems. In In Healthcare Recommender Systems (pp. 221–237). https://doi.org/DOI: 10.1007/978-3-031-80056-6_10

Ward, P. J., Rock, P. J., Slavova, S., Young, A. M., Bunn, T. L., & Kavuluru, R. (2019). Enhancing timeliness of drug overdose mortality surveillance: A machine learning approach. *PLoS One*, *14*(10), e0223318. DOI: 10.1371/journal.pone.0223318 PMID: 31618226

Xue, J., Min, F., & Ma, F. (2020). Research on Diabetes Prediction Method based on Machine learning. *Journal of Physics: Conference Series*, *1684*, 012062. DOI: 10.1088/1742-6596/1684/1/012062

ADDITIONAL READING

Al Nahian, M. S., Delcher, C., Harris, D., Akpunonu, P., & Kavuluru, R. (2025). Large language models for drug overdose prediction from longitudinal medical records. *Preprint, arXiv*.

Corso, A., Asariah, J. S., Park, K.-P., Corso, N. A., & Lee, E. L. (2025). A DSR approach for geospatial AI: Prediction of drug overdoses. *AMCIS 2025 Proceedings*.

KEY TERMS AND DEFINITIONS

DDORS (Dynamic Drug Overdose Response System): An AI-powered system designed to predict, prevent, and respond to drug overdoses in real-time by integrating data from sources like EMS calls, hospital records, and social media to enable faster and smarter interventions.

Overdose Hotspot Prediction: A machine learning–based method for identifying geographical areas with a high likelihood of future drug overdoses, enabling targeted deployment of resources such as naloxone and community outreach.

Continuous Glucose Monitoring (CGM): A method of tracking blood glucose levels throughout the day and night using a sensor placed under the skin, providing detailed data trends used in both diabetes management and AI-driven health monitoring systems.

Natural Language Processing (NLP): A branch of artificial intelligence that enables computers to interpret and analyze human language. In DDORS, NLP is used to analyze unstructured text data such as EMS reports and medical examiner documents to detect overdose patterns.

Medication-Assisted Treatment (MAT): A treatment approach for substance use disorders that combines behavioral therapy with medications like buprenorphine or methadone. AI-enabled systems can personalize and optimize MAT dosing based on individual data.

Chapter 12
Investigation on Data Driven Modelling and Estimation of Concentrations in Three-Compartment Model for the Benchmark Pharmacokinetic System

V. Sujatha
https://orcid.org/0000-0002-8123-7733
SRM Institute of Science and Technology, India

ABSTRACT

In the three-compartment model of the pharmacokinetic system, the estimation of blood concentration is examined in this chapter. The compartmental models describe the dynamic behaviour of blood concentration in blood tissues. The dynamics of the five pharmacokinetic parameter sets using first-principles method, model is derived. MATLAB is used to estimate the concentrations in each of the three compartments. This study estimates concentrations for each of the five pharmacokinetic parameter sets in each of the three compartments. The experimental value is used to validate the estimated concentration in each of the three compartments. Data driven machine learning algorithms are also employed for prediction of concentrations in three compartment model. The quality of estimation has been verified based on the validation of experimental values with the estimated concentration values in all the three compartments. Quantitative comparison is also done based on the computation

DOI: 10.4018/979-8-3373-2043-4.ch012

and comparison of square relative error, root mean square error, r squared and Mean Absolute Percentage Error.

INTRODUCTION

The study of dynamic behaviour of drug concentrations in blood tissues are called as Pharmacokinetics. This behaviour is described using the compartmental models. This study employs the widely utilized 3-compartment model. Compartment 1 is utilized to represent blood plasma, and it is assumed that the medicine is administered directly into the same compartment. Well-perfused tissues (such as the brain and muscles) and residual tissues (such as bones) are represented by compartments two and three. Additionally, it is anticipated that the medication can diffuse between compartments 1 and 2, respectively. For the three-compartment model, the transfer parameters are $K_{10,}$ K_{12}, K_{13}, K_{21}, K_{31}. In this compartment model, it is difficult to achieve desired concentration with intravenous drug delivery. In practice, physicians recommend the intravenous delivery of drugs dose per kilogram of body weight by manually controlled infusion pumps. In this work, all five benchmark pharmacokinetic models' concentrations in compartments 1, 2, and 3 are estimated. This estimation will enable the clinician to explore about the drug concentration in blood as well as to administer the intravenous delivery of drugs based on pharmacokinetic models. With the help of computer simulation, one can estimate the blood-drug concentration thereby allowing the anaesthesiologist to deliver the intravenous drugs to a subject.

The performance of the computer-controlled infusion of propofol in female patients is analyzed in (Jaap Vuyk et al 1995), which presents comparison sets of propofol pharmacokinetic parameters. The pharmacokinetic three compartment model referenced in Wayne Bequette (2002) is the source of the modelling equations used in this work. A straightforward model was created and validated to assess the plasma concentration in the study conducted in Sara Cascone et al. 2013 by employing the three-compartment modelling approach for the pharmacokinetics of remifentanil. (Al Rifai et al. 2016) proposed that for pharmacokinetics model inter-individual variability represents a challenging aspect in Total I.V. Anaesthesia, hence care must be taken to ensure that the expected clinical response is actually obtained. (Kartono et al 2020) estimated the parameters of the pharmacokinetic model using particle swarm optimization (PSO) algorithm. An approach that helps pharmacometricians to determine a theoretical method to establish compatibility between the models in Hyo Jeong Ryu et al, 2022. The optimal model for propofol infusion is not yet available.

The framework for compartmental modeling utilizing a system of ODEs derived from first principles is established by Gabrielsson & Weiner (2016). Under the assumption of linear dynamics, these models shed light on drug kinetics. In order to take into consideration both intra- and inter-subject variability, population pharmacokinetics developed nonlinear mixed-effects (NLME) models (Bonate, 2011). Quantification of uncertainty is made possible via Bayesian inference, however its application can be costly and susceptible to presumptions. The advent of machine learning (ML) and data-driven techniques to supplement or replace conventional PK models has been highlighted in recent publications. It has been studied how to learn system dynamics directly from data using methods like neural ordinary differential equations (neural ODEs) (Chen et al., 2018), Gaussian Processes (GPs) (Hernández-Lobato et al., 2014), and sparse identification of nonlinear dynamics (SINDy) (Brunton et al., 2016). Real-time monitoring is possible using ML-based methods, which also provide flexibility in managing nonlinearities and adaptability to new patient data. Hybrid modeling, which combines data-driven layers with mechanistic models, is a promising approach. Semi-parametric models and physics-informed neural networks (PINNs), for instance, are becoming more and more popular for simulating physiological systems. Applications in PK are still in their infancy, and many research lack the interpretability mechanisms, uncertainty quantification, and strong validation frameworks that are essential for clinical decision-making.

Liu et al. (2024) used machine learning in a three-compartment framework to create a data-driven pharmacokinetic model for propofol, showing better prediction accuracy than conventional techniques. For patients with extremely high BMI, Rasmussen, Pedersen, and Smith (2024) created a three-compartment population pharmacokinetic model for propofol that included sex and weight descriptors as covariates. In order to improve automated anesthetic delivery systems, Kumar, Jones, and Patel (2024) investigated the integration of deep learning and control techniques with three-compartment pharmacokinetic models. An LSTM-based model for real-time propofol concentration tracking was created by Zhao, Li, Wang, and Chen (2024) utilizing a four-compartment PK/PD framework that was verified in swine models. A hybrid data-driven and mechanistic modeling approach to propofol pharmacokinetics utilizing deep neural networks within a three-compartment framework is presented by Fernandez et al., 2023. Smith, Nguyen, and Banerjee (2023) created a deep reinforcement learning–based strategy for propofol dosing, led by simulations from a three-compartment pharmacokinetic/pharmacodynamic model, highlighting greater adaptability in clinical dosing techniques. The study He et al (2023) proposed a hybrid Transformer and LSTM model to predict depth of anesthesia during propofol infusion, leveraging pharmacokinetic principles within a three-compartment framework to enhance real-time estimation accuracy. Koren, van der Walt, and Eleveld (2022) automated covariate modeling in pharmacokinetics using symbolic regression techniques; they particularly used a propofol three-compartment model to illustrate their approach. A clinical validation of a covariate-based propofol pharmacokinetic model under target-controlled infusion in surgical patients was carried out by Zong, Wang, and Lin in 2022. A convolutional neural network with self-attention mechanisms was constructed by Wu, Chen, and Feng (2022) to predict the depth of anesthesia after propofol administration.

This article aims to make the clinicians to be familiar with the model which matches the characteristics of the patient among the usual patient population. However, all the existing pharmacokinetic models are having inherent assumptions which lead to inaccuracy in the estimated model. Hence, the role of anaesthetist is to have the close clinical monitoring of the patient under treatment. This article focusses on the mathematical modelling of pharmacokinetic models with no assumption. Clinicians and pharmacologists can develop more precise and customized treatment plans by using data-driven modeling techniques to estimate drug concentrations within a three-compartment pharmacokinetic system. These strategies include: enhanced dose optimization, real-time therapeutic drug monitoring, improved understanding of drug behaviour, simplifying drug development, and integration with electronic health records.

The objective of this chapter is to provide a mathematical model and estimate the blood plasma concentration for the benchmark pharmacokinetic models in each of the three compartments. The rest of the chapter is organized as follows: section 2 discusses three compartment model in pharmacokinetic model, the five benchmark Pharmacokinetic model for propofol infusion and modelling of the pharmacokinetic model. The solution and recommendation is explained in section 3. Section 4 presents the future research directions. After analysing the concentration in each of the three compartments for each of the five pharmacokinetic models and a conclusion of the chapter is given in the last section.

BACKGROUND

1. Pharmacokinetic Model – Three-Compartment Model

A basic method for measuring the absorption, distribution, metabolism, and excretion (ADME) of medications within a biological system is pharmacokinetic (PK) modeling. PK models offer important insights into drug behavior and therapeutic efficacy by explaining how drug concentrations vary over time inside various bodily compartments. The creation of dosage regimens, customized therapy, toxicity evaluation, and regulatory decision-making are only a few of the stages of drug development and clinical practice where these models are crucial. Conventional compartmental models, including one-, two-, and three-compartment models, capture the fundamental dynamics of drug transit through the body while simplifying physiological processes. Data-driven methods have surfaced in recent years to supplement traditional PK modeling and, in certain situations, outperform it in terms of adaptability and predictive power. It is essential to comprehend the state of these models today and recognize their shortcomings in order to improve drug development pipelines and pharmacokinetic analysis.

The pharmacokinetic model is used for examining the behaviour of intravenous delivery of drugs to the subject. In this chapter, three-compartment models are used to estimate the blood concentration in all the compartments. Figure 1 represents the three-compartment model.

Figure 1. Three compartment model

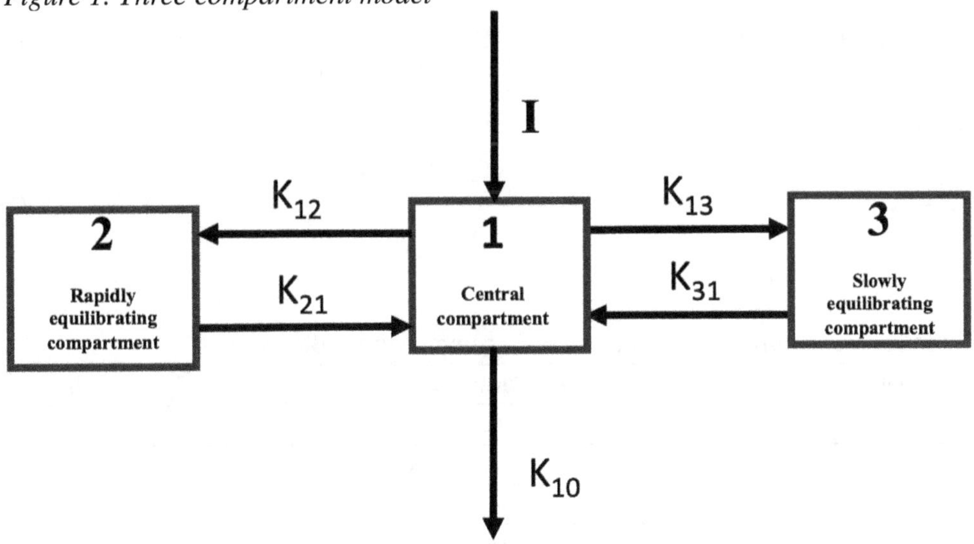

In the pharmacokinetic model, it is mandatory to derive the mathematical models in order to estimate the blood concentration. The mathematical models in bio-chemical systems are non-linear in nature. The commonly used models are five pharmacokinetic models are taken for study.

Let I be the Mass infusion rate of the drug (mass/unit time), then the mass balance equations are represented as:

$$\frac{dM_1}{dt} = -\left(K_{12} + K_{13} + K_{10}\right)M_1 + K_{21}M_2 + K_{31}M_3 + I \tag{1}$$

$$\frac{dM_2}{dt} = K_{12}M_1 - K_{21}M_2 \tag{2}$$

$$\frac{dM_3}{dt} = K_{13}M_1 - K_{31}M_3 \tag{3}$$

Drug concentrations must be given greater consideration than the overall quantity of the drug. The blood plasma concentration can therefore also be connected using the formula C1=M1/V1. It is also possible to express the mass balance equation of the three-compartment model in terms of blood plasma concentration, whose parameters are listed in table 1:

$$\frac{dC_1}{dt} = -(K_{12} + K_{13} + K_{10})C_1 + K_{21}C_2 + K_{31}C_3 + \frac{1}{V_1}I \tag{4}$$

$$\frac{dC_2}{dt} = K_{12}C_1 - K_{21}C_2 \tag{5}$$

$$\frac{dC_3}{dt} = K_{13}C_1 - K_{31}C_3 \tag{6}$$

$$C_1 = C_1 \tag{7}$$

Table 1. Description of parameters in Bergman Minimal Model

SYMBOL	DESCRIPTION	UNIT
I	Mass infusion rate	Mass/time
C_1	Blood plasma concentration in compartment 1	µg/ml
C_2	Blood plasma concentration in compartment 2	µg/ml
C_3	Blood plasma concentration in compartment 3	µg/ml
K_{10}	Rate constant for drug elimination from central compartment	min^{-1}
K_{12}	Rate constant between 1 and 2	min^{-1}
K_{21}	Rate constant between 2 and 1	min^{-1}
K_{13}	Rate constant between 1 and 3	min^{-1}
K_{31} V_1	Rate constant between 3 and 1 volume of the blood plasma compartment	min^{-1} litres

2. Five Pharmacokinetic Model For Propofol Infusion

The differential equations governing the pharmacokinetic model can be modelled using MATLab simulation tools. The input and output variables are drug infusion rate and blood plasma concentration in compartment 1, 2 and 3 respectively. The parameter values for the five pharmacokinetic models are tabulated in table 2 and the same were implemented during simulation.

Table 2. Parameter values of five benchmark pharmacokinetic models for propofol infusion

Parameters	Gepts et al	Shafer et al	Kirkpatrick et al.	Cockshott et al.	Tackley et al.
I	3	1.5	2.5	2	3
K_{10}	0.1190	0.152	0.077	0.1058	0.0870
K_{12}	0.1140	0.207	0.2460	0.1440	0.1050
K_{21}	0.0550	0.092	0.0597	0.0640	0.0640
K_{13}	0.0419	0.040	0.0391	0.0282	0.0220
K_{31}	0.0033	0.0048	0.0019	0.0034	0.0034
V_1	16.2	12	26.3	17.5	22.4

3. Mathematical Modelling of Benchmark Pharmacokinetic Models:

Simulink was used to implement the pharmacokinetic minimum model. The parameter values of the five benchmark Pharmacokinetic model for propofol infusion are obtained through simulation. Using ODE solver in MATLab, the blood plasma concentration in three compartments is estimated for the normal individual.

3.1 Gepts et al

The pharmacokinetic model proposed by Gepts et al. (1987) has been taken for study.

Figure 2. Plot of concentration C1 for Gepts et al. pharmacokinetic models

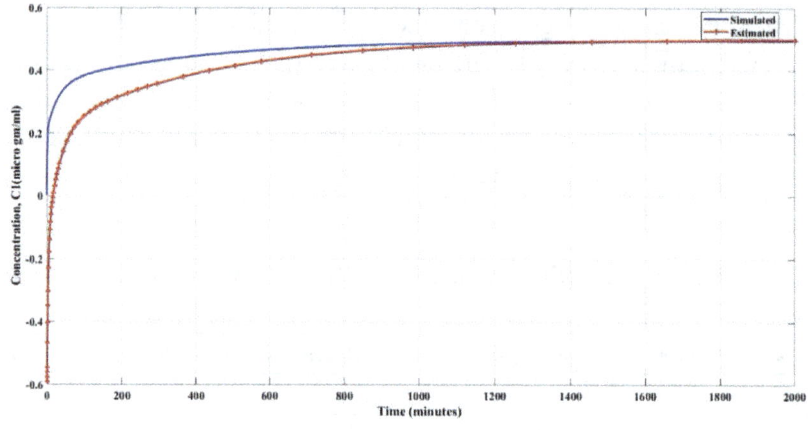

Figure 3. Plot of concentration C2 for Gepts et al. pharmacokinetic models

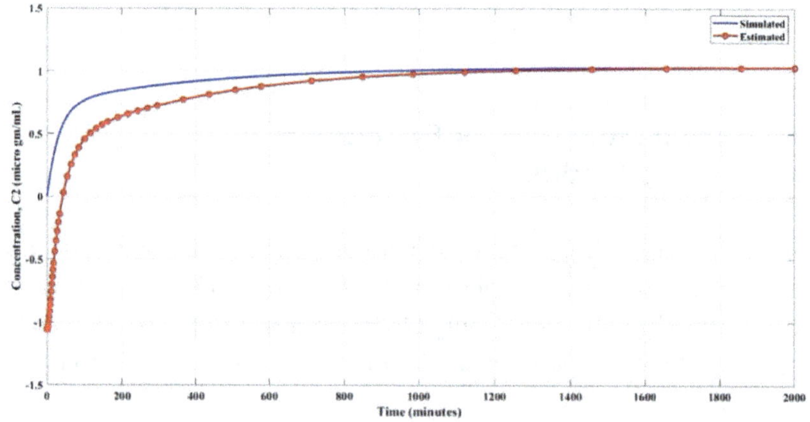

Figure 4. Plot of concentration C3 for Gepts et al. pharmacokinetic models

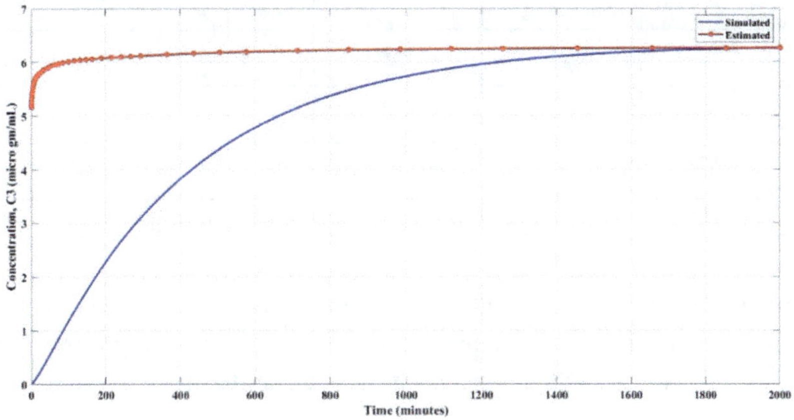

It is evident from figures 2, 3, and 4 that the estimated concentration values and the simulated concentrations are rather close. To justify how the estimated value is close to the true or actual value, it is required to compute the relative error using the following:

$$\text{Relative error} = \frac{\mathbf{C} - \widehat{\mathbf{C}}}{\mathbf{C}}$$

Where C is the simulated concentration value.
$\widehat{C}$ is the estimated concentration value obtained using solver.

Table 3. Simulated and Estimated values of Concentration for Gepts et al.

C_1	$\widehat{C}_1$	**Relative error**	C_2	$\widehat{C}_2$	**Relative error**	C_3	$\widehat{C}_3$	**Relative error**
0.33	0.011	0.966667	0.6	0.07	0.883333	0.24	4.54	-17.9167
0.41	0.196	0.521951	0.9	0.52	0.422222	1.52	4.58	-2.01316
0.46	0.347	0.245652	1.0	0.7	0.3	2.9	4.57	-0.57586
0.48	0.397	0.172917	1.03	0.8	0.223301	4.09	4.56	-0.11491
0.51	0.46	0.098039	1.08	0.97	0.101852	4.15	4.56	-0.0988
0.53	0.50	0.056604	1.16	1.08	0.068966	4.3	4.56	-0.06047

continued on following page

Table 3. Continued

C_1	$\widehat{C}_1$	Relative error	C_2	$\widehat{C}_2$	Relative error	C_3	$\widehat{C}_3$	Relative error
0.54	0.52	0.037037	1.19	1.15	0.033613	4.34	4.56	- 0.05069
0.546	0.536	0.018315	1.21	1.20	0.008264	4.50	4.55	- 0.01111
0.547	0.537	0.018282	1.229	1.22	0.007323	4.48	4.55	- 0.01562
0.547	0.547	0	1.23	1.23	0	4.55	4.55	0

Both the simulated and estimated concentration values in all the three compartments along with the relative error are given in table 3. It was found from the relative square error that the estimated concentration is closer to the true value.

4. Data Driven Modelling Using Machine Learning Approach For Benchmark Pharmacokinetic Model:

Machine learning is one of promising tool to predict the concentrations in pharmacokinetic model. Several machine learning algorithms can be employed for prediction and estimation. In this article, supervised learning- based classification MATLab based machine learning algorithms have been used to predict the concentrations. First step is to predict the concentration in compartment 1 and followed by compartment 2 and 3 respectively. Algorithms like linear regression and support vector machine are used for estimating the concentration in all the compartments.

Figure 5. Linear regression based estimation of C1

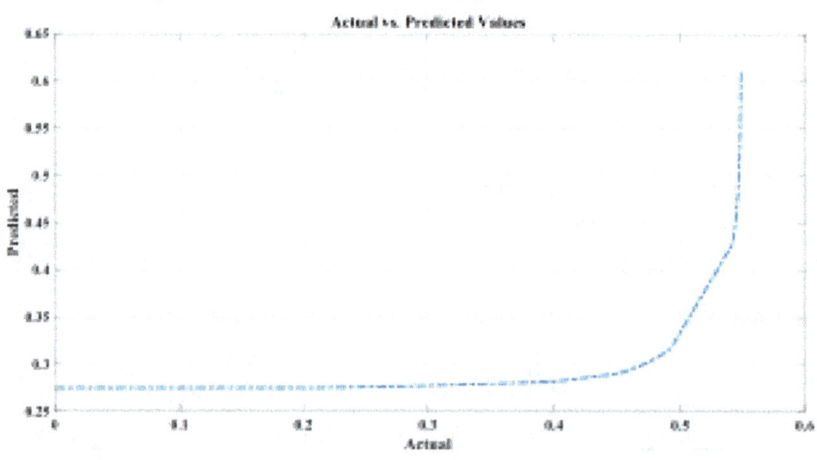

Figure 6. SVM based estimation of C1

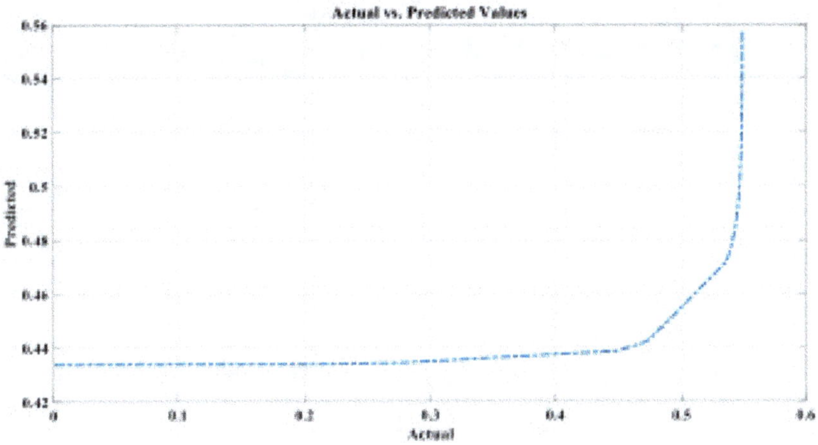

Figure 7. Linear regression based estimation of C2

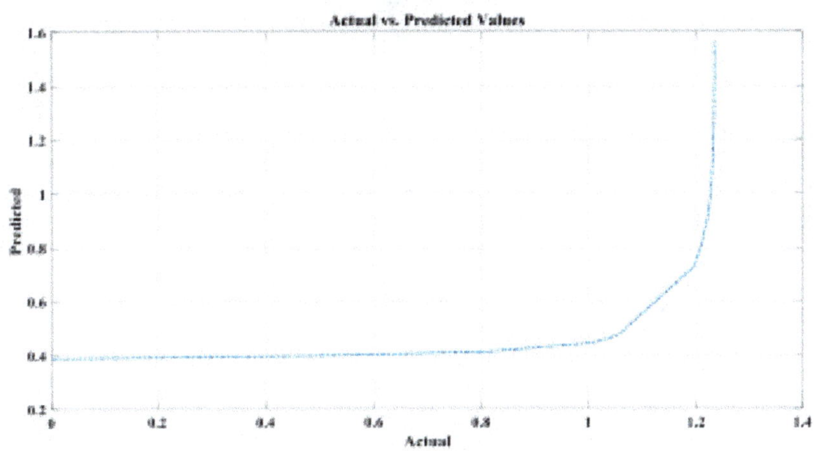

Figure 8. SVM based estimation of C2

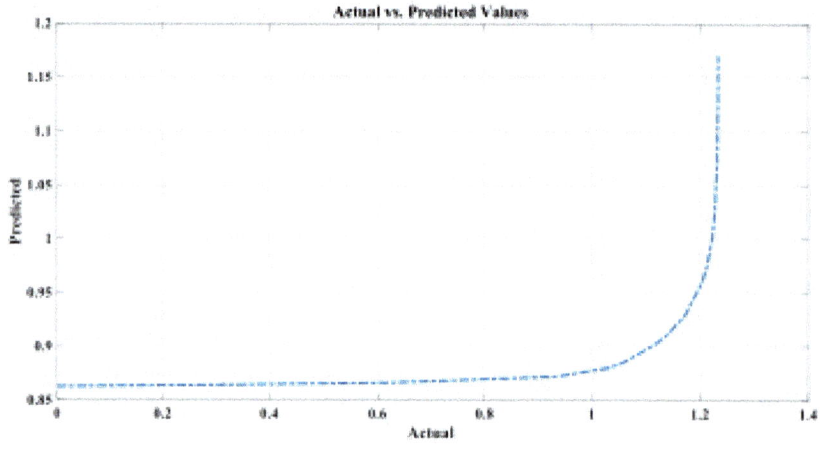

Figure 9. Linear regression based estimation of C3

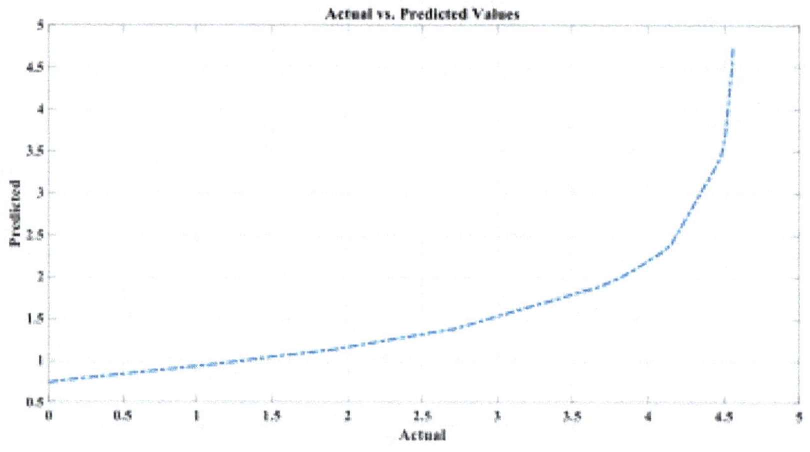

Figure 10. SVM based estimation of C3

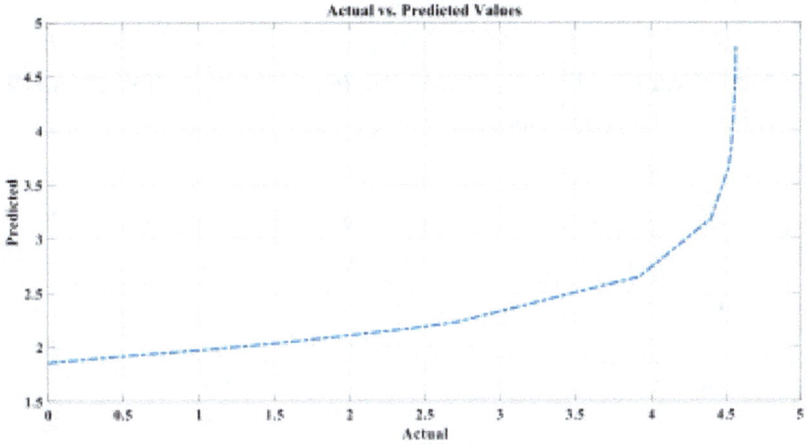

Fig. 5, 7 and 9 qualitatively estimate the concentration C1, C2 and C3 using linear regression-based machine learning algorithms.

Similarly, Support Vector Machine based qualitative estimation of concentration C1, C2 and C3 are shown in fig. 6, 8 and 10 respectively.

Linear regression and support vector machine are analysed for benchmark system, both the machine learning algorithms are predicting the concentration in all the three compartments. Quantitative measure of concentrations can be computed based on Root Mean Square Error, R squared and Mean Absolute Percentage Error.

Root Mean Square Error (RMSE) can be computed by taking square root of the average of the squared errors using the formula:

$$RMSE = \sqrt{\frac{\sum_{i=1}^{n}\left(C_1 - \widehat{C}_1\right)^2}{n}} \tag{8}$$

Due to squaring operation in RMSE, big errors are magnified while small ones are ignored.

R squared is calculated using the formula:

$$\text{Rsquared} = 1 - \frac{SS_{res}}{SS_{total}} \tag{9}$$

Where SSre is residual sum of squares and SStotal is total sum of squares. The more the value of R squared near 1, the better the model is.

Mean Absolute Percentage Error (MAPE) is the mean of all absolute percentage errors using the formula:

$$MAPE = \frac{1}{no.ofpredictions}\sum\left(\frac{\lfloor C_1 - \widehat{C_1}\rfloor}{P_m}\right) \tag{10}$$

Lower MAPE value indicates accurate prediction whereas higher MAPE value indicates less accurate prediction.

Table 4. Quantitative performance measure for pharmacokinetic model

Machine learning algorithms	RMSE	R Squared	MAPE
Linear Regression for C1	0.1359	0.4508	Inf
SVM for C1	0.2020	0.0373	4.4673e+03
Linear Regression for C2	0.3516	0.5844	Inf
SVM for C2	0.4582	0.2023	9.9366e+07
Linear Regression for C3	0.9799	0.7364	Inf
SVM for C3	1.4472	0.4118	Inf

From Table 4, the quantitative performance of C1, C2 and C3 are computed using linear regression and Support Vector Machine. This can be concluded that Support Vector Machine offers enhanced performance by accurately predicting concentration using AI techniques.

SOLUTIONS AND RECOMMENDATIONS

The concentration in all the three compartments is analysed for all the five pharmacokinetic models in figure 11, 12 and 13 respectively. It is evident from the response that C1's concentration is lower than that of C2 and C3. Similarly, the concentration in compartment C_2 is lesser than $C_{3.}$

Figure 11. Plot of concentration C1 for five pharmacokinetic models

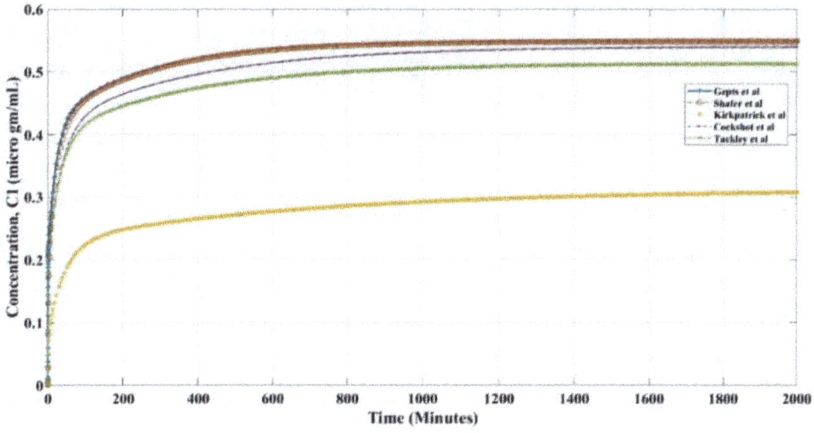

Figure 12. Plot of concentration C2 for five pharmacokinetic models

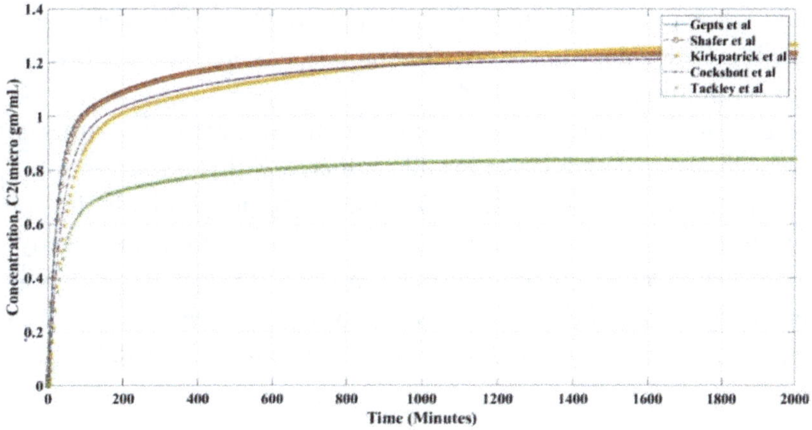

Figure 13. Plot of concentration C3 for five pharmacokinetic models

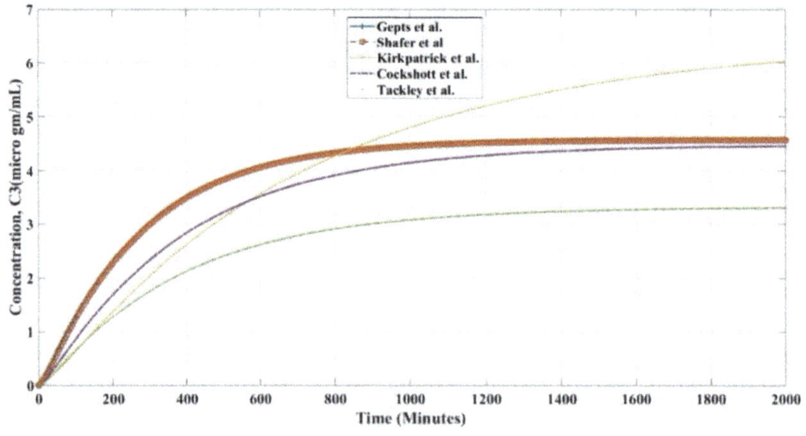

Hence it is clear that the drug concentration is high in residual tissues in slowly equilibrating compartment compared to the well perfused tissues in rapidly equilibrating compartment for all the five pharmacokinetic models. From the plot, the traversing of drug concentration from one compartment to other compartment can be obtained. It is also used to analyse the stability of concentration level by using the common three compartment model.

Based on comparison of concentrations in all the three compartments for the five pharmacokinetic models given in table 5, it is clear that concentration C_1 in the central compartment remains stable at 0.5 micro gm/mL. Similarly, it is observed that concentration C_2 in the slow equilibrium compartment remains steady state at 1.2 micro gm/mL and in rapid compartment reaches steady state at 4.5 micro gm/mL respectively. Hence the estimated values of the concentration in all the three compartments remains same for all the five pharmacokinetic models.

FUTURE RESEARCH DIRECTIONS

Although machine learning (ML) has considerable potential for modeling intricate pharmacokinetic (PK) systems, there are a number of significant obstacles that make it difficult to integrate ML into clinical pharmacology and drug development. First, PK data quality and availability are frequently inadequate; clinical datasets are often sparse, noisy, and imbalanced, which compromises ML models' ability to generalize, especially in underrepresented populations. Second, a lot of machine learning algorithms, particularly deep learning, are not interpretable like classic mechanistic PK models, which lowers clinical trust and regulatory approval. Another major problem is overfitting, whereby machine learning models readily adjust to noise in short datasets, resulting in subpar performance on unknown data. Furthermore, ML models frequently function without including accepted physiological principles, which could result in medically implausible outputs unless they are limited by hybrid or physics-informed frameworks. Significant obstacles are also presented by regulatory and validation issues, since clinical acceptance of ML models requires that they satisfy strict requirements for robustness, explainability, and reproducibility. The absence of established pipelines for creating and evaluating ML-based PK models further contributes to the field's varied approaches and challenges in duplicating outcomes.

Table 5. Comparison of Concentrations in all three compartments for the five pharmacokinetic models

Five Pharmacokinetic Models	Concentration C_1 in compartment 1	Concentration C_2 in compartment 2	Concentration C_3 in compartment 3
Gepts et al.	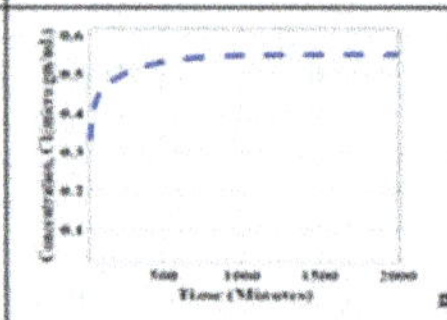	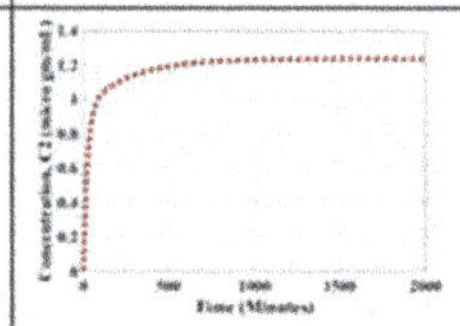	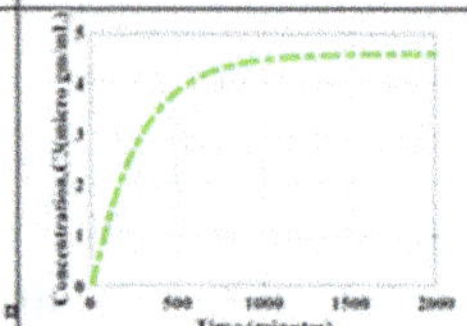
Shafer et al	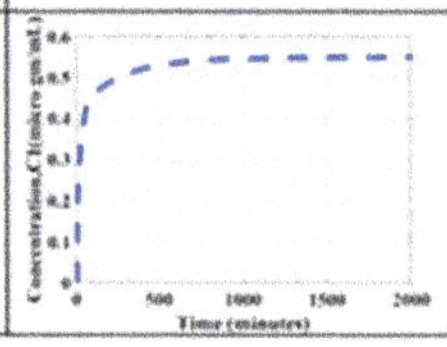	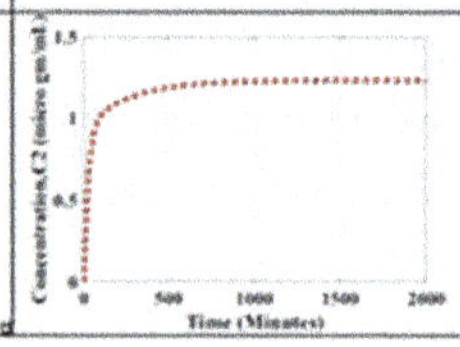	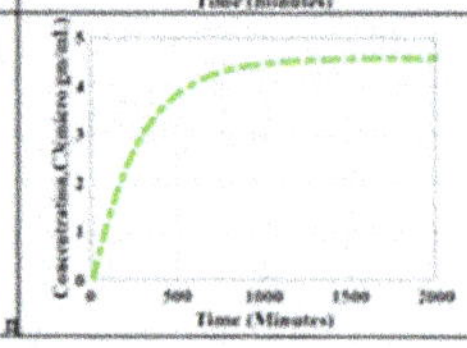
Kirkpatrick et al.	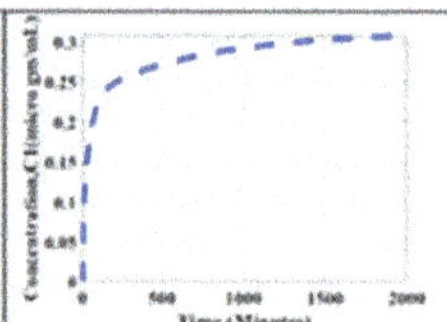	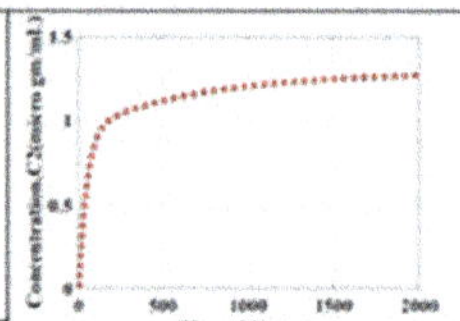	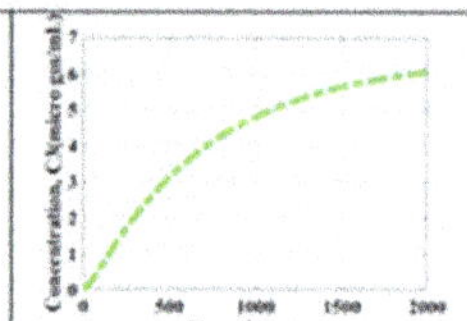
Cockshott et al.	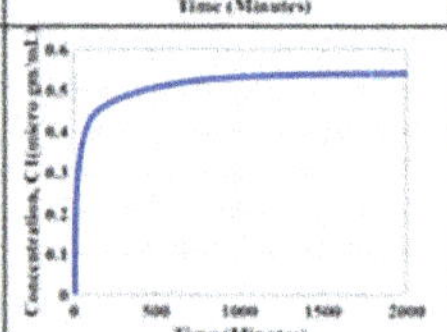	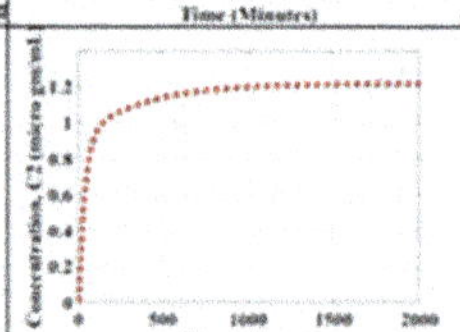	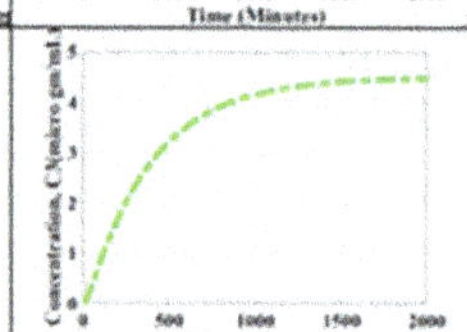
Tackley et al.	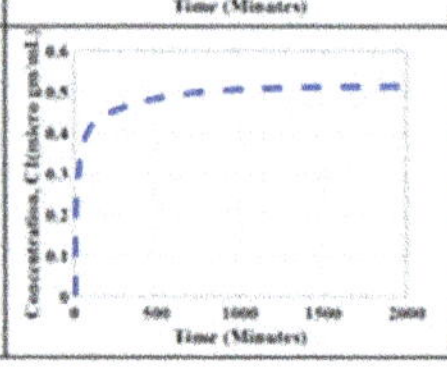	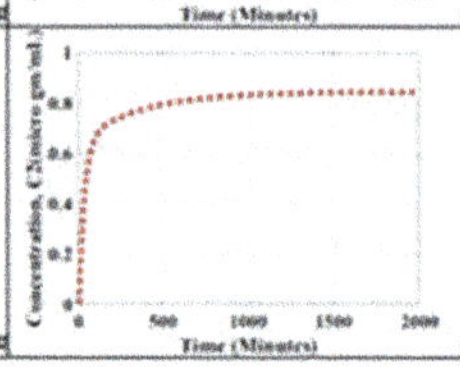	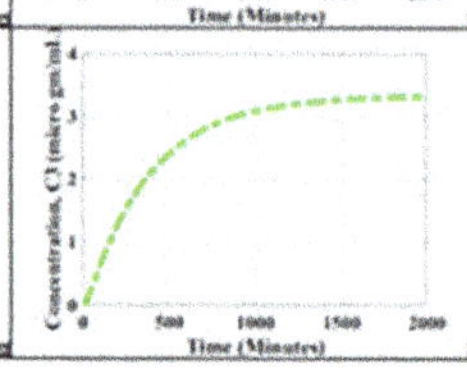

CONCLUSION

The concentration is estimated by the pharmacokinetic model using a three-compartment model. Three compartment models are non-linear having mass infusion rate as single input and three outputs as blood concentration in compartment 1, 2 and 3. This non-linear system has been modelled as non-square system having one input and three output system. This system is modelled using the first principles approach, and its parameters are computed using an ODE solver. For the five pharmacokinetic models, the concentration values in each of the three compartment models are estimated. Also, the estimated concentration values are compared with the simulated values by calculating relative square error. All the results in this chapter reveals that there is minimum relative square error for all the subject of study and hence enhanced performance has been obtained for the pharmacokinetic models. Overall based on computer simulation using machine learning algorithms like linear regression and SVM, both the clinician and anaesthesiologist will be explored to not only estimate the drug concentration in blood but also to administer the intravenous delivery of drugs to the subjects. Support vector machine accurately predicts the concentration in all the three compartments of pharmacokinetic models.

REFERENCES

. Wayne Bequette. (2002) Process Control: Modeling, Design, and Simulation. Prentice Hall PTR, 769.

Bonate, P. L. (2011). *Pharmacokinetic-Pharmacodynamic Modeling and Simulation* (2nd ed.). Springer. DOI: 10.1007/978-1-4419-9485-1

Brunton, S. L., Proctor, J. L., & Kutz, J. N. (2016). Discovering governing equations from data by sparse identification of nonlinear dynamical systems. *Proceedings of the National Academy of Sciences of the United States of America, 113*(15), 3932–3937. DOI: 10.1073/pnas.1517384113 PMID: 27035946

Cascone, S., Lamberti, G., Titomanlio, G., & Piazza, O. (2013). Pharmacokinetics of Remifentanil: A three-compartmental modeling approach. *Translational Medicine @ UniSa*, 18–22. PMID: 24251247

Chen, R. T. Q., Rubanova, Y., Bettencourt, J., & Duvenaud, D. (2018). *Neural ordinary differential equations.* In *Advances in Neural Information Processing Systems* (NeurIPS 2018), 31.

Cockshott, I. D., Douglas, E. J., & Prys-Roberts, C. (1987). Pharmacokinetics of propofol during and after intravenous infusion in man. *British Journal of Anaesthesia, 59*, 941.

Fernandez, J. M., Choi, D., Ahmed, N., & Gupta, R. (2023). Hybrid data-driven and mechanistic modeling of propofol pharmacokinetics in three compartments using deep neural networks. *IFAC-PapersOnLine*, *56*(10), 850–857.

Gabrielsson, J., & Weiner, D. (2016). *Pharmacokinetic and Pharmacodynamic Data Analysis: Concepts and Applications* (5th ed.). CRC Press.

Gepts, E., Camu, F., Cockshott, I. D., & Douglas, E. J. (1987). Disposition of propofol administered as constant rate infusions in humans. *Anesthesia and Analgesia, 66*(12), 1256–1263. DOI: 10.1213/00000539-198712000-00010 PMID: 3500657

He, X., Zhao, Y., & Kumar, R. (2023). Transformer and LSTM hybrid model for depth-of-anesthesia prediction under propofol infusion. *IEEE Transactions on Biomedical Engineering*, *70*(7), 1980–1991.

Hernández-Lobato, J. M., Houlsby, N., Ghahramani, Z., & Herbrich, R. (2014). *Probabilistic backpropagation for scalable learning of Bayesian neural networks.* In *Proceedings of the 32nd International Conference on Machine Learning* (ICML 2014), 1861–1869.

Hyo Jeong Ryu, Won ho Kang, Taeheon Kim, Jae Kyoung Kim, Kwang-Hee Shin, Jung-woo Chae, Hwi-yeol Yun. (2022). A compatibility evaluation between the physiologically based pharmacokinetic model and the compartmental PK model using the lumping method with real cases. *Frontiers in Pharmacology*, 13. PMID: 36034786

Kartono, A., Anggraini, D., Wahyudi, S. T., Setiawan, A. A., & Irmansyah, . (2021). Study of Parameters Estimation of The Three-Compartment Pharmacokinetic Model using Particle Swarm Optimization Algorithm. *Journal of Physics: Conference Series*, *1805*(1), 012032. DOI: 10.1088/1742-6596/1805/1/012032

Kirkpatrick, T., Cockshott, I. D., Douglas, E. J., & Nimmo, W. S. (1988). Pharmacokinetics of propofol (Diprivan) in elderlv patients. *British Journal of Anaesthesia*, *6O*, i46–i150. PMID: 3257879

Koren, Y., van der Walt, J., & Eleveld, D. J. (2022). Symbolic regression for automated covariate modeling in pharmacokinetics: Application to a propofol three-compartment model. *CPT: Pharmacometrics & Systems Pharmacology*, *11*(12), 1441–1453.

Kumar, R., Jones, S., & Patel, N. (2024). Advances in automated anesthesia control: Integrating deep learning and control methods over three-compartment PK models. *Anesthesiology & Perioperative Science*, *5*(1), 34–49.

Liu, Y., Zhang, H., Chen, X., Wang, Q., & Li, M. (2024). Data-driven pharmacokinetic modeling for propofol using machine learning approaches in a three-compartment framework. *European Journal of Pharmaceutical Sciences*, *190*, 106464. DOI: 10.1016/j.ejps.2023.106464

Rasmussen, M., Pedersen, J., & Smith, L. (2024). A three-compartment population pharmacokinetic model for propofol in very-high-BMI patients: Weight descriptors and sex as covariates. *Acta Anaesthesiologica Scandinavica*, *68*(3), 210–221. DOI: 10.1111/j.1399-6576.1975.tb05243.x PMID: 1101602

Shafer, A., Doze, V. A., Shafer, S. L., & White, P. F. (1988). Pharmacokinetics and pharmacodynamics of propofol infusions during general anesthesia. *Anesthesiology*, *69*(3), 348–356. DOI: 10.1097/00000542-198809000-00011 PMID: 3261954

Smith, A. L., Nguyen, P. T., & Banerjee, S. (2023). Deep reinforcement learning–based propofol dosing guided by three-compartment PK/PD simulations. *Journal of Clinical Pharmacology*, *63*(4), 367–379.

Tackley, R. M., Lewis, G. T. R., Prys-Roberts, C., Boaden, R. W., Dixon, J., & Harvey, J. T. (1989). Computer-controlled infusion of propofol. *British Journal of Anaesthesia*, *62*(1), 46–53. DOI: 10.1093/bja/62.1.46 PMID: 2783854

Vuyk, J., Engbers, F. H. M., Bum, A. G. L., Vletter, A. A., & Bovill, J. G. (1995). Performance of Computer-Controlled Infusion of Propofol: An Evaluation of Five Pharmacokinetic Parameter Sets. *Anesthesia and Analgesia*, *81*, 1275–1282. PMID: 7486116

Wu, Q., Chen, Y., & Feng, S. (2022). A convolutional neural network with self-attention for depth-of-anesthesia prediction under propofol anesthesia. *Computers in Biology and Medicine*, *148*, 105801. DOI: 10.1016/j.compbiomed.2022.105801

Zhao, H., Li, X., Wang, Y., & Chen, L. (2024). LSTM-based real-time concentration tracking of propofol using a four-compartment PK/PD model in swine. *Frontiers in Medical Engineering*, *10*, 112.

Zong, Z., Wang, H., & Lin, J. (2022). Clinical validation of a covariate-based propofol pharmacokinetic model under target-controlled infusion in surgery patients. *Journal of Clinical Anesthesia*, *80*, 110886.

ADDITIONAL READING

. Ahmadi Daryakenari, N., Wang, S., & Karniadakis, G. (2024). CMINNs: Compartment model informed neural networks – unlocking drug dynamics. *Preprint, arXiv*.

Nasim, I., & Nasim, A. (2024). Discovering intrinsic multi-compartment pharmacometric models using physics-informed neural networks. *International Conference on Scientific Computing and Machine Learning (SCML2024)*.

KEY TERMS AND DEFINITIONS

Pharmacokinetic (PK) Modeling: A method used to study how a drug is absorbed, distributed, metabolized, and excreted (ADME) in the body. It helps in understanding drug concentration changes over time within various compartments.

Three-Compartment Model: A pharmacokinetic model dividing the body into three compartments—central, rapidly equilibrating peripheral, and slowly equilibrating peripheral—to simulate drug distribution and elimination more accurately.

Propofol: A short-acting intravenous anesthetic commonly modeled using multi-compartment pharmacokinetic systems for safe and effective infusion control during surgery.

Data-Driven Modeling: An approach that uses machine learning and statistical methods to model and predict system behavior based on empirical data, without relying solely on predefined equations or parameters.

Machine Learning (ML): A subset of artificial intelligence involving algorithms that learn from and make predictions based on data. In pharmacokinetics, ML can predict drug concentration levels across compartments.

MATLAB: A high-level programming and simulation environment used extensively in engineering and scientific research for modeling dynamic systems such as pharmacokinetic processes.

Simulink: A MATLAB-based graphical environment for modeling, simulating, and analyzing dynamic systems, including pharmacokinetic models with differential equations.

ODE Solver: A numerical tool in MATLAB used to solve ordinary differential equations, which are essential for simulating drug concentration changes in pharmacokinetic models.

Support Vector Machine (SVM): A supervised machine learning algorithm used for classification and regression tasks, capable of modeling non-linear relationships in PK prediction.

Linear Regression: A basic predictive algorithm used in machine learning to model the linear relationship between input variables (e.g., drug infusion rate) and output responses (e.g., drug concentration).

Chapter 13
AI Driven Pharmacovigilance Case Study:
Predicting Adverse Effects of Drugs Using NLP and Patient Feedback

Ruchi Jakhmola Mani
https://orcid.org/0000-0001-9264-867X
Amity University, Noida, India

Manan Garg
https://orcid.org/0009-0009-3593-9871
Amity University, Noida, India

Barsha Rani Bora
Amity University, Noida, India

Kusala Vanam
Amity University, Noida, India

Nureen Amin
Amity University, Noida, India

Snigdha Debashis Bhattacharjee
Vivekanand Education Society Institute of Technology, Mumbai, India

ABSTRACT

Adverse drug reactions (ADRs) due to drug toxicity pose serious risks, often leading to severe health complications or fatalities. Current pharmacovigilance systems rely on clinical trials and post-market surveillance but lack real-time patient insights. This study presents an NLP-based predictive model to identify lethal and severe drug toxicities using real-world patient feedback and online drug databases. By leveraging unstructured text from patient reviews, medical forums, and electronic health records, the model detects early ADR signals. Data is collected from public drug databases and patient forums, then preprocessed using tokenization, stop word removal, lemmatization, and Named Entity Recognition (NER). Sentiment

DOI: 10.4018/979-8-3373-2043-4.ch013

analysis and deep learning models (BERT, LSTM) analyze patient sentiment and toxicity patterns. Machine learning classifiers (Random Forest, SVM, XGBoost) predict high-risk drug pairs. This approach enhances pharmacovigilance, helping healthcare professionals mitigate drug-related risks.

INTRODUCTION

Pharmacovigilance (PV) deals with the surveillance and evaluation of the safety of drug products, an essential element of healthcare systems globally (Lyton, 2018). Its contribution to public health is that it is capable of identifying and analysing adverse drug reactions and guaranteeing overall safety and effectiveness of medicines. Pharmacovigilance in the past has been based on patient care experience, text estimation, and post-mortem study of data from single case writings, epidemiological studies, and analytical trials. However, there were conditions on the efficiency, scalability and vulnerability to biases and human failure of these methods. Automation with AI has started a transformation in the domain of pharmacovigilance by applying ML algorithms, NLP, and modern algorithms to consider large bulk of physical world reports quickly and effectively origin.

AI connections have been found to be capable to shift over social platform updates, negative event responses, medical studies, computerised health publications, and interactions and inconsistencies that can signal novel security matters or adverse acknowledgement (Young et al., 2020). Moreover, using NLP, AI powered mechanization can infer from already tough-to-analyse unregulated data origin like analytical notes, patient details, and administrative documents. This functionality increases the accuracy, rapidity, and capability of conflicting event detection and characteristic detection platforms by sanctioning better proactive and broad liability control. While automation powered by AI can be a game-changer, there are some restraints and difficulties that should be met. These are the requirement to lend heavily in framework, computing capabilities, and administrative consent.

The accuracy, reliability of AI-based connections are still to be ensured with ongoing algorithmic verification, monitoring, and improvement. But since secure and extra efficient drugs take on character, the promise of AI in PV to enhance drug defense examination, administrative choice-making, and patient responsibility is emphasized. This will basically enhance overall human health. This aims to provide a complete view of the ways in which AI is transforming human health safeguard and drug defense study through a discussion of the ethical and legal concerns, the course and forthcoming significance of AI-based PV. This research hopes to contribute to the ongoing debate about the liable and successful implementation of mechanization in the pharmaceutical and healthcare sectors, focusing on enhancing patient safety and maximizing treatment effects, through investigation of the applications of AI in pharmacovigilance.

Phase IV of drug review lasts for several years after a drug is granted a marketing license. In this stage, the drug is studied under real-world circumstances to evaluate its efficacy, safety, and how it is utilized by sizable populations (O'Neill et al., 2007). Confirming that the drug's advantages outweigh any risks and that it actually functions as expected in routine clinical practice is the aim. Researchers also examine if its authorized usage need to be restricted or increased.

Pharmacovigilance involves a drug's effects can be categorized into pharmacodynamic effects and side effects. Pharmacodynamic effects refer to the intended therapeutic actions of a drug— how it helps treat a disease (Reiner et al., 2011). For example, a medication may lower uric acid levels to manage gout or reduce inflammation to alleviate pain. These effects are studied at various stages of drug development. Initially, they are tested in animals, followed by Phase I and Phase II trials in humans, and finally, Phase III clinical trials to confirm their effectiveness. As long as the dosage is appropriate, pharmacodynamic effects occur in all individuals. During drug development, researchers identify the most clinically relevant pharmacodynamic effect, which becomes the focus of Phase III trials. These trials evaluate how well the drug achieves its intended effect, such as relieving pain or treating gout. The results help regulatory agencies determine the drug's approved medical uses. Side effects, on the other hand, arise from the drug's pharmacological properties beyond its primary therapeutic action. These effects can be beneficial or harmful. Additionally, drugs can have harmful effects, which occur when a person is subjected to a high dose. Toxicovigilance refers to the monitoring and investigation of these toxic effects (Roux et al., 2015). On the other hand, pharmacovigilance focuses on ADRs—undesirable side effects that may show risks to patient safety.

Figure 1. Pharmacovigilance process overview

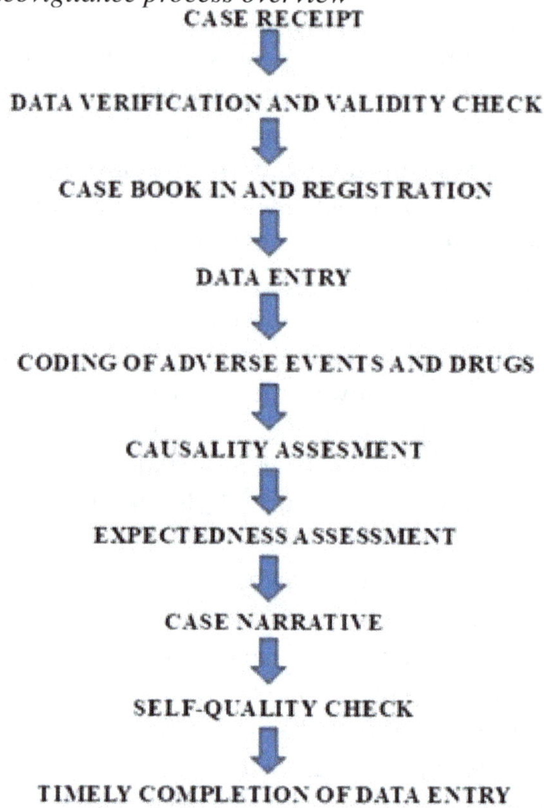

BACKGROUND

History of Pharmacovigilance

Pharmacovigilance, the art and science involved in the discovering, estimation, knowing, prevention of ADRs and any other drug-related issue, has a fascinating and long history, spurred by medical progress and public health protection needs. Initially, drug safety was mainly evaluated on a trial-and-error basis. Before the advent of modern medicine, treatments were based on herbal drugs and chemicals with not much understanding of their potential harms. With an increase in knowledge of medicine came an increase in care about the need for safety, though the process was still simple.

One of the most important milestones was in 1961, when the thalidomide medicine, marketed as a safe sedative, caused thousands of newborn babies to be born with birth defects, and to cause widespread outrage across the world. The disaster had pointed to a demand for a system of orderly monitoring of drug safety (Boulos, 2004). Drug control agencies, reacting to this, started to increase their attention to drug safety, and the idea of pharmacovigilance started gaining acceptance. This global movement enabled nations to exchange information about ADRs and gave a platform to comprehend the global effect of drugs on different populations. (22nd Sylvester O'Halloran Meeting, 2014). WHO's efforts in harmonizing the reporting of ADRs across nations were a breakthrough toward patient protection. Advances in the next decades with digital technologies and complex databases improved pharmacovigilance. Development of systems for the assembling and study of information on ADRs, such as the United States' FDA Adverse Event Reporting System (AERS), expanded the ability for identifying safety issues rapidly. The increase in global usage of medicines, combined with higher standards of testing and reporting, made continual enhancement of drug safety monitoring necessary.

\Pharmacovigilance took speed with the 2000s' introduction of Risk Management Plans (RMPs), which today are a component of drug approval. They mandate manufacturers to track long-term drug effects and act on them in case new risks come to light after a drug has been introduced into the market. Nowadays, pharmacovigilance is a built-in feature of the healthcare system across the globe, placing maximum stress on transparency, patient protection, and teamwork among regulatory authorities, physicians, and the drug industry. All this collaboration has taken us a long distance from the pre-reform days of unsafe drugs on sale in an unregulated atmosphere. Pharmacovigilance continues, with the new directions being focused on customized medicine and evidence-based monitoring of safety, indicating the path towards a safer, better-enlightened future of drug management.

Adverse Drug Reaction (ADRs)

ADRs are unwanted effects that may arise when a drug is applied according to the prescription, whether it is for the prevention, treatment, or diagnosis of a disease (Haber et al., 2009). ADRs, in contrast to problems brought on by excessive use or improper drug use, can occur even when a medication is used as prescribed. These reactions have the potential to cause hospitalization, chronic health issues, or even death in certain situations, which makes them a major healthcare concern. The fact that ADRs account for 3.6% of all hospital admissions raises concerns (Tasaka et al., 2018). Unintentional re- dispensing or re-prescribing of the medications is the reason behind about 27% of ADR cases that occur within 6 months after the initial incident. For patients in hospitals 16.88% of patients had ADRs, 6.7% had major ADRs, and 0.32% were fatal. An exciting opportunity for the study of digital pharmacovigilance has been created by the rise of "big healthcare data," which is defined by tremendous volume, complexity, and velocity. Thus, social media has emerged as a source that facilitates the identification and prediction of ADRs to enhance pharmacovigilance, in addition to existing traditional data platforms. Numerous current studies employ various approaches to identify ADRs by evaluating the correlation between a medication and its side effects.

However, in practice, there are other cause elements that might contribute to the occurrence of ADRs, therefore identifying the multiple components that cause ADRs is important. The range of PV to enhance the safety of patients encompasses identification and reporting of ADR events, drug errors, spurious and substandard drugs, ineffectiveness of drugs, misuse and/or abuse of drugs, and drug–drug interactions. ADRs are still the major target of PV activities. Spontaneous reporting system (SRS) is the most used system in the world to report adverse reactions by healthcare professionals, drug firms, or patients themselves to the national authorities controlling PV activities in the nation. Reporting System would enhance the safety profile of a specific drug through informing and identifying ADRs that might not have been identified while premarketing or even post marketing clinical trials. Hence, it can be used as a means of detection for novel, uncommon or severe ADR events. A major strength of SRS is that it applies to all medications throughout its lifecycle and not confined to a period of investigation. SRS of ADR is also not free of limitations. Low quality of reports, recognized reactions, and failure to develop causal relationship are some of the characteristics of SRS which are reported most often. Furthermore, SRS restricts the ability to calculate the rates because of missing numerator data and unreliable denominator. Additionally, SRS has been linked with underreporting that may impact new drugs and serious reactions. Although it is limited, SRS is regarded as the most cost-effective technique in monitoring drug safety.

Classification of ADRs

Originally, there were two primary categories for ADRs. Exaggeration of the drug's recognized pharmacological effects causes type A ADRs, which are dependent on dose and likely to be predictable. Orthostatic hypotension brought on by antihypertensive drugs is one case. On the other hand, Type B ADRs are uncommon, unpredictable dose-independent, and frequently affected by patient-specific factors. A tiny percentage of people have these side effects, which have nothing to do with the primary way that the drug works. Hypersensitivity (allergic) reactions are included in this category (Hopkins et al., 2021). Other categories were added over time: ADRs of Type C (chronic), which are associated with both dosage and length of usage; Type D, which show up long due to exposure to drug; and Type E, which arise as a result of withdrawal; and Type F (failure) ADRs, which include a sudden lack of impact from treatment. Approximately 80% ADRs in hospitalized patients or those who need hospitalization are Type A, according to studies, and are typically known and preventable (Table 1). The most common pharmaceuticals linked ADRs in adults include opioids, NSAIDs, anticoagulants, antineoplastic and immunosuppressive treatments, cardiovascular medications, and adrenal corticosteroids (Houssari et al., 2017). The drug classes most implicated in children include immunizations, respiratory medicines, and anti-infective treatments.

Table 1. 13 Types of ADRSs

Reaction Type (Mnemonic)	Characteristics	Examples	Administration
A: Dose related (Augmented)	-Standard Exaggerated -Pharmacologic response is linked with the drug's pharmacologic effect. -Consistent -Minimal death rate	-Tricyclic antidepressants and dry mouth; opioids and respiratory depression; warfarin and serotonin-induced haemorrhage SSRI-associated syndrome and digoxin toxicity	-Lower dosage or stop taking the medication -Think about the consequences of simultaneous treatment.
B: Non–dose related (Bizarre)	-Rare -Unrelated to how the medication works pharmacologically -Inconsistent -High death rate	-Immunologic responses: penicillin anaphylaxis Idiocentric responses: using general anaesthetics for malignant hyperthermia	-Avoid and withhold in the forthcoming.
C: Dose related and time related (Chronic)	-Rare -Associated with the total dose	-Jaw osteonecrosis and corticosteroid- induced inhibition of the hypothalamic pituitary-adrenal axis using bisphosphonates	-Lower the dosage or stop it altogether; withdrawal could need to be extended
D: Time related (Delayed)	-Rare -Typically related to dose -Dose-related -Takes place or becomes noticeable after using the medication.	-The development of cancer Tardive dyskinesia the process of Teratogenesis using leucopenia and lomustine	-Frequently unreachable

continued on following page

Table 1. Continued

Reaction Type (Mnemonic)	Characteristics	Examples	Administration
E: Withdrawal (final use)	-Rare -Occurs shortly after stopping the medicine.	-Withdrawal symptoms from opiates or benzodiazepines, such as anxiety or insomnia	-Slowly remove and reintroduce the medicine.
F: Unexpected therapeutic failure (Failure)	-Standard -Typically related to dose -Frequently brought on by drug interactions	-When used with an enzyme inducer, an oral contraceptive at an inadequate dosage antimicrobial agent resistance	-Raising the dosage -Examine the results of concurrent treatment.

How ADRs Differ From Other Drug-Related Issues

Even if drugs are given according to the diagnosis, treatment, or prevention prescriptions, ADRs can still occur. ADRs are the harmful and unwanted reactions to a drug at typical doses (Paananen et al., 2019). In contrast with the expected side effects, which generally are mild and well-known, ADRs can be severe, unpredictable, and life-threatening ones. This is a major problem in the medical field which requires careful monitoring and early intervention. Adverse drug reactions are common in the population and are usually mild. The point is that they are already identified before the drug is marketed and the symptoms are common for drowsiness, nausea, or headaches, which, although are unpleasant, do not always require stopping the medication. Nevertheless, ADRs can be responsible for the severe forms of diseases, such as organ damage, allergies, or life- threatening events like anaphylaxis. ADRs are different from the toxicity which is a condition when a medicine has too high a concentration in the patient's system as a result of an overdose, metabolic disorder, or drug interaction. One of the mutual activities of medication errors and ADR is that these two often result in life-threatening conditions whereas medication errors like prescription errors or dose errors, are not ADRs but drug errors (though medication errors). Surveillance is the main key to pharmacovigilance which is extremely important to guide medical staff in assessing the safety of the drug, to predict the potential risks and to prescribe only the drugs that are safe and evidence-based so that they can provide patient safety.

1. **ADRs vs. side effects:** Despite their frequent confusion, side effects and ADRs differ significantly. The unwanted consequences of a drug that accompany its intended therapeutic advantages are known as side effects (Goodwin et al., 2016). Usually predictable and dose- dependent, these effects show consistently based on the dosage of the medicine. Most of the time, adverse consequences are

minor or even advantageous. Commonly used to treat allergies, antihistamines, for example, frequently result in sleepiness, which some people find undesirable but beneficial for those who suffer from insomnia. In a similar vein, some blood pressure drugs offer a calming impact in along with controlling hypertension, which may help some people suffering from anxiety. The well-known ADR example included the pain reliever rofecoxib (Vioxx), which was originally advised for arthritis. The medication was taken off the market because it was discovered that continuous use of the drug raised the risk of heart attacks and strokes, despite its effectiveness in treating pain.

2. **ADRs vs. toxicity:** Although negative effects generated by drugs are a common feature of both drug toxicity and ADRs, their methods of action differ. When too much drug is consumed, whether by mistake or on purpose, toxicity develops, which can have serious as well as fatal consequences. The toxicity increases with the dose because it is strongly dose dependent. On the other hand, ADRs are not always related to dosage and might happen even when a medication is taken at the recommended rate. ADRs might not be caused by drug abuse, but rather by things like immune system reactions, individual metabolism, or genetic susceptibility. Digoxin, a drug used to treat heart failure, is a real-world example of drug toxicity (Ponikowski et al., 2016). Strict dose monitoring is necessary because high doses of digoxin can cause severe toxicity, resulting in life-threatening cardiac rhythm disturbances. However, due to differences in individual sensitivity to the medicine, some people may develop ADRs such as nausea and visual issues even while taking the recommended dosage.
3. **ADRs vs. allergic reactions:** Although they have different underlying mechanisms, allergic reactions and ADRs are both undesirable pharmacological side effects. ADRs can be caused by toxicity, drug interactions, or specific patient sensitivity. ADRs are described as any unpleasant or unexpected reaction to a medication at normal dosages. Acetaminophen-induced liver damage in certain people is an example of an unanticipated side effect, while NSAID-induced stomach ulcers are an example of a predictable one. An allergic reaction, which occurs when the immune system confuses a treatment for a dangerous substance, is one kind of adverse drug reaction (Fatima et al., 2016). In reaction, the body's immune system releases histamine, which can result in symptoms including rash, swelling, itching, or, in extreme situations, anaphylaxis. Changing the medication or dosage will help you control ADRs; allergic reactions need stopping the drug straight away and might demand for the use of antihistamines, corticosteroids, or epinephrine. Though allergic reactions are always unexpected and immune-driven, different non- immune routes could lead to ADRs.

Importance of Monitoring Adverse Drug Reactions

Pharmaceutical side effects (ADRs) play a role, in ensuring the effectiveness and safety of drugs and are essential for proper patient care management." While medications aim to treat illnesses without causing harm to patients" unforeseen side effects can sometimes go unnoticed initially." These adverse reactions range from issues like skin rashes nausea to more severe complications such, as organ damage or even fatalities " presenting a diverse array of symptoms." Medical professionals can detect issues by monitoring ADRs and then make necessary adjustments, to the medication schedule or treatment plan to protect the patient's well-being effectively while also ensuring that the therapy remains safe and effective as intended. Monitoring drug reactions (ADRs) holds importance as it enhances the overall understanding of medicine, in general by examining how groups of individuals, like those with existing conditions or specific genetic traits (Arundel et al., 2010). React to treatments through the accumulation of data health authorities can ensure that medications are safe and effective for a broad range of users rather than just a select few.

Monitoring drug reactions (ADRs) fosters transparency and trust, in the relationship between patients and healthcare providers, by assuring patients that their drug responses are being closely monitored, and any potential risks are being promptly addressed for their well-being and safety assurance. The pharmacovigilance mission, in addition to ensuring health among all at-risk patient populations, by regulating the use of drugs, also implies the monitoring of ADRs (Bellazzi et al., 2016). ADR surveillance protocol also benefits medical professionals in making the right calls for long-term hazards posed by drug use, hence flourishing client's health over the period of time. One of the main success factors of ADR monitoring is early detection. Although many ADRs are detected through clinical trials, some can become apparent only when a drug is being tested among a wide range of people, which includes those with comorbidities, different ages, or genetic differences. Therapeutic interventions can be thus changed by the healthcare system posing great flexibility of prescription recommendations, dosages, and even the removal of a pharmaceutical from the market through post-marketing surveillance, in addition to revealing the otherwise latent side effects. The affinity for treatments of ADRs is another means by which the quality of treatment is improved.

Through the collection of real-world performance data on the treatment of each individual, healthcare professionals can afford to administer the perfect treatment that best suits every patient's needs and, therefore, minimize side effects. For instance, using pharmacogenetic data, one can appropriately prescribe individuals who are more likely to have particular reactions to a certain drug. This is not without the significant gains that contribute to the minimization of negative drug interactions or the shots in the arm which, otherwise, are engendered by inappropriate prescription patterns. The drug safety and efficacy corpus are, moreover, approved by the continuous ADR monitoring, which is the backbone of innovation for drug development. Along with the progress of monitoring activities, health authorities and pharmaceutical companies can adjust drug labels, you may stop reading and allow better treatment regimens and inform medical practitioners of the latest safety issues as they get more information from the continuous monitoring programs. Consistently, this everlasting method sustains the best patient outcomes and also enhances the confidence in pharmaceutical goods by constantly equipping the medical sector with the latest secure-using data and information.

Case Study Based on Our Own Work

As the world population increasingly depends on medicines to manage acute and chronic illnesses, drug safety has never been more important. Patients often post about their treatment online — reporting symptoms, side effects, and concerns in unstructured language (Fig 3). Such valuable data sources are not used by traditional monitoring systems. This case study speaks about why I undertook the research: an imperative to design a proactive, AI-powered pharmacovigilance system that is capable of extracting adverse drug reactions straight from patients' narratives. Using Natural Language Processing methods, my goal is to identify and label adverse events within high-volume patient reviews and complaints, in an effort to speed up safety signals detection earlier on and help alleviate patient harms.

Database: RxList

RxList is by far an authentic and comprehensive online medicinal resource devoted to providing precise, detailed, and timely pharmaceutical-related information regarding brand-name and generic medicines. Starting in 1995 with an experienced pharmacist team, it emerged as one of the foremost sources for drug-related information known on the Internet. Over the years, RxList has also earned its spark as an organization providing excellent, evidence-based information so that healthcare professionals, patients can make well-informed decisions regarding their medications and their safe use. The joining of forces with WebMD, another giant in online health information, in 2004 kick-started its growing credibility and prominence.

It is unique in the strict peer-review and editorial processes carried out by in-house experts. Articles and information on drugs are written and reviewed by professionals under pharmacy and medicine for the sake of producing accurate and informative content. The three pillars of high standard used by RxList are the US FDA, Cerner Multum, and First Databank, Inc. These sources are reliable because they provide recent drug information such as prescription information, adverse effects, interactions, dosing, and contraindications. By updating with the most recent regulatory changes, safety alerts, and clinical updates, RxList affords their clients with the most current relevant information.

Ease is a hallmark of RxList, and convenience allows visitors to search for what they may want. One helpful tool for moving about this website is Drugs A-Z, which is organized alphabetically by brand-name and generic medications. An advanced search function is positioned at the top of each page in RxList (Fig 2). The user types in the generic or brand name of a drug in the search box, and comprehensive information about that drug pops up immediately. This speed-search function contributes to further convenience by providing both consumers and health professionals important drug information in just seconds. Providing multiple browsing and searching means offers RxList a versatile response to the different needs of its large constituency from clinical-information investigation health care professionals to regular consumers seeking layman explanations for medication queried. With a blend of expert-reviewed content, trusted data sources, and a simple interface, RxList is a real boon to web-goers looking for reliable databases for drug information.

Figure 2. Homepage of RxList

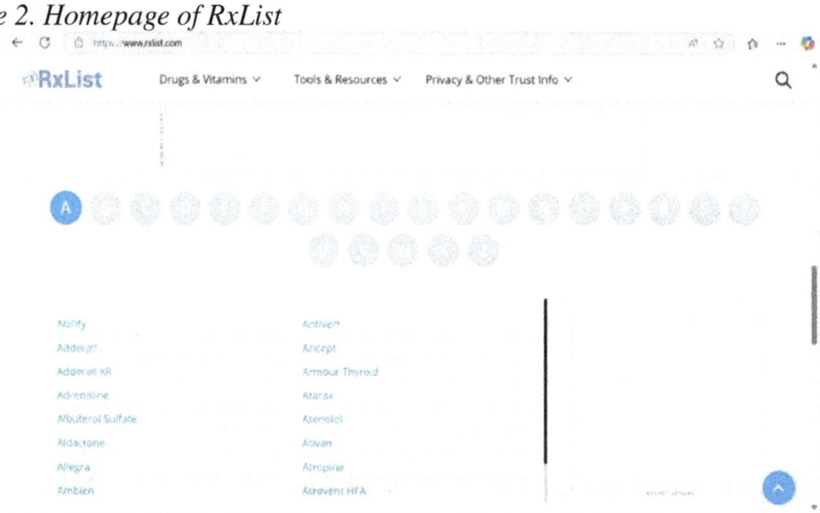

Figure 3. Patient reviews

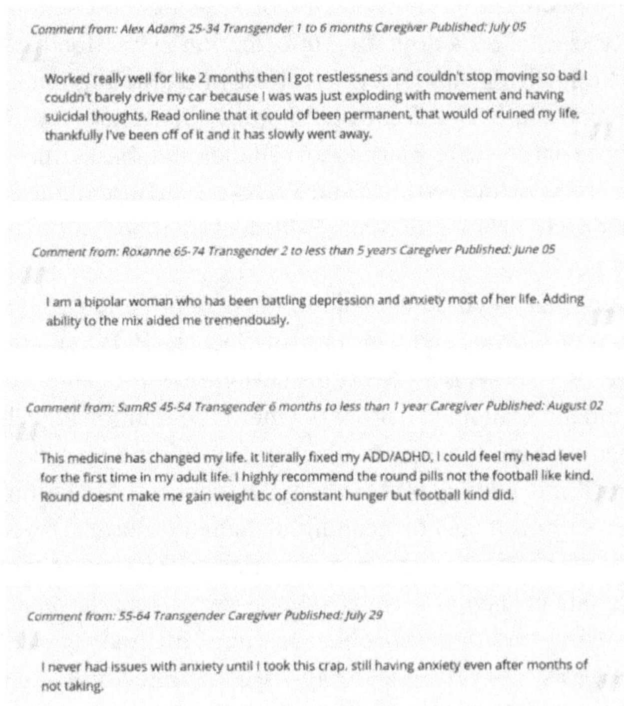

Comment from: Alex Adams 25-34 Transgender 1 to 6 months Caregiver Published: July 05

Worked really well for like 2 months then I got restlessness and couldn't stop moving so bad I couldn't barely drive my car because I was was just exploding with movement and having suicidal thoughts. Read online that it could of been permanent, that would of ruined my life, thankfully I've been off of it and it has slowly went away.

Comment from: Roxanne 65-74 Transgender 2 to less than 5 years Caregiver Published: June 05

I am a bipolar woman who has been battling depression and anxiety most of her life. Adding ability to the mix aided me tremendously.

Comment from: SamRS 45-54 Transgender 6 months to less than 1 year Caregiver Published: August 02

This medicine has changed my life. It literally fixed my ADD/ADHD, I could feel my head level for the first time in my adult life. I highly recommend the round pills not the football like kind. Round doesnt make me gain weight bc of constant hunger but football kind did.

Comment from: 55-64 Transgender Caregiver Published: July 29

I never had issues with anxiety until I took this crap. still having anxiety even after months of not taking.

SOLUTIONS AND RECOMMENDATIONS

Common Pharmacovigilance AI Approaches

1. **Natural Language Processing (NLP):** One of AI subfields is NLP, allowing computers to fully comprehend and make use of human language. Like humans, it mixes languages, computers, and machine learning to translate words and speech. Think about how we get our messages across by voice messages, texts, emails, and even social media posts. Machines can analyze this information, find meaning, and respond wisely due to NLP. NLP is applied, for instance, when you query Siri about the weather or when Google suggests search terms as you type. It works by processing text, recognizing syntax, identifying key words, and even detecting thoughts. NLP assists in extracting and processing useful information from unstructured text data like electronic health records (EHRs), social media, patient feedback, and scientific articles. It supports ADR identification through

drug name, side effect, and symptom extraction employing methods such as Named Entity Recognition (NER). Case processing automation is also an area in which NLP is used for automating information extraction from Spontaneous Reports to diminish manual effort involved in extracting data. It also aids in signal discovery and evaluation of temporality/causality from insights gained upon analyzing large-scale pharmacovigilance databases like FAERS (FDA Adverse Event Reporting System) and WHO's VigiBase for detecting potential safety signals more efficiently than traditional methods.

There are many NLP techniques behind these applications. Tokenization split the text into words or phrases and then Part-of-Speech (POS) tagging to label each word in nouns, verbs, or adjectives to get the structure of the sentence. The next step is to apply Dependency parsing A process where the relationships between words can be established making it easier to identify causation between drug intake and side effects. Algorithms like Latent Dirichlet Allocation (LDA) for topic modelling enable researchers to group text into meaningful thematic clusters, revealing emerging safety issues. Another important method is text classification, in which reports are assigned discrete labels such as serious vs. non-serious based on a predefined list of labels, either using traditional machine learning methods (e.g. Support Vector Machines (SVM)) as well as deep learning-based architectures such as BERT and BioBERT. Sentiment analysis is commonly used for a variety of analysing products or drugs' feedback from the patients to identify whether the experience with the drugs is positive or negative (Schot et al., 2018).

There are a range of NLP-based tools and models that support pharmacovigilance activities. These are domain-specific pretrained models such as BERT, BioBERT, and SciBERT for biomedical text, domain-specific frameworks such as SpaCy, and NLTK for basic NLP features. Two examples of NLP pipelines that are used in the process of automated data extraction/web scraping (Fig 4) and analysis of drug regulatory documents are tailored databases like MedDRA (Medical Dictionary for Regulatory Activities) and PubMed. Example: Patient Review: "I began taking Metformin last week, and I am feeling really nauseous and dizzy." With NLP, the system would identify that the drug name is Metformin, adverse events are the nausea and dizziness, and the sentiment is negative, would extract the drug name Metformin, would extract the adverse effects nausea and dizziness, would classify the sentiment as negative Organizing such information enables pharmacovigilance teams to identify new signals.

2. **Machine Learning (ML):** Machine learning is totally changing the game in pharmacovigilance. It's like having a superpower to spot and handle those scary drug safety issues way faster than we ever could before. Back in the day, we had

to rely on humans to sift through all this data, which was obviously a slow and sometimes messy deal because, let's face it, we're not perfect. But now, we've got computers with brains that can chew through a ton of data like its candy – they can look at stuff like health records, patient stories, and even the boring stuff from clinical trials and regulations, and boom! They find out if a drug might not be playing nice with our bodies quicker and more accurately than we ever could. These ML algorithms are like the Sherlock Holmes of the drug world, uncovering patterns that our human brains might miss. They're trained with old data about drug safety to guess what might happen next with new drugs. And get this – there are two main ways they do it: supervised learning, where they learn from examples, like a kid with a flashcard, and unsupervised learning, where they just explore data on their own and find weird stuff we didn't know about. It's like teaching them to recognize when something's not quite right before it turns into a big problem. And then there's NLP, which is basically AI that helps us read and understand all that messy human talk. It sifts through the jumble of words in online reviews and doctor notes to see if anyone's mentioning anything fishy about a drug. It's like having a gossip network for side effects, but it's totally science-y and helpful. What's even cooler is that it doesn't just stop at finding things; it actually makes the whole process of dealing with these safety issues easier. It's like having a robot assistant that can do all the tedious stuff like sorting cases and figuring out if a drug's causing problems. This means that when something does go wrong, the people who are in charge of our health can jump on it faster and keep us all safer.

3. **Deep Learning (DL):** Deep Learning, is a fascinating range of AI. It's actually inspired by how our brains function. So, it uses these things called neural networks—think of them like layers of connected nodes, or virtual neurons, if you will. These networks are designed to handle vast amounts of data and find patterns that might not be obvious at first glance. What's really cool about deep learning is that it can automatically learn features from raw data. This means it doesn't always need a human to point out what to look for, which is a big deal. Take pharmacovigilance, for instance. Here, deep learning can dive into complex medical texts, patient records, and even social media chatter to spot ADRs or to predict potential safety risks. Unlike the old-school methods that might just rely on specific keywords, deep learning gets context. This comes in handy, especially when patient reports are written casually or when you need to tease out subtle links between symptoms and medications. Then you've got models like BERT and BioBERT, which are built on this deep learning framework. They're already helping researchers and regulators comb through tons of safety data much more efficiently.

4. **Sentiment analysis:** Computers are able to understand the emotional tone or attitude of a text better using a method known as sentiment analysis. The aim of this NLP method is to establish whether the target emotions conveyed in a sentence, paragraph, or text are neutral, negative, or positive. To help researchers, drug companies, and regulators understand the true sentiments of patients toward their drugs, sentiment analysis lies at the heart of pharmacovigilance. I did sentiment analysis on the patient reviews from Rxlist showing how we can apply this technique in real-world (Fig 5). In electronic health records, product review sites, internet health forums, and social networking sites, patients often post. To assess these enormous amounts of unstructured content, sentiment analysis automatically analyzes whether the sentiment is neutral, negative, or positive in aggregate. For instance, sentiment analysis may detect an unfavorable trend and alert about a potential issue of safety if numerous patients are reporting to have developed intense headaches upon consumption of a certain prescription. But it is likewise probable that one may capture positive sentiment in case patients are praising a medication for improving their life quality. This approach is very useful as it identifies the context and tone behind individuals' reports of their experience, for instance, relief, sarcasm, or frustration, instead of only looking for keywords. Pharmacovigilance teams are able to enhance overall drug safety by enhancing risk assessments, enabling more patient-centric decisions, and detecting new signals of safety earlier by monitoring real- world patient feedback in real-time. Fundamentally, sentiment analysis guarantees patient experiences result in safer drugs through the closure of the gap between drug safety surveillance and patient voices.
5. **Signal detection** and **causality assessment:** Signal detection and causality assessment are two important processes in pharmacovigilance that help to guarantee the safety of drugs after they have been marketed. Signal identification is the process of detecting early warning signs, or "signals," that a drug may be having unexpected or otherwise unrecognized side effects. Signals are hints that something unusual may be occurring and need further investigation, but do not necessarily mean that the medicine is unsafe. These signals can occur in many locations, such as internet discussion boards or social media, scientific literature, electronic health records, and unexpected adverse event reports (from patients, doctors, or drug companies). Because there is so much data available, modern pharmacovigilance depends almost exclusively on artificial intelligence and machine learning algorithms to scan automatically various sources and look for patterns, clusters of identical reports, or statistical disproportions that can signal a new safety problem. Detection of such signs should be early as it enables the authorities and the pharmaceutical companies to respond in good time, something that may mean modifying safety data, carrying out additional

research, or, in extreme cases, suspending treatment. Once a potential signal is identified, assessment of causality is carried out. The aim of this step is to establish whether the adverse event was indeed caused by the drug or whether it was likely caused by another prescription, a pre- existing condition, or even lifestyle. The WHO-UMC Causality Assessment System is one of the accepted procedures and tools that experts use to examine the evidence. They consider the timing of the event, whether the patient recovered following suspension of the treatment, and if similar cases were reported.

Scraped reviews results

Figure 4. Scraped reviews of the drug Abacavir, Dolutegravir, and Lamivudine

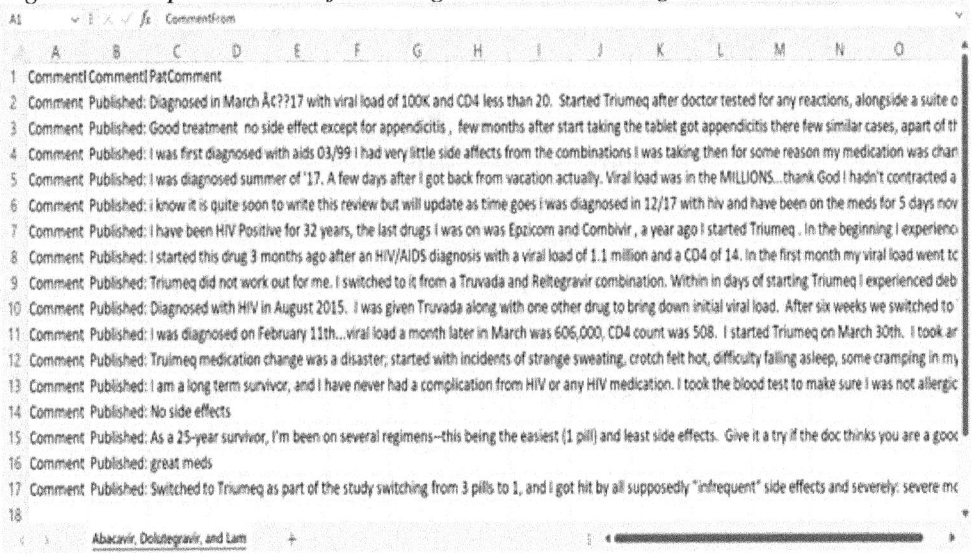

A1 CommentFrom

	A	B	C
1	CommentI	CommentI	PatComment
2	Comment	Published:	Diagnosed in March Âc??17 with viral load of 100K and CD4 less than 20. Started Triumeq after doctor tested for any reactions, alongside a suite o
3	Comment	Published:	Good treatment no side effect except for appendicitis , few months after start taking the tablet got appendicitis there few similar cases, apart of tl
4	Comment	Published:	I was first diagnosed with aids 03/99 I had very little side affects from the combinations I was taking then for some reason my medication was char
5	Comment	Published:	I was diagnosed summer of '17. A few days after I got back from vacation actually. Viral load was in the MILLIONS...thank God I hadn't contracted a
6	Comment	Published:	i know it is quite soon to write this review but will update as time goes i was diagnosed in 12/17 with hiv and have been on the meds for 5 days nov
7	Comment	Published:	I have been HIV Positive for 32 years, the last drugs I was on was Epzicom and Combivir , a year ago I started Triumeq . In the beginning I experienc
8	Comment	Published:	I started this drug 3 months ago after an HIV/AIDS diagnosis with a viral load of 1.1 million and a CD4 of 14. In the first month my viral load went tc
9	Comment	Published:	Triumeq did not work out for me. I switched to it from a Truvada and Reltegravir combination. Within in days of starting Triumeq I experienced deb
10	Comment	Published:	Diagnosed with HIV in August 2015. I was given Truvada along with one other drug to bring down initial viral load. After six weeks we switched to
11	Comment	Published:	I was diagnosed on February 11th...viral load a month later in March was 606,000, CD4 count was 508. I started Triumeq on March 30th. I took ar
12	Comment	Published:	Truimeq medication change was a disaster; started with incidents of strange sweating, crotch felt hot, difficulty falling asleep, some cramping in my
13	Comment	Published:	I am a long term survivor, and I have never had a complication from HIV or any HIV medication. I took the blood test to make sure I was not allergic
14	Comment	Published:	No side effects
15	Comment	Published:	As a 25-year survivor, I'm been on several regimens--this being the easiest (1 pill) and least side effects. Give it a try if the doc thinks you are a gooc
16	Comment	Published:	great meds
17	Comment	Published:	Switched to Triumeq as part of the study switching from 3 pills to 1, and I got hit by all supposedly "infrequent" side effects and severely: severe mc
18			

Abacavir, Dolutegravir, and Lam

Sentiment analysis result

Figure 5. Sentiment analysis of the drug Abacavir, Dolutegravir, and Lamivudine

A1 fx CommentFrom

	A	B	C	D	E
1	Comment	Comment	PatComm	Sentiment	
2	Comment	Published:	Diagnosec	1	
3	Comment	Published:	Good trea	-1	
4	Comment	Published:	I was first	-1	
5	Comment	Published:	I was diag	1	
6	Comment	Published:	i know it is	1	
7	Comment	Published:	I have bee	1	
8	Comment	Published:	I started tl	1	
9	Comment	Published:	Triumeq d	1	
10	Comment	Published:	Diagnosec	-1	
11	Comment	Published:	I was diag	1	
12	Comment	Published:	Truimeq n	-1	
13	Comment	Published:	I am a lon	1	
14	Comment	Published:	No side ef	-1	
15	Comment	Published:	As a 25-ye	1	
16	Comment	Published:	great med	1	
17	Comment	Published:	Switched t	-1	

FUTURE RESEARCH DIRECTIONS

AI integration in Pharmacovigilance

Pharmacovigilance has been rapidly revolutionized by artificial intelligence (AI), which makes it possible to monitor and assess adverse drug responses more precisely and effectively (Nassiri et al., 2024). AI's proactive approach to discovering possible safety issues with drugs is best demonstrated by predictive modelling, which improves safeness of patient through initially identifying adverse practices. AI enables the estimation and finding of massive amounts of data from various originations like EHRs along with social media, entirely detecting possible drug reaction signals and enabling rapid response where necessary. Despite its revolutionary potential, AI integration into pharmacovigilance has been slowed by issues of confidentiality of data and adjustment of regulatory framework. But the apparent benefit of enhancing drug safety as well as patient outcomes underscores the need for ongoing research and development. The union of AI and pharmacovigilance is a revolution in monitoring drug safety with early identification of drug safety problems and simplification of investigation of adverse drug reactions.

Pharmacovigilance solutions for the use of AI incorporate natural language processing for withdrawing intelligence from disorganised sources of data and data that can be predicted for anticipating adverse events based on progressions in the data. Applications of AI in pharmacovigilance in real life include automating the detection and classification of ADRs from varied sources of data and monitoring social media for potential defence warnings, saving resources and time required during enhancing firmness and efficiency. AI-fortified pharmacovigilance promises the two opportunities as well as challenges such as data privacy concerns and model regulation. Coming evolution in AI-based drug safety estimation scheme can give assurance proactive patient-centred approaches by advancing modernization along with advancement. Reports indicate the capabilities of AI programs in detecting safety notices at earliest and general outcomes of patient safeness. Use of AI in pharmacovigilance is the dawn of new proactive, evidence-based strategies in monitoring drug safety, with unrealized potential for enhancing patient results and healthcare governance.

Potential Advantages of Combining AI with Pharmacovigilance

1. **Advanced data mining methods:** Pharmacovigilance experts are able to use artificial intelligence in order to utilize modern mining of data methods, like NLP and ML algorithms, in order to pull out important understanding from different sources of information. By implementing these tools, one is able to recognize patterns, trends, and relationship related to drug safety by evaluating huge data sets like adverse practice records, medical articles, social media, and computerized health condition reports.
2. **Semantic analysis of reports of adverse events:** Pharmacovigilance scientists can specially control or grasp the content of reported adverse response with the help of AI-driven semantic analysis tools that evaluate adverse event record meaning and content. Semantic evaluation enhances the general quality of pharmacovigilance methods by developing importance and efficiency of adverse practice findings.

3. **Signal detection in actual time**: Artificial intelligence systems can identify patterns in approaching data streams in actual time to find arising progression and safeness alerts. AI-driven connections are capable of rapidly identifying any safety concerns by consistently data consideration from various different origins, confining social media websites, healthcare information, and regulatory documents. This facilitates rapid response and proactive risk control interventions.
4. **Integration of wearable devices**: Artificial intelligence (AI) coupled with wearable technology facilitates continuous monitoring of patient health parameters, including vital signs, activity, and medication adherence. AI-based solutions can collect actual-time information from wearable sensors in an effort to detect initial signs of negative reactions and provide individualized safety monitoring according to the needs of each patient.
5. **Monitoring of population health:** Population health surveillance systems powered by artificial intelligence (AI) monitor health trends and patterns at the community level, and it becomes feasible to detect potential drug safeness issues and collection of adverse event knots. AI facilitates initial acknowledgement and detection to new health issues by assessing pooled abstracts from numerous origins, including registries of human health, databases demand, and electronic well-being responses.
6. **Augmented risk-benefit analysis:** Through considering a wide range of criteria, such as patient preferences, treatment, disease harshness, and patients distinctives, AI allows for major complete risk-benefit analyses. AI-enabled platforms support more knowledgeable ruling regarding drug and medical intervention use by integrating clinical trial, empirical evidence, and patient-reported data.
7. **Drug safety predictive modelling:** Predictive modelling approaches based on artificial intelligence (AI) estimate the likelihood of side effects associated with specific medications or drug combinations. Predictive models help identify high- risk situations and offer direction for decision-making in drug development, regulatory assessment, and clinical practice by analyzing historical information regarding drug exposures, patient profiles, and adverse event reports.
8. **Electronic Health Record (EHR) integration**: Integration with EHR capabilities allows to obtain and process information related to the PV of the patient. The AI solution in the EHR area would contribute to enhancing signal detection, risk estimation and safety activity tracking/conducted by electronically importing EHR associated information into an EHR (i.e., history of prescribing, lab tests, diagnosis codes).
9. **A computer-automated literature review:** Locating scientific literature for pertinent safety information is eased by artificial intelligence-based literature review tools. Artificial intelligence (AI) systems spot applicable studies, summarize key conclusions, and distil the cumulative evidence on medication safety

and side effects by mining vast quantities of biomedical literature, including journal articles, conference proceedings, and regulatory documents.

10. **Coding and semantic annotation**: Artificial intelligence (AI) tools enhance data compatibility and pharmacovigilance procedures by simplifying it to code and annotate adverse event reports semantically. AI offerings bring consistency and accuracy in adverse event reporting and analysis by classifying incidents automatically according to pre-defined coding systems, including MedDRA (Medical Dictionary for Regulatory Activities).

Benefits of Pharmacovigilance AI Integration

1. Integration of AI makes it easy to gather pharmacological adverse effect reports from various sources (Thieme et al., 2020). Due to the gathering of data from multiple sources, we are in a position to achieve a perfect consideration of the possible uncertainty and advantages of a drug.
2. It allows us to process much information quickly. Consequently, we can analyze multiple reports and find patterns or trends quicker.
3. AI makes it easier to organize and understand the information we collect. To enhance our drug safety decision making, this allows us to recognize trends or data associations.
4. Security of information and loss avoidance are provided by integrated mixed Artificial Intelligence systems. This also ensure that patient private information is only available to individuals which are authorized.
5. The time needed for processing and entry of data has been reduced with integration of AI. It is able to create templates for common data and identify voices and handwriting.
6. Following observation of past history and trend detection, AI will help us in reading probable issues safeness. In this, we are able to control problems before things spiral too far out of hand.

Role of AI and NLP in Pharmacovigilance

AI and NLP are developing the area of pharmacovigilance, or the practice of medicine safety control. AI and NLP are providing positivity to improving the way we identify, evaluate, and assess the dangers of medicine. AI and NLP are aiding healthcare professionals and official authorities in effectively protecting public health by increasing efficiency, accuracy, and speed (Dwivedi et al., 2019). AI, particularly with machine learning, is great at managing big volumes of information everything from reports of harmful events to the results of clinical trials and electronic medical records. AI can acknowledge patterns and trends that may indicate safety issues by demonstrating this data. This is a huge gap from conventional methods, which tend to dominate these subtleties. One of the most significant benefits of AI in pharmacovigilance is that it can predict possible ADRs prior to them becoming global. Amid the study of previous data and finding key trends about various types of drugs, patient characteristics, and illnesses, AI can alert risks in prior. This enables medical professionals to act preventatively before severe issues starts. Also, AI assists in simplifying much of the work that goes into pharmacovigilance, including the analysis and collation of ADR reports. This helps human experts of the responsibility, allowing them to give their attention to more details of safety surveillance and planning.

NLP, one of the most major fields of AI, is especially useful for cleaning unstructured data like clinical notes, patient feedback, social media updates, and scholarly studies. Such data are usually rich sources of information on drug safety but difficult to explain manually since they occur in casual and free form. NLP assists by pulling out salient information, such as names of drugs, symptoms, dosages, and patient demographics, from the enormous unstructured database (Cattaneo et al., 2024). It also organizes and structures the information, facilitating ease of use in incorporating the data into safety repositories. In addition, NLP can examine patient sentiment and understand how people feel regarding a drug—a fact that can reveal the drug's effect further than mere clinical symptoms. NLP can also identify drug-drug interactions or low-frequency ADRs by reading from medical literature and clinical reports and finding side effects or interactions that otherwise could go unseen. This capability is instrumental to delivering comprehensive drug safety. NLP also makes processes within the regulatory reporting process more streamlined, so that required data is collected, in proper form, and sent in alignment with regulatory processes. Not only is the process quicker, but also accuracy and compliance with safety protocols are increased.

Overall, AI and NLP are reengineering pharmacovigilance such that drug safety monitoring becomes faster, accurate, and on-time. These technologies enable quicker detection of adverse events, more data processing, and decision making based on information, all of which are required in order to determine that pharmaceutical products are safe as well as effective for the population. In addition to the benefits of AI and NLP in pharmacovigilance summarized above, these technologies are also providing the gateway to more innovative solutions for monitoring drugs and safety. Firstly, AI can be applied to predict long-term safety outcomes of drugs based on previous history, trial results, and patient records to make predictions about probable health hazards not easily detectable. Second, NLP is also required for the derivation of real-world evidence from varied sources like computerized health records, scientific information, and social media, enabling estimation of drug safety in a broader range of different patient populations. Through the revelation of trends in colossal datasets, NLP and AI can also aid in the detection of subgroups at risk, i.e., uncommon comorbidities, which may be subjected to previously unknown adverse effects. This customized strategy enables earlier risk identification in the drug life cycle, thereby enabling improved preventive action and facilitating intervention by targeted regulatory actions. Additionally, combining these technologies has the potential to move towards predictive pharmacovigilance where not only is the adverse drug reaction detected earlier but also the potential concerns are pre-empted and addressed proactively. AI models are able to learn and improve constantly from streaming data, enhancing their ability to predict, and enable pharmaceutical firms and healthcare organizations to make better choices. As the increasing dependency on AI and NLP propels the future of pharmacovigilance, its future is directed towards an increasingly dynamic, efficient, and patient-centric system for monitoring and ensuring drug safety worldwide.

Ethical Issues in AI Driven ADR Prediction

1. **Fairness and biases in ADR prediction:** Artificial Intelligence models are just as fine as the data upon which they were skilled. Skilled datasets that don't represent various populations—racial and ethnic minorities, women, older patients, or patients from low-income communities—then may not make predictions about ADRs that hold for such groups. For instance, if an AI model is primarily trained on clinical trials from Western nations, it can miss how some drugs interact with individuals of Asian or African descent. Moreover, AI models can miss rare but severe adverse effects if they happen to appear very infrequently in the data. This can result in erroneous or incomplete predictions, perpetuating healthcare disparities. To enhance equity, AI engineers should make sure that datasets are comprised of varied patient populations and implement methods that identify and minimize bias in ADR detection. Regulatory bodies should also require testing for bias and validation prior to deployment of AI-based drug safety models in actual practice.
2. **Using social media data ethically:** Ethical Use of Social Media Data Numerous ADR monitoring systems powered by AI scour social media sites such as Twitter, Reddit, Facebook, and health forums online to detect possible adverse drug reactions that do not get reported conventionally. But the exercise is fraught with important ethical issues. To begin with, insufficient informed consent is a significant problem—most social media users who post comments on the sites have no idea that their posts will get mined, analyzed, and utilized for pharmacovigilance. Second, there is a lot of misinformation present on social media, and AI systems can find it difficult to distinguish between actual ADR reports and alarming or fictitious reports. For instance, a viral Twitter post stating that

one certain drug has serious side effects might not be backed by clinical research, but an AI system can accidentally label it as an established ADR. To guarantee ethical usage of social media information, AI models must incorporate fact-checking protocols to eliminate unreliable details, and developers must outline strict data collection policies to guarantee that privacy legislation and moral standards are observed.

3. **Possibility of abuse (Pharmaceutical Conflicts of Interest):** Pharmaceutical firms worldwide have strong economic motives to market their products and reduce adverse publicity. If drug firms develop or manipulate AI- based ADR detection systems, the potential exists for drug firms to distort AI models, so they underreport side effects or present only positive results selectively. Because AI systems are trained on data, an incomplete or biased dataset will cause the predictions to be biased, confusing healthcare providers and regulators alike. Without independent monitoring, AI systems might be used to advance corporate interests at the cost of patient safety. To avoid such conflicts of interest, AI-based ADR monitoring should itself be audited by third parties, and training datasets should be open to public access for independent validation. Governments and regulatory agencies must also compel pharmaceutical corporations to publish AI methods and have safety evaluations carried out in transparent ways.
4. **Problems with ethics in automatic decision-making:** While AI can significantly augment identification and prediction of ADRs, there is a risk of overdependence on computer-based decision-making in medicine. If AI models are given full autonomy to label drugs as safe or unsafe without human oversight, errors will have catastrophic outcomes. For instance, if an AI system makes a false prediction that a life-saving drug has harmful side effects, it can be removed from the market unnecessarily, denying patients an effective drug. Conversely, if an AI model fails to detect a severe ADR, patients can be injured before regulatory action. To reconcile automation with ethical decision- making, AI should be employed as a tool and not a replacement for human judgment. Healthcare professionals should retain the final say in ADR classification, and AI predictions should always be validated by experts before any meaningful regulatory action is initiated.
5. **Insufficient clinical validation and real-world experiments:** Some AI models forecasting ADRs are developed and validated in controlled experimental settings using retrospective clinical trial data or patient records. Few are appropriately validated in real-world settings prior to their use in real- world healthcare settings. A model that trains well on data may not perform well in real-world clinical application for lack of patient histories, unstructured physician remarks, or unexpected drug-drug interactions. Until AI-identified ADRs are properly authenticated in real-world settings with heterogeneous environments, they are

subject to misclassification, leading to false positives (identification of non-existent ADRs) or false negatives (overlooking true ADRs). Ethical concerns are generated when AI models are rolled out with inadequate clinical trials, peer review, and approval by regulatory bodies. Healthcare agencies must ensure AI-powered ADR systems are scientifically validated in real-world settings prior to high-stakes clinical choices being made.

Challenges and Limitations of AI and NLP in PV

PV is the science and actions related to finding, understanding, estimation and prohibition of ADRs or any problems related to drug throughout the life cycle of drug and identifying, estimating, understanding and preventing effects which are other than the intended therapeutic effects. As the healthcare system, drug development, and patients become more complex, risk monitoring and management of drug safety becomes less feasible. Traditional pharmacovigilance systems including but not limited to spontaneous reporting schemes are now increasingly supported by AI and NLP technologies, which will improve the accuracy of signal detection, but also risk assessment and post-marketing surveillance. However, with all the potential these technologies have, there are also some challenges and limitations associated with them.

1. **Consistency and quality of data**: AI and NLP algorithms heavily rely on data for training as well as operation. In pharmacovigilance, such data typically come from heterogeneous sources of data such as medical history, adverse event reports, clinical trial findings, social media, and scientific literature. Heterogeneity and low-quality pose one of the largest issues with this kind of information. Adverse event reports are often incomplete, vague, or misreported, for instance, which can undermine the operation of AI models based on tidy, structured data. NLP, whose main aim is to extract useful information from unstructured data such as social media posts or free text reports, generally faces difficulty in handling variability of the data. Usage of unwanted jargon words and abbreviations employed in the medical vocabulary or reports can be tricky in extracting the meanings and oftentimes in vague or complex contexts. Also, diverse regions and agencies may use diverse terminologies, formats, or reporting classification systems, thereby complicating data integration and analysis even further.
2. **Bias in AI models**: Historical information is practiced preparing the models of AI, and such information may have built biases due to initial procedures, patient populations, or giving mechanisms. The models could be mimicking or even amplifying such biases if not taken into account at the development or deployment phases. For example, specific population segments may have been

underreported in adverse events and thus AI models would not take specific risk factors for those populations into account. Bias in pharmacovigilance results in false risk assessment or a one-sided picture of a drug's safety profile. Models may overlook side effects that affect some populations more intensely, thus causing an undue sense of safety for those patients. In addition, AI algorithms are usually "black boxes" whose working is not clear, so stakeholders cannot easily spot and correct biases, which also hinders their uptake in highly regulated areas such as healthcare and pharmacovigilance.

3. **Interpretability and transparency**: Another big disadvantage while implementing NLP and AI based solutions in pharmacovigilance is that the issue of interpretability. Most of the AI models, especially the deep learning models, work in a non-transparent way for humans. This renders it difficult when AI-based decisions need to be justified to regulatory authorities, clinicians, or patients (Hacker et al., 2020). For example, if an AI system flags a potential safety signal, it should be able to explain why it did so. In pharmacovigilance, where there are sensitive regulation and accountability, the inability to interpret and explain the findings from AI, as well as interpret and supplement what human experts might gain from the AI, could hold back the widespread adoption of such systems.
4. **Resource intensiveness:** Development, training, and deployment of AI and NLP systems are extremely resource-intensive in terms of computational resources and human capability. The models require training on vast high-quality data, which consumes a great deal of time and capital (Yeager et al., 2019). AI models also require constant updating and tuning so that they are as accurate and efficient as they need to be. In pharmacovigilance, when the environment of medicine safety information is varying continuously, AI systems should be able to develop with new trends, new uprising risks, and developing principles. Moreover, AI and pharmacovigilance talent is poor. This creates a talent and technical skill barrier that can work against the use of AI and NLP tools. Associations must invest time and economic resources guiding employees, which lifts the cost of jobs and slows down employment.

CONCLUSION

Adverse drug reactions continue to challenge global healthcare systems, often resulting in critical outcomes that traditional pharmacovigilance methods struggle to detect early enough. This chapter explored how artificial intelligence—particularly natural language processing (NLP) and machine learning—can transform pharmacovigilance by shifting the focus from reactive, post-market reporting to proactive, real-time surveillance. By tapping into rich, unstructured data sources like patient forums, electronic health records, and online drug reviews, AI-powered models offer a more nuanced and timely understanding of drug toxicity and patient sentiment. Through techniques such as Named Entity Recognition, sentiment analysis, and deep learning models like BERT and LSTM, the proposed framework demonstrates the potential to identify early warning signs of severe or lethal drug reactions. Predictive tools like Random Forest, SVM, and XGBoost further strengthen risk detection by pinpointing high-risk drug combinations. While challenges around infrastructure, regulatory compliance, and algorithm validation persist, the promise of AI in improving patient safety and decision-making in pharmacovigilance is undeniable. Ultimately, as the pharmaceutical industry embraces digital transformation, AI-driven pharmacovigilance stands out as a vital advancement—one that not only enhances drug safety monitoring but also empowers healthcare professionals to act faster and more effectively to protect patients.

REFERENCES

22nd Sylvester O'Halloran Meeting 2014. (2014). Irish Journal of Medical Science (1971 -), 183(S1), 1–69.

Boulos, M. N. K. (2004). Towards evidence-based, GIS-driven national spatial health information infrastructure and surveillance services in the United Kingdom. *International Journal of Health Geographics*, *3*(1).

Arundel, A., Sawaya, D., & Valeanu, I. (2010). Human Health Biotechnologies to 2015. *OECD Journal General Papers*, *2009*(3), 113–207.

Bellazzi, R., De Quiros, F. G. B., Koch, S., Kulikowski, C., Lovell, N., Maojo, V., Park, H., Sanz, F., Sarkar, I., Tanaka, H., & Al-Shorbaji, N. (2016). Discussion of "The New Role of Biomedical Informatics in the Age of Digital Medicine.". *Methods of Information in Medicine*, *55*(05), 403–421. DOI: 10.3414/ME15-12-0005 PMID: 27524112

Cattaneo, A., Vitali, A., Regazzoni, D., & Rizzi, C. (2024). A sustainable approach to telerehabilitation in Europe: Patients are ready, but caregivers are essential. *Studies in Health Technology and Informatics*. Advance online publication. DOI: 10.3233/SHTI240014 PMID: 38682507

Dwivedi, Y. K., Hughes, L., Ismagilova, E., Aarts, G., Coombs, C., Crick, T., Duan, Y., Dwivedi, R., Edwards, J., Eirug, A., Galanos, V., Ilavarasan, P. V., Janssen, M., Jones, P., Kar, A. K., Kizgin, H., Kronemann, B., Lal, B., Lucini, B., & Williams, M. D. (2019). Artificial Intelligence (AI): Multidisciplinary perspectives on emerging challenges, opportunities, and agenda for research, practice and policy. *International Journal of Information Management*, *57*, 101994. DOI: 10.1016/j.ijinfomgt.2019.08.002

Fatima, N., & Nayeem, N. (2016). Toxic effects as a result of herbal medicine intake. In InTech eBooks. DOI: 10.5772/64468

Goodwin, G., Haddad, P., Ferrier, I., Aronson, J., Barnes, T., & Cipriani, A. Coghill, Fazel, S., Geddes, J., Grunze, H., Holmes, E., Howes, O., Hudson, S., Hunt, N., Jones, I., Macmillan, I., McAllister-Williams, H., Miklowitz, Morriss, R., & Young, A. (2016). Evidence-based guidelines for treating bipolar disorder: Revised third edition recommendations from the British Association for Psychopharmacology. Journal of Psychopharmacology, 30(6), 495–553.

Haber, P., Lintzeris, N., Proude, E., & Lopatko, O. (2009). Guidelines for the treatment of alcohol problems [Dataset]. In *PsycEXTRA Dataset.*

Hacker, P., Krestel, R., Grundmann, S., & Naumann, F. (2020). Explainable AI under contract and tort law: Legal incentives and technical challenges. *Artificial Intelligence and Law*, *28*(4), 415–439. DOI: 10.1007/s10506-020-09260-6

Hopkins, C., Surda, P., Walker, A., Wolf, A., Speth, M., Jacques, T., Hox, V., Van Gerven, L., Santamaria-Gadea, A., Segboer, C., Lourijsen, E., Turri-Zanoni, M., Huart, C., Rennie, C., Green, R., Society, N. S., Kelly, C., Knill, A., Lund, V., & Fokkens, W. (2021). EPOS 4 patients. *Rhinology*, *0*(0), 1–57. DOI: 10.4193/Rhin20.950 PMID: 34762718

Houssari, M., Boukhalfa, I., Henry, J., Mulder, P., Richard, V., Brakenhielm, E., Nili, R., Amet, D., Vidil, F., Beller, C. L., Pedard, M., Totoson, P., Demougeot, C., Salem, J., Germain, M., Hulot, J., Marie, C., Abudoureheman, A., Wuliya, Y., & Zhou, W. (2017). Discussed poster abstracts. *Fundamental & Clinical Pharmacology*, *31*(S1), 21–50. DOI: 10.1111/fcp.12272

Layton, D. (2018). Developments and Future Directions of Prescription-Based Observational Cohort Pharmacovigilance. In Methods in pharmacology and toxicology (pp. 105–134). DOI: 10.1007/978-1-4939-8818-1_6

Nassiri, K., & Akhloufi, M. A. (2024). Recent advances in large language models for healthcare. *BioMedInformatics*, *4*(2), 1097–1143. DOI: 10.3390/biomedinformatics4020062

O'Neill, J., Bartlett, J., & Mignone, J. (2007). Best practices in intercultural health.

Paananen, J., & Fortino, V. (2019). An omics perspective on drug target discovery platforms. *Briefings in Bioinformatics*, *21*(6), 1937–1953. DOI: 10.1093/bib/bbz122 PMID: 31774113

Ponikowski, P., Voors, A. A., Anker, S. D., Bueno, H., Cleland, J. G. F., Coats, A. J. S., Falk, V., González-Juanatey, J. R., Harjola, V., Jankowska, E. A., Jessup, M., Linde, C., Nihoyannopoulos, P., Parissis, J. T., Pieske, B., Riley, J. P., Rosano, G. M. C., Ruilope, L. M., Ruschitzka, F., & Van Der Meer, P. (2016). 2016 ESC Guidelines for the diagnosis and treatment of acute and chronic heart failure. *European Heart Journal*, *37*(27), 2129–2200. DOI: 10.1093/eurheartj/ehw128 PMID: 27206819

Reiner, Z., Catapano, A. L., De Backer, G., Graham, I., Taskinen, M., Wiklund, O., Agewall, S., Alegria, E., Chapman, M. J., Durrington, P., Erdine, S., Halcox, J., Hobbs, R., Kjekshus, J., Filardi, P. P., Riccardi, G., Storey, R. F., Wood, D., Bax, J., & Zamorano, J. L. (2011). ESC/EAS Guidelines for the management of dyslipidaemias: The Task Force for the management of dyslipidaemias of the European Society of Cardiology (ESC) and the European Atherosclerosis Society (EAS). *European Heart Journal*, *32*(14), 1769–1818. DOI: 10.1093/eurheartj/ehr158 PMID: 21712404

Roux, G. L., Bruneau, C., Lelièvre, B., Deguigne, M. B., Turcant, A., Harry, P., & Boels, D. (2015). Recreational phenethylamine poisonings reported to a French poison control center. *Drug and Alcohol Dependence*, *154*, 46–53. DOI: 10.1016/j.drugalcdep.2015.05.048 PMID: 26205314

Schot, J., & Steinmueller, W. E. (2018). Three frames for innovation policy: R&D, systems of innovation and transformative change. *Research Policy*, *47*(9), 1554–1567. DOI: 10.1016/j.respol.2018.08.011

Tasaka, Y., Tanaka, A., Yasunaga, D., Asakawa, T., Araki, H., & Tanaka, M. (2018). Potential drug-related problems detected by routine pharmaceutical interventions: Safety and economic contributions made by hospital pharmacists in Japan. *Journal of Pharmaceutical Health Care and Sciences*, *4*(1), 33. DOI: 10.1186/s40780-018-0125-z PMID: 30564432

Thieme, A., Belgrave, D., & Doherty, G. (2020). Machine learning in mental health. *ACM Transactions on Computer-Human Interaction*, *27*(5), 1–53. DOI: 10.1145/3398069

Yeager, D. S., Hanselman, P., Walton, G. M., Murray, J. S., Crosnoe, R., Muller, C., Tipton, E., Schneider, B., Hulleman, C. S., Hinojosa, C. P., Paunesku, D., Romero, C., Flint, K., Roberts, A., Trott, J., Iachan, R., Buontempo, J., Yang, S. M., Carvalho, C. M., & Dweck, C. S. (2019). A national experiment reveals where a growth mindset improves achievement. *Nature*, *573*(7774), 364–369. DOI: 10.1038/s41586-019-1466-y PMID: 31391586

Young, J. C., Mitchell, C., & Redpath, S. M. (2020). Conservation Research, policy and practice. In *Cambridge University Press eBooks*.

ADDITIONAL READING

Choi, J., Palumbo, N., Chalasani, P., Engelhard, M. M., Jha, S., Kumar, A., & Page, D. (2024). *MALADE: Orchestration of LLM-powered agents with retrieval-augmented generation for pharmacovigilance. arXiv*. https://doi.org//arXiv.2408.01869DOI: 10.48550

Dimitsaki, S., Natsiavas, P., & Jaulent, M.-C. (2024). Applying AI to structured real-world data for pharmacovigilance purposes: Scoping review. *Journal of Medical Internet Research*, *26*, e57824. DOI: 10.2196/57824 PMID: 39753222

Golder, S., Xu, D., O'Connor, K., Wang, Y., Batra, M., & Hernandez, G. G. (2025). Leveraging natural language processing and machine learning methods for adverse drug event detection in electronic health/medical records: A scoping review. *Drug Safety*, *48*(4), 321–337. DOI: 10.1007/s40264-024-01505-6 PMID: 39786481

KEY TERMS AND DEFINITIONS

Adverse Drug Reactions (ADRs): Undesired and harmful effects caused by a medication when used correctly for prevention, diagnosis, or treatment, often leading to hospitalization or serious health complications.

Big Healthcare Data: Massive, complex datasets derived from electronic health records, social media, and clinical databases, offering new opportunities for ADR detection using AI technologies.

Machine Learning Classifiers: Algorithms like Random Forest, SVM, and XGBoost that categorize or predict outcomes—in this case, identifying high-risk drug interactions from data.

Named Entity Recognition (NER): A text analysis technique in NLP that identifies and classifies key information such as drug names, diseases, or adverse effects from unstructured text sources.

NLP (Natural Language Processing): A branch of artificial intelligence that enables computers to understand, interpret, and generate human language, used in this study to analyze patient feedback and detect drug toxicity.

Pharmacovigilance: The science and activities related to the detection, assessment, understanding, and prevention of adverse effects or other drug-related problems to ensure patient safety.

Phase IV Trials: The post-marketing stage of drug testing that assesses the drug's safety, effectiveness, and usage in large, real-world populations over extended periods.

Sentiment Analysis: An AI-based method that evaluates the emotional tone in text, used here to assess patients' attitudes toward drug effects and identify early warning signs of toxicity.

Spontaneous Reporting System (SRS): A passive pharmacovigilance tool allowing healthcare providers and patients to report suspected ADRs, useful for post-marketing drug surveillance.

Toxicovigilance: The monitoring and evaluation of toxic effects caused by drugs, especially due to overdose or exposure beyond therapeutic levels, complementing pharmacovigilance efforts.

Chapter 14
Building a Knowledge Network of Drug–Drug Interactions Using Natural Language Processing and Graph Databases:
Drug–Drug Interaction and Graph Networks

Ruchi Jakhmola Mani
https://orcid.org/0000-0001-9264-867X
Amity University, Noida, India

Harsh Lalwani
https://orcid.org/0009-0002-0539-5841
Amity University, Noida, India

Angamba Meetei Potshangbam
Discovery Boulevard, Imphal, India

Shikha Rani
Discovery Boulevard, Imphal, India

Kriti Katare
Discovery Boulevard, Imphal, India

Abhishek Chauhan
Chaudhary Charan Singh University, Meerut, India

ABSTRACT

Drug-drug interactions (DDIs) are a critical healthcare concern, often causing adverse effects and poor treatment outcomes. While many studies address DDIs, integrating this knowledge in a structured, accessible format remains a challenge. This study proposes a data-driven method using Natural Language Processing

DOI: 10.4018/979-8-3373-2043-4.ch014

(NLP) and graph networks to extract and analyze DDI patterns. PubMed articles related to a specific drug are mined using Python, and interacting compounds are extracted from abstracts via Named Entity Recognition (NER) and text mining. These mentions form a curated DDI dataset used to build a knowledge network illustrating co-prescribed drugs, studied interactions, and reported effects. The resulting graph enables visual and query-based exploration of known and potential DDIs. Graph analytics help identify frequent drug pairs, interaction trends, and research gaps. This platform aids biotech and pharma R&D professionals in visualizing past DDI studies and planning future research efficiently, emphasizing the value of automated literature mining.

INTRODUCTION

Drug-Drug Interactions (DDIs)

In today's world, modern medicine has made it possible to treat many diseases that were once untreatable. Doctors often prescribe more than one medicine to a patient, especially when the person is suffering from multiple health problems. For example, an elderly person may take medicines for blood pressure, diabetes, and joint pain, all at the same time. This practice is called polypharmacy (*Polypharmacy and Drug Adherence in Elderly Patients*, n.d.). While taking multiple medicines is sometimes necessary, it also brings risks. One major risk is that the medicines may interact with each other in unexpected or harmful ways. This is known as a Drug-Drug Interaction. A DDI happens when the effect of one drug changes because of the presence of another drug in the body. This can lead to reduced effectiveness of the drug, increased side effects, or even dangerous health outcomes. For example, let's say a person is taking medicine for heart disease and then starts a new antibiotic. If those two drugs interact, the antibiotic may reduce the effect of the heart medicine, putting the patient at risk. In some cases, drug interactions can even be life-threatening. Drug interactions are especially important in sensitive groups like elderly people, pregnant women, and patients with chronic diseases. That is why doctors, pharmacists, and researchers must be very careful while combining drugs. To prevent harmful interactions, many drug labels and medical guidelines include known DDIs. However, the problem is that new interactions are being discovered all the time. The amount of medical information available today is massive, and it keeps growing every day. It is not possible for a human being to read all the scientific papers and keep track of every new drug interaction.

THE CHALLENGE OF TRACKING DRUG INTERACTIONS

There are thousands of research articles, clinical trials, case reports, and drug labels that mention drug interactions. This information is usually written in free text form i.e. in full sentences and paragraphs. For example, a research paper may say, "The combination of warfarin and aspirin increases the risk of bleeding." This is a useful piece of information, but it's hidden inside a paragraph. Now imagine that there are millions of such articles. If a researcher or doctor wants to find whether two specific drugs interact, they would have to search through huge amounts of text. This is not only time consuming but also very inefficient. Sometimes, important interactions are missed just because the information was not easily accessible or searchable. Also, the same drug might be written with different names in different articles. For example, "Paracetamol" and "Acetaminophen" are two names for the same medicine. This creates more confusion when trying to gather and connect information. All these challenges point to one big problem that we need a better way to collect, organize, and access information about drug interactions.

Impact of Choosing Bad Drug-Drug Partners

Adverse drug reactions are major public health issues, with more than 29 million cases since 2011 and resulting in millions of emergency department visits and hospitalizations annually. There are several examples in the recent literature for ADRs, such as undesirable interactions between warfarin, an anticoagulant drug, and nonsteroidal anti-inflammatory drugs (NSAIDs), emphasizing mechanisms and clinical relevance. It highlights that all NSAIDs are effective in extending the time of bleeding by inhibiting platelet function, which poses risk to patients on warfarin. Aspirin in the high doses has a direct hypoprothrombinemia effect, which can complicate the control of anticoagulation. Additionally, its analogues potentiate the hypoprothrombinemia action of warfarin through interaction at the level of pharmacokinetics by inhibiting its metabolism in the liver. Mefenamic acid has also been reported to be a drug enhancing warfarin's anticoagulant action, but its mechanism of action is not known (Chan, 1995). A classic example of a very important one would be the combination of selective serotonin reuptake inhibitors (SSRIs) and monoamine oxidase inhibitors (MAOIs) that cause serotonin syndrome, which is a life-threatening disease. This interaction is one of the ways that some drug combinations can result in adverse effects that are severe and need monitoring and control in an alert manner. The FDA invites healthcare providers to report ADRs to further enhance safety and surveillance. Furthermore, advances in pharmacogenomics indicate that preemptive testing can prevent ADRs, representing a shift toward personalized medicine for healthcare. The AGS Beers Criteria also focuses on mindful prescribing, especially in the elderly, to exclude potentially inappropriate medications.

Overall, ADR resolution by reporting and individual measures is most critical with respect to maintaining patient safety, Computation Methods for DDI detection are being implemented in the healthcare system to make the process of ADRs reporting and data analysis faster, safer, and easier. A reporting database system may be developed to report and identify the upcoming ADRs in the population such as spontaneous reporting database of Veneto Region, Italy, which would identify and characterize severe ADRs by employing real DDIs. For the case study of Italy, serious ADR reports excluding for vaccines, from January 2015 to May 2020 were considered. It was called as DRUGDEX® system which was utilized to study drug pair reports which can be composed of possible negative, neutral or positive interaction. The research was then co-related with the ADR reports that led to description of interaction effects on which basis actual DDIs were formed. Total ADR reports studied were 31.604 including 2,195 serious ones involving minimum two drugs. 55% (1,208 reports) had a minimum of one possible DDI, and 17.4% (381 reports) proved to be with actual DDIs.

Warfarin was the most frequently reported interaction for ADRs such as gastrointestinal and cerebral hemorrhage. Out of all the DDIs the most frequently occurring were the drugs of proton pump inhibitor and the second one was platelet aggregation inhibitor. The results of this research were confirmatory in the sense that approximately one-third of the DDI-exposed patients had ADR. With this case study we can envision how much importance spontaneous reporting databases carry particularly when there is a direct co-relation of DDI to their respective ADRs. This relationship can also be examined on further results like which pathway is being activated by which DDI and through which bio-pathways it is inducing ADR. Hence, we can suspect the role, limitation and the advancement of a new drug. In cases like polypharmacy there is a requirement of continuous pharmacovigilance to reduce the risk induced by DDIs. Therefore, by incorporating ADRs links into DDIs we can improve our drug safety levels and are able to make well-informed clinical choices.

Clinical Data Repositories (CDRs)

There is a critical role of clinical data repositories (CDRs) in identifying drug-drug interactions, particularly those involving statins. It is especially important to note that traditional web-based DDI databases may not provide comprehensive or up-to-date information, as evidenced by the discovery of several potential statin-drug interaction drugs that were absent from the original sources. The limitation on relying only on existing databases for DDI extraction got highlighted by the identification of drugs such as lysine and ketotifen. Therefore, the role of CDRs becomes to aggregate vast amounts of real-world data from electronic health records which can offer a more reliable and thorough approach to identifying clinically significant interactions. The integration of CDRs into clinical practice has ensured the handling of patient safety and optimization of medication management, particularly in populations at risk of polypharmacy. This approach could lead to better surveillance of adverse drug events and improve patient outcomes in healthcare settings (Kiogou & Adam, 2023a) .

EXISTING AND ADVANCED APPROACHES FOR DDI DETECTION

Existing approaches involve the classification of DDI prediction methodologies as classical and advanced. Two main approaches included in the classical methods were frequency-based approaches and Bayesian techniques which are the foundation of DDI research. In case of advanced methods there are latest statistical techniques which use machine learning, network analysis and deep learning, the results of advanced methods are more accurate and highly efficient. Still there is always the need to continue research in the computational approaches to enhance the DDI prediction capabilities. Continued innovation will be essential for improving drug safety and efficacy in clinical settings (Tian, 2022) .

Challenges with Traditional Methods

Traditional approaches for detecting drug-drug interactions (DDIs) rely heavily on manual curation, clinical trials, and bibliometric analysis. While these methods have historically been effective, they face significant limitations in the context of modern biomedical data volumes. Some of the limitations are discussed below.

1. **Labor-Intensive Manual Curation**: Manual curation is a process where individual studies or reports are hand-screened by specialists to detect DDIs. It is time-consuming and susceptible to human error, particularly with the explosive increase of biomedical literature daily. PubMed, for instance, adds thousands of articles monthly, hence it is nearly impossible for researchers to keep pace manually (Celebi et al., 2019).
2. **Limited Scope of Clinical Trials**: Clinical trials typically focus on specific drugs or combinations under controlled conditions, which limits their ability to identify rare or unforeseen DDIs in real-world settings. Trials often exclude populations such as older adults or patients with polypharmacy, where DDIs are more prevalent (Celebi et al., 2019).

3. **Static and Incomplete Databases**: Traditional web-based DDI databases are often static and may not include emerging interactions or newly approved drugs. For example, studies have found that several statin-drug interactions were absent from existing databases(Celebi et al., 2019).
4. **Inability to Manage Big Data:** The sheer volume of unstructured biomedical data spanning journal articles, electronic health records (EHRs), and adverse event reports renders traditional methods inefficient (Rohani & Eslahchi, 2019). Analysis using bibliometric software's was able to quantify the trends, but the limitation was that it failed to extract the complex relationship between drugs which diluted the efficiency in the insights of DDI. (Celebi et al., 2019).

How Computational Methods Address These Limitations

Computational methods help in several ways. First is automation of Text Mining wherein NLP techniques automate the extraction of DDIs from vast repositories like PubMed etc., reducing reliance on manual labour while improving accuracy (Rohani & Eslahchi, 2019). Named Entity Recognition (NER) identifies key entities like drug names and interaction types from unstructured text, enabling faster processing of biomedical literature (Rohani & Eslahchi, 2019). Another important role is the Integration of Real-World Data. Computational methods can incorporate real-world evidence from EHRs and adverse event reporting systems (e.g., spontaneous reporting databases), providing a more comprehensive view of DDIs in diverse patient populations (Rohani & Eslahchi, 2019). For example, a study analysing ADR reports in Italy identified serious DDIs using computational tools that matched reported interactions with expected effects described in Micromedex. where drugs are represented as nodes and interactions as edges. Such a structure facilitates effective querying and visualization of intricate relationships.

Graph-based predictions also allow researchers to explore new interactions and confirm hypotheses by conducting network analysis. Computational method have evolved with the incorporation of data science and Artificial intelligence to create an Advanced Predictive Models using Machine Learning (ML) and Deep Learning (DL) algorithms trained on structured datasets predict potential DDIs with high accuracy (Pan et al., 2024). Hybrid approaches combining text-mining techniques with graph neural networks (GNNs) have demonstrated success in uncovering molecular interactions for complex disorders like insomnia[REMOVED HYPERLINK FIELD] (Pan et al., 2024). The last but not the least is the Scalability and Real-Time Updates we can acquire on computational frameworks that can be scaled to manage large datasets while providing real-time updates on emerging DDIs and thus enhancing pharmacovigilance efforts (Pan et al., 2024). For instance, NLP-based systems can continuously monitor adverse drug reactions reported in EHRs or literature databases, ensuring timely identification of high-risk interactions(Rohani & Eslahchi, 2019)

Motivation for Data-Driven DDI Analysis

Advancements in AI have introduced computational techniques for DDI identification, including the use of Machine Learning (ML) & Deep Learning (DL) Algorithms trained on structured datasets that predict potential drug interactions. While Natural Language Processing (NLP) extracts DDIs from unstructured text sources such as PubMed, improving real-time detection and reducing manual labor. NLP-based techniques, although promising, require ongoing refinement to address challenges like entity disambiguation and contextual interpretation.

Role of NLP and Graph Databases in Biomedical Knowledge Extraction

Biomedical knowledge extraction is a critical task for advancing drug discovery, pharmacovigilance, and clinical decision-making. Natural Language Processing (NLP) and graph databases play complementary roles in this process, enabling efficient data mining and relationship mapping.

a) **Natural Language Processing (NLP)**

Natural Language Processing is a part of artificial intelligence (AI) that helps computers understand and work with human language. NLP allows computers to read texts like research papers, clinical notes, and drug labels and identify useful information from them. For example, NLP can help a computer scan through an abstract and find drug names, side effects, and mentions of interactions. It can also help identify sentences where two drugs are discussed together, which often suggests an interaction. NLP tools like Named Entity Recognition (NER) are especially useful. NER can detect and label specific types of words like drug names, diseases, or chemical compounds in a sentence. Once the computer knows which words are drugs, it can start linking them to find interaction patterns.

NLP techniques are essential for processing the vast amount of biomedical literature published daily. They enable the extraction of key drug interaction in an artificial simulation environment which contributes to drug safety and efficacy. The information on gene-drug relationships is scattered across numerous publications and research papers. A unified algorithm using NLP and ML is a necessity of hour which will integrate every data set available thus allowing researchers to analysis and extract the required data relationship with each other or to the new object. Some studies (Table 1) have used an automated text mining approach to extract gene drug intraction from medline abstracts resulting in the high accuracy in gene identification and nature of its relationship. (Ben Abdessalem Karaa et al., 2021; Ben et al., 2021)

Table 1. This table shows different approaches done by various researchers with their method, relation, and the used corpus(Ben et al., 2021)

Used method	Type of relation	Used corpus
Neural network	Cure, only dis., only treat, prevent, vague, side effect, no cure	MEDLINE 2001
Linear SVM	Cure, prevent, side effect	MEDLINE 2001
NLP, BOW, biomedical concepts, and UMLS concepts	Cure, prevent, side effect	MEDLINE 2001
Cooccurrence analysis, NLP, BOW, biomedical and UMLS concepts, inductive logic techniques, Bloom filter	Cure, prevent, side effect	MEDLINE 2001
Pattern, UMLS	Inducement, treatment	Abstracts from PubMed

Natural Language Processing (NLP) is one of the major enablers of model-informed drug development (MIDD) since it optimizes different steps like drug discovery, clinical trials, and pharmacovigilance. Core functionalities like named entity recognition, relation extraction, and topic modeling play a crucial role in optimizing steps like gene-disease mapping and patient-trial matching. Advanced deploys these days utilize transformer models and pre-trained neural networks such as those in hugging face and sparkNLP libraries. Still, issues of reproducibility and sparsity remain, suggesting a requirement for further progress in NLP application in MIDD. The research tackles the difficulties arising from the rapid increase in biomedical literature, wherein it is difficult for researchers to remain updated. It points out the limitations of conventional text-mining approaches and the disadvantages of deep-learning models, including high computation requirements and low interpretability. To address these issues, the authors suggest a hybrid solution that uses text-mining methods along with graph neural networks (GNNs) and fine-tuned large language models (LLMs). This process will improve biomedical knowledge graphs and provide explanations for predicted interactions. The method was implemented to experimentally validate protein interactions with a Matthews correlation coefficient (MCC) of 0.772 and successfully predicted unknown interactions associated with insomnia, thereby illustrating its usefulness in discovering molecular interactions for multifactorial diseases. These methods integrate textual data with graph-based predictions to provide context-aware insights. By combining NLP with graph databases, researchers can build comprehensive biomedical knowledge graphs. These graphs facilitate tasks like predicting novel DDIs and validating hypotheses through network analysis.

b) Graph Databases and Knowledge Networks

After extracting drug interaction data using NLP, we need a smart way to store and explore this information. That's where graph databases come in. Traditional databases store data in rows and columns (like Excel), which is fine for simple data. But drug interactions are all about relationships for example, "Drug A interacts with Drug B," or "Drug C is frequently prescribed with Drug D." Graph databases store information in the form of nodes (points) and edges (connections between points). In our case, each node is a drug, and each edge is an interaction. This format is perfect for showing how different drugs are connected. The result is a knowledge network which is a web of connected drugs that shows how they interact. This network is not just useful for visualizing data; it can also be searched and analysed using special queries. For example:

- Which drugs are involved in the most interactions?
- What are the common interaction partners for a specific drug?
- Are there any unknown or less studied drug pairs?

Using this kind of system, researchers can quickly find useful patterns without having to read hundreds of articles manually.

The combination of NLP and graph databases provides an effective way of structuring and analyzing sophisticated drug interaction information to construct dynamic knowledge networks that significantly improve a variety of areas in pharmaceutical research and medicine. An arguably most useful application is pharmacovigilance, where NLP-triggered drug interaction knowledge is dynamically updated online in a graph database so real-time tracking of adverse drug reactions (ADRs) can be ensured. Through extensive analysis of enormous biomedical literature, clinical trial reports, and patient data, the system helps regulatory agencies and clinicians in early identification of potential safety issues, resulting in timely intervention and enhanced drug safety. In contrast to relational databases based on static tabular representations, graph databases offer a dynamic and networked formulation of drug interactions, enabling scientists to uncover hidden associations between drugs, biological mechanisms, and disease processes. The system can then predict new drug interactions that are relevant to drug repurpose and speed up the discovery of more effective treatments using graph-based machine learning models.

Benefits of a Data-Driven Approach

Creating a knowledge network of drug interactions using NLP and graph databases offers many advantages:

- Time-saving: Computers can read thousands of papers in a short time and extract useful information automatically.
- Structured data: Instead of scattered text, we get organized information that is easy to search and understand.
- Better research planning: Scientists can find gaps in research and plan studies based on what is already known.
- Clinical safety: Doctors can check if two drugs have known interactions before prescribing them.
- Scalability: As new research comes out, the system can be updated easily with more data.

This approach is especially helpful for researchers in India and other developing countries where access to expensive databases may be limited. A locally developed system based on open-access data and open-source tools can make drug interaction knowledge available to everyone.

The main aim of this chapter is to build a knowledge network of drug-drug interactions by using natural language processing and graph databases. The steps include:

1. Collecting abstracts from PubMed related to specific drugs
2. Using NLP to extract drug names and interaction information
3. Cleaning and curating the extracted data
4. Building a graph-based network to represent drug interactions

This system can be used by students, researchers, doctors, and people in the pharmaceutical industry to explore DDIs in an easy and visual way.

METHODOLOGY

Data Collection

PubMed was queried by using keywords like "Levodopa AND combination" or "Levadopa AND co-administration". The extracted data with its code can be seen in Figure 1. The query was divided into date wise categories. Further, the challenge was that not all the extracted articles were having abstracts thus sorting and data cleaning was performed. The total number of articles extracted was 5224 and post cleaning the dataset had 4617 entries.

Figure 1. Showing the algorithm and the data generated from scraping PubMed.

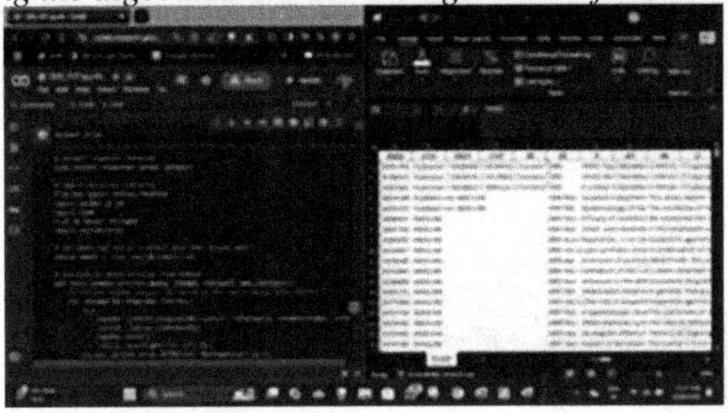

Preprocessing of unstructured text for NLP Analysis.

Techniques Used in Preprocessing

Preprocessing is a critical step in Natural Language Processing (NLP) that ensures the data is clean, structured, and ready for analysis. Figure 2 shows us the preprocessing of text results.

The following steps are commonly followed:

1. Tokenization involves splitting text into smaller units, such as words, phrases, or sentences. Let's take an example of a sentence "Drug A interacts with Drug B", this sentence is one string which contain many tokens(words), these tokens are needed to be separated first so that NER analysis can then be applied on each token.
2. Another removal will be of the stop words like (and the, is) as these words don't add anything sentimentally significant to the data. Removal of these words will improve the accuracy of the ML model.
3. To reduce the words to their root form stemming and lemmatization will be done where the words like "interacting" becomes "interact". This will make the uniformity in the text representation to the model which will clear the noise.
4. Then name entity recognition (NER) will be performed which will further classify the drugs as names, disease and symptoms inside the unstructured text. For this we called Rxnorm API which will send every token to the databases and will return the matched word with the drug database.

5. There is always a context to the interaction of tokens withing the sentence, these interactions will get make out uniformly using part-of-speech tagging.
6. To identify meaningful phrases or clauses using the grammatical relationships between drugs we did dependency parsing
7. There was a need to standardize the text for example converting all text into lower case letters and deleting special characters or spelling correction. This is termed as text normalization.

Figure 2. Preprocessing of unstructured text for NER analysis.

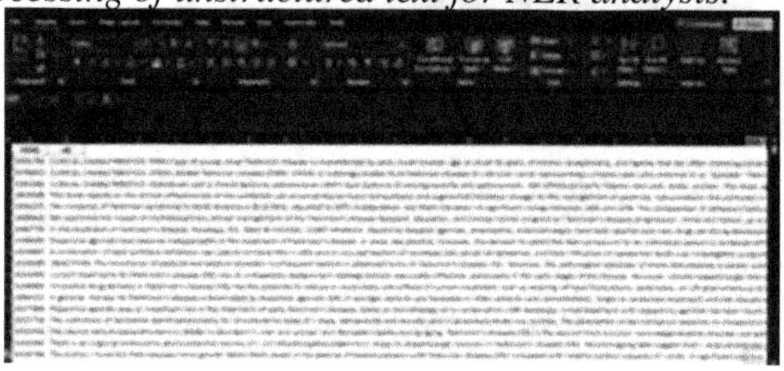

Challenges in Preprocessing

1. There are several ambiguous terms which are the words that have multiple meanings which change the context of the text. for example, "ACE" which can be a drug class in a particular drug related text or can be a card game in un-related context. Hence, there is a need to disambiguate such words which require more awareness.
2. In biomedical text there are complex sentences which contain nested clauses which are difficult to parse. This can be in the case where multiple drug names are mentioned in a line but with a single relationship defining token.
3. In any medical document a word or drug can have multiple abbreviations or synonyms which make lots of variation in the terminology of the same drug making it difficult to understand the context of the data. Database systems Rxnorm can unify the variation but on a large data set the efficiency reduces significantly.
4. There can also be the presence of noisy data which may contain irrelevant information or data in an unstructured format, this will make the NLP model misunderstand the context making the NER less efficient. Example of this can be the section of "Acknowledgments" in a biomedical text which are contribution nothing to the sentiment of the literature thus is noise to the NLP model.

5. Imbalanced data types like the overrepresentation of a certain type of drug making other rare and misleading the data. Example can be that aspirin drug has most common drug interactions available that doesn't mean it as the only interaction in the biomedical text.
6. Without the use the advanced transformer-based architecture (BERT) we will not be able to find the context in which a particular token has been used in the text, like the token "interaction" can have different meaning depending upon the context of the background that you are talking about drug or some other non-biological materials.
7. Scalability Issues as Processing large-scale biomedical datasets requires significant computational resources and efficient algorithms. These issues can be solved using distributed computing techniques or an NLP cloud-based environment, but this will add complexity in the results.

NLP-Based DDI Extraction

Implementation of Named Entity Recognition (NER) using Rxnorm API

Now we will be discussing the implementation of NER technique to our framework using the Rxnorm API in the python environment and using libraries like pandas and requests. This will standardize the drug entities from text data, a very important step toward the building of a knowledge network.

Core Implementation Steps

1. **Preparation and Data Loading –** This will start with the loading of extracted articles from excel file using pandas. The articles extracted contain a column containing text which will be read into the list
2. RxNorm API Interaction:
    - The core of our NER implementation lies in the get_drug_name_from_rxnorm(text) function. This function takes a text string as input (typically a word from the article text) and queries the RxNorm API.
    - It uses the requests library to make a GET request to the RxNorm API endpoint: "https://rxnav.nlm.nih.gov/REST/rxcui.json".
    - The name parameter is passed to the API, which is the drug name we are trying to resolve.
    - Error Handling: The try...except block handles potential network errors (requests. RequestException) during the API call, ensuring the process doesn't terminate unexpectedly.

- Response Parsing: The function parses the JSON response from the RxNorm API. If the API returns a valid rxnormId within the 'idGroup', it extracts and returns a list of RxCUI (RxNorm Concept Unique Identifier) codes. RxCUI is RxNorm's unique identifier for a concept.

3. Drug Information Extraction:
   - The extract_drug_info(text) function tokenizes the input article text into individual words.
   - For each word, it calls the get_drug_name_from_rxnorm () function to check if it's a recognized drug entity.
   - Identified drug names are added to a set (drug_info) to avoid duplicates.
   - The function returns a comma-separated string of unique drug names found in the text.
4. Processing in Chunks:
   - To handle large datasets and prevent memory issues (especially in environments like Google Collab), the articles are processed in chunks.
   - The tqdm library provides a progress bar to monitor the processing of each chunk.
   - The results from each chunk are appended to the extracted_drugs list.
5. **Saving Results:**
   - The extracted drug names are added as a new column (Drugs_Retrieved) to the original pandas DataFrame.
   - Data frame got updated and saved as a new excel file.

Challenges and Considerations

1. **API Rate Limiting:** Every API has its own request rate limits. This is to avoid all the requests from the robot or from the time of the over calling. This limit may slow down the process, specifically when you are working with a lot of data. We can add pauses or conjugate the methods in the NLP, to encounter these limits.
2. **Ambiguity and Context:** Some medications fall within a longer phrase in the biomedical text which can cause them to become misspelled by the model. Techniques such as fuzzy matching or context-aware should be explored to mitigate this limitation.
3. **Handling of negotiations:** The detection of negation, like “does not” is not included in the default code of the NLP increasing the ambiguity of the biomedical text creating noise for the model.

4. **Scalability:** When dealing with the extremely large amount of data, it has been seen that chunking does not help much in improving the speed of the process, thus parallel processing or distributed computing can be done to improve the efficiency of the model.
5. **Missing Synonyms:** Very few of the drug's use their synonyms rather than the original one, so while requesting NER API (such as Rxnorm), we can make that function query more advanced by including unknown synonyms of the drugs.

Improvements and Future Directions

To further improve our drug-drug interaction (DDI) extraction model, we outline some key improvements and future directions below:

1. Fuzzy Matching for Drug Name Extraction

Applying fuzzy string-matching libraries like the FuzzyWuzzy library or RapidFuzz would enhance drug name detection that could be slightly different because of typographical mistakes, abbreviations, or name variant conventions. By fuzzy matching, our system will correctly match drug names with their proper entities even in the case of a misspelling or variant spelling. This will enhance recall rates and the strength of entity recognition in biomedical literature and clinical reports.

2. Contextual Named Entity Recognition

By employing pre-trained transformer models in the Hugging Face Transformers library, like BioBERT, SciBERT, or ClinicalBERT, we will be able to attain great contextualization of the entity recognition. These are biomedical text trained and can identify better drug entities even with complex sentence structures. Secondly, through fine-tuning our models on our dataset, we can improve precision and versatility towards drug name identification in various kinds of biomedical text.

3. Relationship Extraction for Drug Interactions

Extending the model from basic entity recognition to relation extraction will enable us to identify the type of drug interaction in the text. We can extract useful relationships between drugs using dependency parsing, attention mechanisms, or relation extraction models (such as BERT-based RE models) such as: Inhibition interactions (such as "Drug A inhibits Drug B"), Enhancement interactions (such as "Drug A enhances the effect of Drug B"), Negative interactions (e.g., "Co-administration of

Drug A and Drug B contributes to risk of toxicity"). This innovation will enhance the density and utility of the derived DDI knowledge graph.

4. Caching Mechanism for RxNorm API Calls

Given that calling the RxNorm API to normalize drugs can cause latency, we suggest that we build a caching system that holds on to previously received results. This will Cut down redundant API calls, improving responses. Enhance processing speed to enable real-time applications to be more efficient. Reduce API usage cost, particularly for processing massive-scale datasets. Redis caching or in-memory storage can be employed to cache and retrieve normalized drug names in an efficient manner.

Requirement of a Drug Synonym Dictionary in DDI Extraction

Drug-drug interaction (DDI) extraction has one of its most critical problems being the inconsistency in drug name conventions across sources. A single drug may have many different names in scientific literature, clinical reports, and prescribing manuals. For example, Paracetamol is referred to as Acetaminophen in the United States, brand name Tylenol, and sometimes shortened as APAP. Variations like these create disparities in text-mining systems, and when there are no inclusions of all possible synonyms, it results in interaction omission. Availability of brand names and trade names is another crucial feature. Most pharmaceutical companies produce the same active pharmaceutical ingredient under various brand names, which can be confusing to natural language processing (NLP) algorithms. In the absence of a formal synonym mapping framework, an NLP algorithm may not be able to identify that various brand names are referring to the same drug and thus may overlook DDI detection. For instance, it might print "Lantus," the brand name for Insulin Glargine, but not say what its generic name is. If the mapping is not appropriate for "Lantus" to "Insulin Glargine," the system can ignore important interactions of this drug. Not including drug synonyms in generating DDI reports results in incorrect negative findings for DDI analysis. If an NLP system fails to recognize various names of the same medication, it may fail to recognize important interactions simply because another variant was used in the document. This can be especially unfortunate when it is required to screen large volumes of literature, where nomenclature variations could hide important safety warnings. Hence, incorporating an exhaustive drug synonym dictionary is critical to enhance the accuracy and consistency of DDI extraction by catching all possible interactions irrespective of name variation.

Implementation Strategy

1. Integration of Drug Bank Synonym Data
   - o Drug Bank provides a comprehensive database of drug synonyms, brand names, and trade names that can be programmatically integrated into the system.
   - o This can be used to map all variations of a drug to a standardized identifier.
2. Enhancing Named Entity Recognition (NER) Models
   - o The synonym dictionary will be integrated into NLP pipelines to improve entity recognition, ensuring that different variations of a drug name are properly identified.
   - o Machine learning models, such as BERT-based biomedical NER models, will be fine-tuned using this enhanced dictionary.
3. Expanding Coverage and Reducing False Negatives
   - o By linking synonyms, abbreviations, and trade names to their corresponding active compounds, the system will extract interactions with higher precision and recall.
   - o This ensures that even if a study mentions a less common drug name, it will still be included in the DDI analysis.
4. Optimization for Scalability and Speed
   - o The pre-mapped synonym dictionary will be stored in an indexed, query-efficient format (e.g., Neo4j graph database, Elasticsearch) for faster lookup and reduced computational overhead.
   - o This approach minimizes the need for real-time synonym resolution, improving the efficiency of large-scale text processing.

The planned system will provide numerous advantages that significantly improve drug interaction analysis, pharmacovigilance, and customized medicine. Enhanced coverage of drug interactions is one of the main advantages because the system provides a full extraction of DDIs from different sources, such as biomedical publications, clinical trials, and drug regulatory files. With the merging of multiple datasets and the utilization of advanced NLP techniques, the system makes the detected interactions more accurate and credible. It also eliminates false negatives with the inclusion of all the trade names, alternative identifiers, and drug names. Recall enhancement ensures that no valid drug interactions are lost by nomenclature differences, and thus the system is stronger in real-world application. Yet another significant advantage is the faster and more scalable performance of the system. Through optimized synonym matching and entity recognition processes, the framework achieves faster processing, which enables it to work with large-scale datasets without loss of accuracy. This makes it highly useful in applications where real-time or high-throughput analysis is sought after. The effect of this increased efficiency is felt in pharmacovigilance and drug safety, where the system helps regulatory agencies, researchers, and clinicians in better estimation and prediction of possible drug interactions. Through ongoing, automated surveillance of biomedical literature, the system offers real-time evidence of adverse drug reactions, which helps in earlier detection and intervention plans. Furthermore, the system is applicable in enabling personalized medicine, as it allows for a customized drug interaction analysis. Through exact mapping of patient prescriptions to active ingredients and using genetic or metabolic factors, the system facilitates patient-specific drug interaction risk assessment. This accuracy is necessary for individualizing treatments, particularly for individuals with special pharmacogenomic profiles, and thus improving the efficacy of treatments and reducing side effects. Overall, these anticipated benefits place the framework as a catalyst of drug safety, personalized medicine, and clinical decision-making, ultimately leading to improved patient outcomes and more advanced research practices in medicine.

With the addition of Named Entity Recognition (NER) and RxNorm API calls to our system, we have been able to significantly enhance accuracy and automation in extracting drug-drug interactions (DDIs) from biomedical text. RxNorm API is a clinical drug database and a normalized nomenclature, which helps us achieve accurate entity linking and removing ambiguity in drug names, usually caused by differences in terms used in different datasets. Our NER model performs well in detecting drug mentions from text data extracted from biomedical literature, clinical trial reports, and electronic health records (EHRs). After detection, entities are mapped to RxNorm identifiers, allowing us to normalize and check drug names for consistency on DDIs extraction. False positives were removed and contextual interpretation of drug interactions enhanced. We have conducted NER analyses on a set of biomedical abstracts, and the resulting output with their corresponding RxNorm mappings is shown in Figure 3. The code implementation for said analyses is also included to show our workflow and technical implementation. This holistic solution not only enhances the efficiency of DDI information extraction but also has other applications in pharmacovigilance, personalized treatment, and precision medicine. By making extraction more structured and scalable, our solution facilitates the early detection of adverse drug reactions, enables personalized treatment recommendations, and aids in building a more comprehensive and credible DDI knowledge network. Moreover, the following enhancements to our approach, i.e., domain-specific fine-tuning of NER models, optimization of RxNorm API query strategies, and the addition of more validation layers will also improve the accuracy and legitimacy of our framework. These enhancements will seek to fix long-standing deficiencies, such as drug entity misclassification, handling polypharmacy situations, and integration with live clinical decision support systems.

Figure 3. Implementation of Named Entity Recognition (NER).

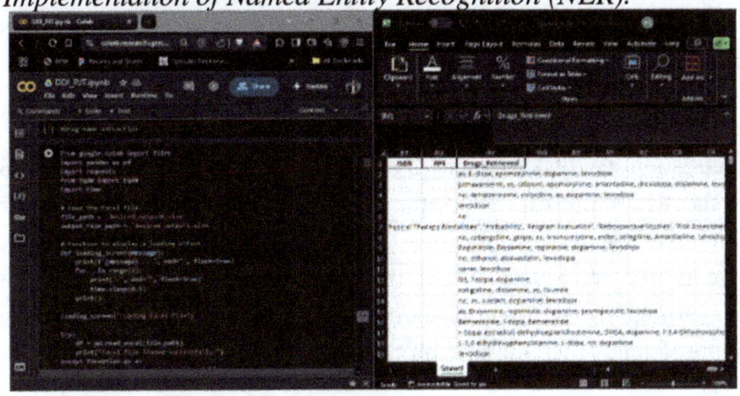

Table 2. Data insights of PubMed scrapping

Total unique drugs retrieved	Top 4 pair of drugs repeated in extraction	Times
838	"dopamine" and "levodopa"	699
	"levodopa" and "mg"	323
	"carbidopa" and "levodopa"	229
	"entacapone" and "levodopa"	150

Based on drug finding research (in the above table), literature review was done for the top 4 drug pair which concluded that-

The repetition of these drug pairs in PubMed research reflects their pharmacological relationships and clinical significance in treating neurological disorders, particularly Parkinson's disease (PD) and inflammation-associated depression. Below is an analysis of each pair with supporting references:

1. "Dopamine" and "Levodopa"

Levodopa is a dopamine precursor that crosses the blood-brain barrier to replenish dopamine levels, addressing motor and motivational deficits in PD and depression (Hardebo & Owman, 1980; Howard et al., 1995; Ovallath & Sulthana, 2017). Dopamine depletion underlies symptoms like bradykinesia in PD and anhedonia in depression. Levodopa's efficacy depends on its conversion to dopamine, making this pairing central to research on dopaminergic therapies (Pan et al., 2024). A 2023 Emory trial showed levodopa reversed inflammation-induced dopamine deficits in depressed patients with high C-reactive protein (CRP), improving reward circuitry connectivity.

2. "Levodopa" and "mg"

Dosage (mg) is usually studied to maximize therapeutic effects with a reduction in side effects such as dyskinesias (Ovallath & Sulthana, 2017; Salat & Tolosa, 2013). The short half-life of Levodopa (~1 hour) requires close dosing regimens. Clinical trials investigate formulations (e.g., duodenal infusion, extended release) to provide steady plasma levels (Ovallath & Sulthana, 2017; Salat & Tolosa, 2013). Comparative clinical trials of levodopa/carbidopa doses (e.g., 100/25 mg vs. 200/50 mg) investigate efficacy in managing motor fluctuations (Ovallath & Sulthana, 2017).

3. "Carbidopa" and "Levodopa"

Carbidopa inhibits peripheral decarboxylation of levodopa, enhancing its central availability (Salat & Tolosa, 2013; Gossard et al., 2021). The combination reduces side effects like nausea and allows lower levodopa dosages. Standard formulations include Sinemet (carbidopa/levodopa) (Gossard et al., 2021; Salat & Tolosa, 2013). A PubMed review notes carbidopa/levodopa combinations improve bioavailability and are first line for early PD(Salat & Tolosa, 2013).

4. "Entacapone" and "Levodopa"

Entacapone prolongs levodopa's effect by inhibiting catechol-O-methyltransferase (COMT), reducing "off" periods in PD (Salat & Tolosa, 2013). Triple therapy which includes (levodopa/carbidopa/entacapone) enhances dopaminergic stability, addressing motor complications(Salat & Tolosa, 2013). In one of the studies Stalevo which includes (levodopa/carbidopa/entacapone) trials demonstrate improved response fluctuations compared to levodopa alone.

Sentiment analysis to classify drug interactions.

The Rationale for Sentiment Analysis in DDI Classification

Sentiment analysis, traditionally used to gauge public opinion or emotional tone in text, might not immediately seem relevant for classifying drug-drug interactions (DDIs). However, when applied thoughtfully, it has the potential to provide valuable information into nature and possible impact of these interactions. The underlying premise is that the language used to describe DDIs in scientific literature often carries an implicit sentiment reflecting the interaction's clinical significance.

Why Sentiment Analysis is Relevant for Classifying Drug Interactions:

Identifying Beneficial vs. Harmful Interactions: Sentiment analysis helps distinguish between DDIs that lead to positive therapeutic outcomes and those that result in adverse effects. The language surrounding beneficial interactions tends to be positive, while harmful interactions are often described with negative terms. As highlighted in the study by Ben Abdessalem Karaa et al. (2021), the integration of NLP and graph databases can provide context-aware insights by combining textual data with graph-based predictions, enabling efficient identification of drug interactions (Kiogou & Adam, 2023b). Prioritizing High-Risk Interactions can be done by quantifying the negative sentiment associated with a particular DDI, healthcare professionals and researchers can prioritize the investigation and management of potentially dangerous drug combinations. A strong negative sentiment may indicate a higher likelihood of severe adverse events. Accordingly analyzing ADR reports can identify serious cases involving potential DDIs, reinforcing the importance of continuous pharmacovigilance to mitigate risks. (Kiogou & Adam, 2023b). Another relevancy of choosing sentimental analysis is the Detection of Subtle Interaction Effects as some DDIs have clear-cut outcomes while others may have more nuanced effects. Sentiment analysis can capture these subtle effects by analyzing the emotional tone of the text describing the interaction. For example, a neutral sentiment might indicate an interaction with minimal clinical significance. Supplementing Traditional DDI with the current DDIs can be done by classifying the Sentiment analysis provides an additional layer of information beyond traditional DDI classification methods, such as pharmacokinetic or pharmacodynamic classifications. It offers a complementary perspective that can enhance the overall understanding of DDIs. This is especially crucial given the limitations of traditional web-based DDI databases, as emphasized by Kiogou & Adam who advocate for the integration of clinical data repositories for a more thorough approach to identifying clinically significant interactions (Kiogou & Adam, 2023b). Contextual Understanding Can also be done by analyzing the sentiment expressed in the surrounding text, the system gains a deeper contextual understanding of the interaction.

Examples of Positive, Negative, and Neutral Interactions:

1. Positive Interaction:

Example: "The combination of entacapone and Levodopa resulted in a significant synergistic effect, leading to enhanced pain relief and improved patient outcomes."

- Sentiment: Positive. Words like "synergistic effect," "enhanced," and "improved" indicate a beneficial interaction.
- Interpretation: This DDI could be intentionally exploited in clinical practice to achieve better therapeutic results.

2. Negative Interaction:

Example: "Concurrent use of haloperidol and Levodopa has been associated with a significantly increased risk of severe gastrointestinal bleeding and cardiac arrest."

- Interpretation: Avoid or closely monitor this DDI because of the possibility of serious adverse effects.
- Interpretation: Exercise caution with or carefully monitor this DDI because of the risk of serious adverse events. As highlighted by Chan (1995), interactions like warfarin with NSAIDs can increase bleeding time, emphasizing the need for careful anticoagulation management (Kiogou & Adam, 2023b).

3. Neutral Interaction:

- Example: "Acetylcholine administration with Levodopa had little effect on plasma levels but did not influence therapeutically significant changes in safety or therapeutic effectiveness. "Sentiment: Neutral. Phrases like "minor alterations" and "no clinically significant changes" suggest a negligible impact.
- Interpretation: This DDI may not require special attention, as it does not appear to pose a significant risk to patients.

Implementation Considerations:

- Sentiment Lexicons: Using sentiment lexicons (e.g., VADER, SentiWordNet) specific to the biomedical domain can improve accuracy.
- Contextual Analysis: Consider the context where the interaction is described. Negations (e.g., "no adverse effects") can reverse the sentiment of a sentence.
- Machine Learning Models: Train machine learning models on labeled sets of DDI descriptions to predict interactions by sentiment. Feature engineering such as bag-of-words, TF-IDF, and word embeddings can be used to improve model performance. For instance, has proposed a hybrid approach combining

text-mining steps with graph neural networks (GNNs) and fine-tuning large language models (LLMs) and has demonstrated its suitability to the detection of molecular interactions for multifactorial diseases.

By integrating sentiment analysis into DDI classification as seen in Figure 4, researchers and clinicians will be able to obtain meaningful information about the nature and potential impact of drug interactions, thereby improving patient safety and treatment outcomes.

Figure 4. Sentiment analysis to classify drug interactions.

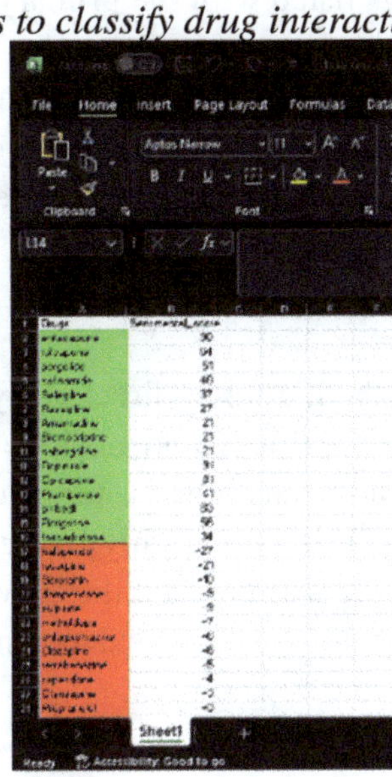

Graph Database Integration to form knowledge map

Knowing about the interaction of drugs with each other is very important in biomedical disease research in diseases such as Alzheimer's or Parkinson's disease. We then went ahead and did this by building a knowledge network with drugs as nodes, and edges showing their interactions, which we mined from scientific literature. We have also assigned each of these interactions with a sentiment score that makes a drug combination positive, negative, or neutral.

1. Constructing the Network Graph

First, we use a graph-based approach to model drug interactions. We treat each drug as a node, and we create an edge between the nodes when two drugs appear together in the scientific literature. We assign as a weight on the edge the sentiment score of the interaction, as determined by Natural Language Processing (NLP) techniques, which would be positive (helpful), negative (harmful), or neutral (uncertain). The data used for this study are extracted drug interactions from PubMed scholarly articles. Each record has:

Drug query – The primary drug of interest.
Drugs – Additional drugs listed with the primary drug.

Sentimental score – A numerical value indicating whether the interaction is good, bad, or neutral. By iterating over the dataset, each pair of drugs is represented as an edge in the graph and given the sentiment score as interaction weight.

2. Network Layout Organization

After the relations are graphed, a force-directed layout is employed to arrange the nodes. Nodes with more interactions (more positive sentiment scores) are drawn closer to each other, whereas nodes with less interactions are driven further apart. This aids in visually detecting clusters of highly connected drugs. A fixed random seed is utilized by the layout algorithm to facilitate reproducibility, i.e., node locations don't change whenever the graph is rendered such that comparison among datasets becomes easier.

3. Edge coloring based on Sentiment

Edges are colored according to their sentiment score for enhancing the interpretability of the visualization: Green for positive edges (indicating synergistic drug combinations). Red for negative edges (for toxic interaction). Gray for the interactions with little or no effect. This color-coding aids the researchers in easily recognizing what drug interactions can possibly be beneficial and which may need caution. Moreover, edge width varies based on the sentiment score. Strong interactions have thicker edges, and weak interactions have thinner edges. The main and peripheral interactions are easier to distinguish.

4. Visualizing the Knowledge Network

To see the network of drug interactions, graph is plotted between nodes and drug names. Nodes are made visible and distinguishable, and their color and thickness indicate the type of interactions they depict. Single drugs are depicted with sky-blue color. The interacting drugs are connected by edges whose thickness and color indicate strength in sentiment. Labels are added to enable researchers to easily learn about drugs. A title is added to give context to the visualization.

This network visualization presents a clear, data-derived picture of drug interactions from sentiment analysis of scientific literature. The knowledge network was created using the python libraries and the result can be seen in the figure-5, Green-clump patches of edges might suggest probable drug combinations, while red-dominated patches might suggest hazardous combinations to steer clear of. Combining network visualization with NLP-activated sentiment analysis makes this technique an extremely valuable research tool for pharmacology that enables researchers to take educated decisions on drug efficacy and safety. Figure 5 illustrates the results of Sentiment Analysis of Interactions of Levodopa Drug.

Figure 5. showing different types of layout formats obtained for a knowledge network graph. 5(A)- spring layout. negative and neutral are concentrated at one place, 5(B)- Equidistant layout, 5(C)- shell layout of graph and 5(D)- spring layout with fixed center.

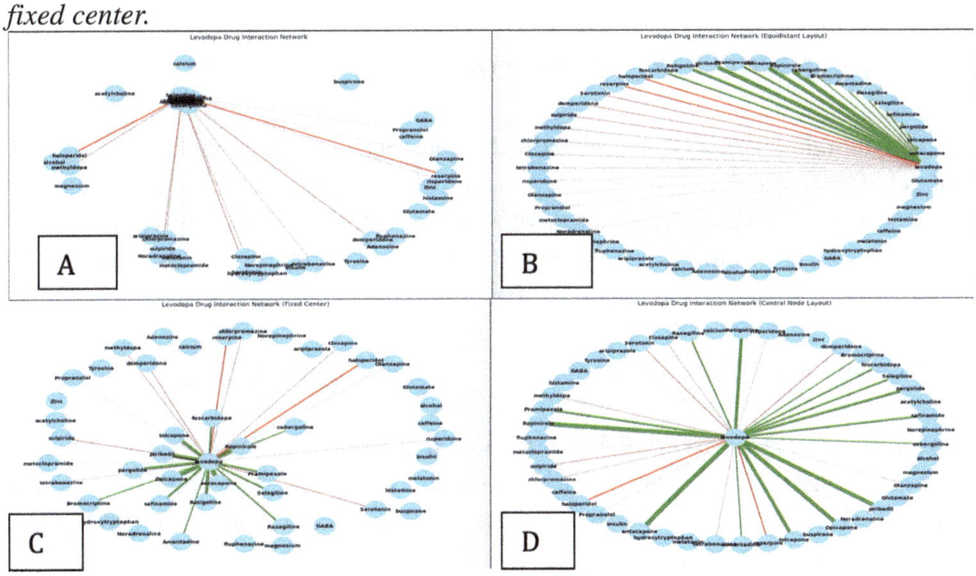

Summary of Key Findings

This chapter outlines a new method using Natural Language Processing (NLP) technologies and graph databases to facilitate totally automated extraction, structuring, and analysis of drug-drug interactions (DDIs) out of the biomedical literature. Applying Named Entity Recognition (NER) and sentiment analysis, the novel method facilitates the effective identification of drug interactions. Knowledge representation also improves through graph databases with the capability in tracing complex relationships for facilitating pharmacovigilance and personalized medicine. Traditional methods for DDI identification such as manual curation, clinical trials, and spontaneous reporting systems are resource-intensive and unable to keep pace with the rapidly expanding body of biomedical literature. Computational techniques like machine learning (ML), deep learning (DL), and statistical modeling have improved prediction accuracy but are at times comes with low interpretability, heterogeneity in data, and too high a computational burden. Compared to previous NLP-based approaches, this study introduces a graph database-powered knowledge network that enhances query efficiency, visualization, and predictive analytics. Unlike static rule-based systems, graph-based models dynamically update relationships, making them particularly valuable for real-time pharmacovigilance applications.

SOLUTIONS AND RECOMMENDATIONS

Our Natural Language Processing (NLP) study of drug interactions from PubMed research papers allowed us to classify Levodopa's interactions as positive, negative, and neutral based on their sentiment scores. These results give us useful information about what drugs would be used for further research and clinical use and which drugs are to be avoided due to side effects.

1. Positive Interaction – Entacapone: A Potential Synergistic Drug

Perhaps the most important discovery was that Entacapone had a positive sentiment score when it was paired with Levodopa. This indicates that scientific research is more than likely to affirm its beneficial effect when combined with Levodopa.

Entacapone works as a COMT inhibitor and prevents the breakdown of Levodopa by the body and subsequently extends its effectiveness. This is done by elevating the dopamine available, allowing Levodopa to be used more effectively to treat Parkinson's disease. Our positive sentiment value is consistent with current clinical thought, confirming our NLP technique for drug interaction analysis to be reliable. As Entacapone is a positive interaction, it offers the chance to explore other drug combinations that are able to synergize with Levodopa. Visualization of the knowledge network revealed some other drugs with green (positive) interactions. These can be tried in combination with Entacapone to produce more effective combination therapies. Drug development and clinical trials can aim at optimizing the dosage and efficacy of this combination. Therefore, Entacapone is an apt candidate to research, and the knowledge network also offers a template to study other synergistic candidates for drugs.

2. Negative Interaction – Haloperidol: Avoid Using

Sentiment analysis indicated that Haloperidol posted a negative sentiment score with Levodopa. This implies that current studies refute their combination and that it may produce unwanted side effects. Haloperidol is an antipsychotic medication which is a dopamine antagonist, or a dopamine receptor blocker. Levodopa is a precursor of dopamine and enhances the levels of dopamine in the brain. Because their modes of action are opposite, both the medications taken simultaneously may result in some ways like Decreased Levodopa effect, with an aggravation of Parkinson's disease symptoms, Augmented motor side effects like rigidity, tremors, and involuntary movement and Amplification of mental problems, perhaps undesirable for patients of neurodegenerative diseases. No more research is necessary on Haloperidol as a combination drug of Levodopa since it already showed side effects in experiments. This discovery is consistent with clinical observations wherein Haloperidol was reported to worsen Parkinson's among some patients. Doctors should exercise caution in prescribing Haloperidol to already pretreated Levodopa patients. Therefore, our affect-based NLP model assists in verifying existing medical information and offering data-driven evidence towards clinical decision-making.

3. Neutral Interaction – Buspirone: Safe Adjunct Treatment

Sentiment analysis also discovered a neutral interaction between Levodopa and Buspirone. A neutral score differs from positive or negative sentiment scores since it describes the absence of decisive evidence to prove positive or adverse effects where these two medicines are administered jointly. Buspirone is basically used in anxiety disorders, and though it does not potentiate or antagonize the effect of Levodopa, its neutrality makes it safe to be administered in combination with Levodopa without the potential enhancement of the risk for adverse effects. Since Buspirone is not interactive with Levodopa, it can be combined with other medications that also have a positive interaction, like Entacapone. It is potentially helpful for treating anxiety or mood disorders in Parkinson's patients, who often experience emotional distress as a result of their disorder. The neutral classification suggests that future research must attempt to examine its long-term consequences when administered in combination with Levodopa, so as to ascertain its safety in different patient groups. Medications such as Buspirone are potential adjunct treatments, i.e., they do not affect the root treatment (Levodopa) directly but can still be applied for supportive treatment.

4. Implications of These Findings on a Larger Scale

The sentiment-driven drug interaction network of Levodopa offers a data-driven and systematic way of looking at drug combinations. Some of the major findings of this study are:

1. Determining Drug Combinations for Further Investigation -Such drugs as Entacapone, with a positive sentiment score, can be further studied to provide improved treatment of Parkinson's. The knowledge network also offers new lines of research by pointing out other drugs that could be used in a synergistic combination with Levodopa.
2. Prevention of Harm through Adverse Combinations of Drugs- Drugs such as Haloperidol, with negative sentiment scores, emphasize the need to avoid conflicting mechanisms of action. The network assists in minimizing trial-and-error in a clinical environment by offering evidence-based advice.
3. Reviewing Neutral Drugs as Safer Additives- Neutral drugs such as Buspirone can be added safely along with positive interactions to offer additional benefits without interrupting major treatments. The findings assist in tailoring patient treatments so that they are given effective as well as safe drugs.

FUTURE RESEARCH DIRECTIONS

The suggested framework has numerous significant applications in drug safety, precision medicine, and clinical decision-making. One of its most significant applications is in pharmacovigilance, where it facilitates the early detection of adverse drug reactions (ADRs) by constantly querying large biomedical literature with high accuracy. Through the application of NLP processes, the system can track drug safety in real time so that regulatory authorities and healthcare centers can avert threats resulting from dangerous drug interactions. The system is also a crucial part of personalized medicine because it can recognize individualized drug interaction risks on the basis of a patient's medication history and genetic background. This makes provision for customized treatment plans that reduce side effects and maximize therapeutic response. Its second significant application is in drug discovery, where the system applies graph-based machine learning models to predict new drug-drug interactions (DDIs). Through the use of structural similarity as well as pharmacological feature analysis of drugs, the system can discover potential, yet unexplored, interactions, thus drug repurposing and synthesis of safer compounds for drugs. Finally, the system improves clinical decision support by leveraging NLP-generated drug interactions to update electronic health records (EHRs) and offer healthcare professionals actionable insights that avoid potentially risky prescriptions and enhance patient outcomes. Apart from application, the suggested framework provides a list of strengths and novel contributions which set it apart from conventional approaches. One of these innovations is automated literature mining, where the NLP pipeline pulls DDIs out of massive, unstructured data sets with minimal human curation and substantially enhancing efficiency and scalability. The system also uses graph databases rather than conventional relational databases, enabling dynamic knowledge representation of drug interaction networks.

Contrary to inflexible relational models, graph databases provide flexible and scalable modeling, making it simpler to uncover intricate relationships between drugs. But another added-value strength is improved interpretability, because the model presents drug interactions in a network structure, so scientists and clinicians can easily explore relationships among various medicinal entities. Although the method is also coupled with multiple benefits, some limitations still have to be tackled. One of them is data quality and bias, as the trustworthiness of predicted interactions considerably relies on biomedical article quality along with employed NLP models. Training set biases may cause misinterpretations, and thus potentially impact the reliability of DDI predictions. Another limitation is entity disambiguation, in which NLP models occasionally are unable to distinguish between drugs with similar names or abbreviations, causing wrong mappings. To minimize this, additional fine-tuning of entity linking approaches is needed. Lastly, computational complexity is a limitation, as graph-based models, although robust, are computationally intensive to handle extensive datasets. Handling huge volumes of real-time drug interaction information demands scalable infrastructure and algorithmic optimizations to prevent falling behind in efficiency at the expense of accuracy. Despite the challenges, ongoing advances in NLP methods, database optimization, and processing capabilities can continue to improve the proposed framework's robustness and worth as a useful resource toward optimizing drug safety, precision medicine, and clinical decision support.

CONCLUSION

In the world of medicine, doctors often give more than one medicine to a patient at the same time. This is called polypharmacy. But sometimes, two or more medicines can react with each other in a bad way. This is called a drug-drug interaction (DDI). DDIs can cause serious problems like side effects, reduced effectiveness of treatment, or even dangerous health conditions. That's why understanding drug interactions is very important. There are many research papers, articles, and clinical reports where drug interactions are discussed. But most of this information is written in text format, scattered across websites and journals. It is difficult for scientists or doctors to read everything and understand the patterns. So, there is a need for a system that can collect this information and organize it properly. In this chapter, we use Natural Language Processing (NLP) and graph network to collect, extract, and show information about DDIs. NLP is a part of artificial intelligence (AI) that helps computers understand human language. A graph network helps visualize connections or relationships between things which in our case is between different drugs. Our goal is to create a knowledge network or a map or web of drug interactions that can help researchers and healthcare professionals explore the available data easily and plan their research better. This work has proven that incorporation of NLP-supported drug interaction extraction into graph-based knowledge networks improves recognition, structuring, and analysis of DDIs. Leveraging graph databases, literature mining, and automation, the strategy brings immense enhancements over the current processes in pharmacovigilance, drug discovery, and clinical decision support. Using NLP-based sentiment analysis, we have been able to map and analyze the drug interactions of Levodopa. From the knowledge network, we have an easy-to-visualize understanding of how various drugs interact with each other, which facilitates drug discovery, clinical decision-making, and future research. Entacapone is worth investigating further because it has a positive interaction with Levodopa. Haloperidol should be avoided because its negative sentiment score indicates that it can cancel out the action of Levodopa. Buspirone is safe to administer since it has a neutral sentiment score, meaning that it does not disrupt the activity of Levodopa. Through the application of sentiment-based drug interaction networks, clinicians and researchers can make informed decisions regarding effective and safe drug combinations, thus optimizing treatment for neurodegenerative diseases. As biomedical literature continues to grow, scalable AI-driven solutions are progressively significant. This study indicates the need for automated knowledge extraction, demonstrating that NLP and graph-based modeling have the potential to give a dynamic, real-time perspective of drug interactions. Subsequent studies must strive to improve model accuracy, minimize data biases, and incorporate patient-specific factors into the DDI prediction pipeline. With ongoing progress in computational methods, researchers can move closer to a fully automated, AI-based pharmacovigilance system, which would render drug therapies safer and more efficient in clinical practice. Overall, this research offers an important step forward in AI-based DDI detection, and further directions are open for further enhancing drug safety and tailored treatment approaches in contemporary medicine.

REFERENCES

Ben, W., Karaa, A., Alkhammash, E. H., & Bchir, A. (2021). *Drug Disease Relation Extraction from Biomedical Literature Using NLP and Machine Learning*. https://doi.org/DOI: 10.1155/2021

Ben Abdessalem Karaa, W., Alkhammash, E. H., & Bchir, A. (2021). Drug Disease Relation Extraction from Biomedical Literature Using NLP and Machine Learning. *Mobile Information Systems*, *2021*(1), 9958410. DOI: 10.1155/2021/9958410

Celebi, R., Uyar, H., Yasar, E., Gumus, O., Dikenelli, O., & Dumontier, M. (2019). Evaluation of knowledge graph embedding approaches for drug-drug interaction prediction in realistic settings. *BMC Bioinformatics*, *20*(1), 1–14. DOI: 10.1186/s12859-019-3284-5 PMID: 31852427

Gossard, T. R., Trotti, L. M., Videnovic, A., & St Louis, E. K. (2021). Restless Legs Syndrome: Contemporary Diagnosis and Treatment. *Neurotherapeutics, 18*(1), <span class=”nowrap”>140-</span>155. DOI: 10.1007/s13311-021-01019-4

Hardebo, J. E., & Owman, C. (1980). Barrier mechanisms for neurotransmitter monoamines and their precursors at the blood-brain interface. *Annals of Neurology, 8*(1), <span class=”nowrap”>1-</span>31. DOI: 10.1002/ana.410080102

Howard, S. T., Hursthouse, M. B., Lehmann, C. W., & Poyner, E. A. (1995). Experimental and theoretical determination of electronic properties in Ldopa. *Acta Crystallogr. B, 51*(3), <span class=”nowrap”>328-</span>337. DOI: 10.1107/S0108768194011407

Kiogou, S. D., & Adam, T. J. (2023a). Clinical Data Repositories: Primary Sources of Drug-to-Drug Interaction Detection and Risk Assessment. *AMIA ... Annual Symposium Proceedings - AMIA Symposium. AMIA Symposium*, *2022*, 625. https://pmc.ncbi.nlm.nih.gov/articles/PMC10148339/ PMID: 37128384

Kiogou, S. D., & Adam, T. J. (2023b). Clinical Data Repositories: Primary Sources of Drug-to-Drug Interaction Detection and Risk Assessment. *AMIA ... Annual Symposium Proceedings - AMIA Symposium. AMIA Symposium*, *2022*, 625. https://pmc.ncbi.nlm.nih.gov/articles/PMC10148339/ PMID: 37128384

Ovallath, S., & Sulthana, B. (2017). Levodopa: History and Therapeutic Applications. *Annals of Indian Academy of Neurology, 20*(3), <span class=”nowrap”>185-</span>189. DOI: 10.4103/aian.AIAN_241_17

Pan, D., Lu, P., Wu, Y., Kang, L., Huang, F., Lin, K., & Yang, F. (2024). Prediction of multiple types of drug interactions based on multi-scale fusion and dual-view fusion. *Frontiers in Pharmacology*, *15*, 1354540. DOI: 10.3389/fphar.2024.1354540 PMID: 38434701

Polypharmacy and Drug Adherence in Elderly Patients. (n.d.). Retrieved April 8, 2025, from https://www.uspharmacist.com/article/polypharmacy-and-drug-adherence-in-elderly-patients

Rohani, N., & Eslahchi, C. (2019). Drug-Drug Interaction Predicting by Neural Network Using Integrated Similarity. *Scientific Reports 2019 9:1*, *9*(1), 1–11. DOI: 10.1038/s41598-019-50121-3

Salat, D., & Tolosa, E. (2013). Levodopa in the treatment of Parkinson's disease: Current status and new developments. *Journal of Parkinson's Disease*, *3*(3), 255–269. DOI: 10.3233/JPD-130186 PMID: 23948989

Tian, J. (2022). A review of methodologies in detecting drug-drug interactions. *AIP Conference Proceedings*, *2511*(1), 020022. Advance online publication. DOI: 10.1063/5.0094306

ADDITIONAL READING

Chen, Z., Liu, H., Wang, X., & Zhao, J. (2024). Integrating Knowledge Graph Embeddings and NLP for Enhanced Drug-Drug Interaction Extraction. *IEEE Transactions on Biomedical Engineering*, *71*, 1104–1115. DOI: 10.1109/TBME.2023.3301237

Li, M., Tang, J., & Li, J. (2023). Drug-Drug Interaction Extraction from Biomedical Text Using Attention-Based Graph Neural Networks. *Bioinformatics (Oxford, England)*, *39*(7), btad238. Advance online publication. DOI: 10.1093/bioinformatics/btad238 PMID: 37402625

Zhang, X., Wang, Y., & Li, J. (2023). Graph Neural Networks for Drug-Drug Interaction Prediction: A Review of Recent Advances. *Briefings in Bioinformatics*, *24*(4), bbac508. Advance online publication. DOI: 10.1093/bib/bbac508

KEY TERMS AND DEFINITIONS

Adverse Drug Reaction (ADR): Unintended, harmful reactions resulting from the use of a medication, which may be caused or worsened by DDIs.

Clinical Data Repository (CDR): A centralized database that aggregates clinical data from various sources such as electronic health records, enabling comprehensive analysis of patient information and drug interactions.

Deep Learning (DL): A type of machine learning that uses neural networks with multiple layers to model complex patterns in large datasets, widely used in biomedical data analysis.

Drug-Drug Interaction (DDI): A situation where the effect of one drug is altered by the presence of another drug, which can lead to changes in drug efficacy or adverse effects.

Graph Neural Networks (GNNs): Advanced machine learning models designed to process data structured as graphs, useful in predicting drug interactions by representing drugs as nodes and their interactions as edges.

Machine Learning (ML): A subset of artificial intelligence involving algorithms that learn from data to make predictions or decisions without being explicitly programmed.

Named Entity Recognition (NER): A Natural Language Processing technique that identifies and classifies key entities, such as drug names or diseases, within unstructured text.

Pharmacovigilance: The science and activities involved in detecting, assessing, understanding, and preventing adverse effects or other drug-related problems.

Polypharmacy: The practice of taking multiple medications simultaneously, especially common among elderly patients or those with multiple health conditions.

Spontaneous Reporting Database: A system for collecting reports of adverse drug reactions from healthcare providers and patients to monitor drug safety in real-world settings

Compilation of References

Abeng, F., Ikpi, M., Ushie, O., Anadebe, V., Nyong, B., Obeten, M., Okafor, N., Chukwuike, V., & Nkom, P. (2021). Insight into corrosion inhibition mechanism of carbon steel in 2 M HCl electrolyte by eco-friendly based pharmaceutical drugs. *Chemical Data Collections, 34*, 100722. DOI: 10.1016/j.cdc.2021.100722

Accenture. (2023). *AI in Pharma Manufacturing: Trends and Market Insights*. Accenture Insights.

Adhiya, J., Barghi, B., & Azadeh-Fard, N. (2024). Predicting the risk of hospital readmissions using a machine learning approach: A case study on patients undergoing skin procedures. *Frontiers in Artificial Intelligence*, *6*, 1213378. DOI: 10.3389/frai.2023.1213378 PMID: 38249790

Ahmed, M., & Barkat Ullah, A. S. (2017, August). False data injection attacks in healthcare. In *australasian conference on data mining* (pp. 192-202). Singapore: Springer Singapore.

Ahmed, S. A., & Pinjari, N. S. (2025). A Review of Sustainable Paradigms in Contemporary Drug Discovery and Development. *Journal of Pharma Insights and Research, 3*(2), 001–018.

Aithal, P. S., & Aithal, S. (2022). Opportunities and Challenges for Green and Eco-Friendly Nanotechnology in Twenty-First Century. *Sustainable Nanotechnology: Strategies, Products, and Applications*, 31–50.

Aithal, S., & Aithal, P. (2021). Green and eco-friendly Nanotechnology–concepts and industrial prospects. [IJMTS]. *International Journal of Management, Technology, and Social Sciences*, *6*(1), 1–31. DOI: 10.47992/IJMTS.2581.6012.0127

Alharbi, H. F., Bhupathyraaj, M., Mohandoss, K., Chacko, L., & Rani, K. R. V. (2023). An overview of artificial intelligence-driven pharmaceutical functionality. *Artificial Intelligence in Pharmaceutical Sciences*, 18–36.

Almeman, A. (2024, May 8). The digital transformation in pharmacy: Embracing online platforms and the cosmeceutical paradigm shift. *Journal of Health, Population and Nutrition, 43*(1), 60. DOI: 10.1186/s41043-024-00550-2 PMID: 38720390

Amabilino, S., Pogány, P., Pickett, S. D., & Green, D. V. S. (2020). Guidelines for recurrent neural network transfer learning-based molecular generation of focused libraries. *Journal of Chemical Information and Modeling, 60*(12), 5699–5713. DOI: 10.1021/acs.jcim.0c00343 PMID: 32659085

Amann, J., Blasimme, A., Vayena, E., Frey, D., & Madai, V. I. (2020). Explainability for artificial intelligence in healthcare: A multidisciplinary perspective. *BMC Medical Informatics and Decision Making, 20*(1), 310. DOI: 10.1186/s12911-020-01332-6 PMID: 33256715

Angwin, J., Larson, J., Mattu, S., & Kirchner, L. (2016). *Machine bias: There's software used across the country to predict future criminals. And it's biased against blacks*. ProPublica. https://www.propublica.org/article/machine-bias-risk-assessments-in-criminal-sentencing

Arabi, A. A. (2021). Artificial intelligence in drug design: Algorithms, applications, challenges and ethics. *Future Drug Discovery, 3*(2), FDD59. DOI: 10.4155/fdd-2020-0028

Arundel, A., Sawaya, D., & Valeanu, I. (2010). Human Health Biotechnologies to 2015. *OECD Journal General Papers, 2009*(3), 113–207.

Arús-Pous, J., Patronov, A., Bjerrum, E. J., Tyrchan, C., Reymond, J. L., Chen, H., & Engkvist, O. (2020). SMILES-based deep generative scaffold decorator for de-novo drug design. Journal of Cheminformatics, 12(1), 38. Artificial Intelligence/Machine Learning (AI/ML)-Based Software as a Medical Device (SaMD) Action Plan. (2021). U.S. Food and Drug Administration. https://www.fda.gov/media/145022/downloadDOI: 10.1186/s13321-020-00441-8

Askin, S., Burkhalter, D., Calado, G., & El Dakrouni, S. (2023). Artificial intelligence applied to clinical trials: Opportunities and challenges. *Health and Technology, 13*(2), 203–213. DOI: 10.1007/s12553-023-00738-2 PMID: 36923325

Aundhia, C., Parmar, G., Talele, C., Shah, N., & Talele, D. (2025). Impact of artificial intelligence on drug development and delivery. *Current Topics in Medicinal Chemistry, 25*(10), 1165–1184. DOI: 10.2174/0115680266324522240725053634 PMID: 39136506

Badwan, B. A., Liaropoulos, G., Kyrodimos, E., Skaltsas, D., Tsirigos, A., & Gorgoulis, V. G. (2023). Machine learning approaches to predict drug efficacy and toxicity in oncology. *Cell Reports Methods*, *3*(2), 100413. DOI: 10.1016/j.crmeth.2023.100413 PMID: 36936080

Bagal, V., Aggarwal, R., Vinod, P. K., & Priyakumar, U. D. (2021). MolGPT: Molecular generation using a transformer-decoder model. *Journal of Chemical Information and Modeling*, *62*(9), 2064–2076. DOI: 10.1021/acs.jcim.1c00600 PMID: 34694798

Bahrin, M. A. K., Othman, M. F., Azli, N. H. N., & Talib, M. F. (2016). Industry 4.0: A review on industrial automation and robotic. *Jurnal Teknologi*, *78*(6), 137–143. DOI: 10.11113/jt.v78.9285

Baig, M. I., Shuib, L., & Yadegaridehkordi, E. (2020). Big data and AI-based marketing strategies in the pharmaceutical industry. *Journal of Business Research*, *131*, 570–580. DOI: 10.1016/j.jbusres.2020.11.014

Baio, G. (2014). Bayesian models for cost-effectiveness analysis in the presence of structural zero costs. *Statistics in Medicine*, *33*(11), 1900–1913. DOI: 10.1002/sim.6074 PMID: 24343868

Bai, X., Xu, Y., & Liu, Y. (2024). Therapeutic effects of DOX-loaded hydrogel MOF nanocarriers on triple negative breast cancer and derivative design via reinforcement learning. *Scientific Reports*, *14*(1), 23946. DOI: 10.1038/s41598-024-75466-2 PMID: 39397066

Baranczak, P. J., Shangari, N. G., Palacios, D. S., Kratz, J. M., & O'Shea, K. (2017). Automated chemistry: A vision for the future. *Journal of Medicinal Chemistry*, *60*(20), 8353–8358. DOI: 10.1021/acs.jmedchem.7b00641

Baskar, K., Venkatesan, G. K. D. P., & Sangeetha, S. (2020). A Survey of Workload Management Difficulties in the Public Cloud. *In Intelligent Computing in Engineering: Select Proceedings of RICE 2019* (pp. 491–499). https://doi.org/DOI: 10.1007/978-981-15-2780-7_54

Bateman, A. W., Gunderson, J., & Mulder, R. (2015). Treatment of personality disorder. *Lancet*, *385*(9969), 735–743. DOI: 10.1016/S0140-6736(14)61394-5 PMID: 25706219

Batra, K., Zorn, K. M., Foil, D. H., Minerali, E., Gawriljuk, V. O., Lane, T. R., & Ekins, S. (2021). Quantum machine learning algorithms for drug discovery applications. *Journal of Chemical Information and Modeling*, *61*(6), 2641–2647. DOI: 10.1021/acs.jcim.1c00166 PMID: 34032436

Beaulieu-Jones, B. K., Finlayson, S. G., Chivers, C., Chen, I., McDermott, M., Kandola, J., Dalca, A. V., & Beam, A. L. (2019). Trends in the adoption of statistical and machine learning methods in biomedical research. *BMC Medical Research Methodology, 19*(1), 162. DOI: 10.1186/s12874-019-0799-4 PMID: 31340753

Bédard, A. C., Adamo, A., Aroh, K. C., Russell, M. G., Bedermann, A. A., Torosian, J., Yue, B., Jensen, K. F., & Jamison, T. F. (2018). Reconfigurable system for automated optimization of diverse chemical reactions. *Science, 361*(6408), 1220–1225. DOI: 10.1126/science.aat0650 PMID: 30237351

Beghi, E., Binder, H., Birle, C., Bornstein, N., Diserens, K., Groppa, S., Homberg, V., Lisnic, V., Pugliatti, M., Randall, G., Saltuari, L., Strilciuc, S., Vester, J., & Muresanu, D. (2021). European Academy of Neurology and European Federation of Neurorehabilitation Societies guideline on pharmacological support in early motor rehabilitation after acute ischaemic stroke. *European Journal of Neurology, 28*(9), 2831–2845. DOI: 10.1111/ene.14936 PMID: 34152062

Begley, C. G., Ashton, M., Baell, J., Bettess, M., Brown, M. P., Carter, B., Charman, W. N., Davis, C., Fisher, S., Frazer, I., Gautam, A., Jennings, M. P., Kearney, P., Keeffe, E., Kelly, D., Lopez, A. F., McGuckin, M., Parker, M. W., Rayner, C., & Sullivan, M. (2021). Drug repurposing: Misconceptions, challenges, and opportunities for academic researchers. *Science Translational Medicine, 13*(612), eabd5524. DOI: 10.1126/scitranslmed.abd5524 PMID: 34550729

Beis, S., & Anandan, J. (1999). Formulary management in an integrated health care system. *Pharmacy Practice Management Quarterly, 18*, 43–49. PMID: 10339067

Bellazzi, R., De Quiros, F. G. B., Koch, S., Kulikowski, C., Lovell, N., Maojo, V., Park, H., Sanz, F., Sarkar, I., Tanaka, H., & Al-Shorbaji, N. (2016). Discussion of "The New Role of Biomedical Informatics in the Age of Digital Medicine.". *Methods of Information in Medicine, 55*(05), 403–421. DOI: 10.3414/ME15-12-0005 PMID: 27524112

Belous, A., Zatolokina, M., Lavrinenko, K., Mal, G., Shevelev, A., & Trubnikova, E. (2016). Trophic changes in the skeletal muscles of rats after therapy with sildenafil and cerebrolysin in the lower limb ischemia model. *Bulletin of Russian State Medical University, 4*(4), 62–66. DOI: 10.24075/brsmu.2016-04-10

Ben Abdessalem Karaa, W., Alkhammash, E. H., & Bchir, A. (2021). Drug Disease Relation Extraction from Biomedical Literature Using NLP and Machine Learning. *Mobile Information Systems, 2021*(1), 9958410. DOI: 10.1155/2021/9958410

Ben, W., Karaa, A., Alkhammash, E. H., & Bchir, A. (2021). *Drug Disease Relation Extraction from Biomedical Literature Using NLP and Machine Learning*. https://doi.org/DOI: 10.1155/2021

Benavides-Hernández, J., & Dumeignil, F. (2024). From characterisation to discovery: Artificial intelligence, machine learning and high-throughput experiments for heterogeneous catalyst design. *ACS Catalysis*, *14*(15), 11749–11779. DOI: 10.1021/acscatal.3c06293

Bhattamisra, S. K., Banerjee, P., Gupta, P., Mayuren, J., Patra, S., & Candasamy, M. (2023). Artificial intelligence in pharmaceutical and healthcare research. *Big Data and Cognitive Computing*, *7*(1), 10. DOI: 10.3390/bdcc7010010

Bhatt, P., Singh, S., Kumar, V., Nagarajan, K., Mishra, S. K., Dixit, P. K., Kumar, V., & Kumar, S. (2024). Artificial intelligence in pharmaceutical industry: Revolutionizing drug development and delivery. *Current Artificial Intelligence*, *2*(1), E051223224198. DOI: 10.2174/0129503752250813231124092946

Bhatt, S., & Sharma, S. (2025). Generative Artificial Intelligence Based Biomedical Applications for Pharmaceutical Industry. In *2025 International Conference on Computational, Communication and Information Technology (ICCCIT)*, 1–6. https://doi.org/DOI: 10.1109/ICCCIT62592.2025.10927855

Biamonte, J., Wittek, P., Pancotti, N., Rebentrost, P., Wiebe, N., & Lloyd, S. (2017). Quantum machine learning. *Nature*, *549*(7671), 195–202. DOI: 10.1038/nature23474 PMID: 28905917

Birjais, R., Mourya, A. K., Chauhan, R., & Kaur, H. (2019). Prediction and diagnosis of future diabetes risk: A machine learning approach. *SN Applied Sciences*, *1*(9), 1112. Advance online publication. DOI: 10.1007/s42452-019-1117-9

Birniwa, A. H., Ali, U., Kutty, S. R. M., Jagaba, A. H., & Noor, A. (2023). Innovative and eco-friendly technologies for the upgradation of pharmaceutical wastewater treatment processes. In *The Treatment of Pharmaceutical Wastewater* (pp. 367–398). Elsevier. DOI: 10.1016/B978-0-323-99160-5.00006-0

Blanco-González, A., Cabezón, A., Seco-González, A., Conde-Torres, D., Antelo-Riveiro, P., Piñeiro, Á., & Garcia-Fandino, R. (2023, June 18). The Role of AI in Drug Discovery: Challenges, Opportunities, and Strategies. *Pharmaceuticals (Basel, Switzerland)*, *16*(6), 891. DOI: 10.3390/ph16060891 PMID: 37375838

Blaschke, T., Arús-Pous, J., Chen, H., Margreitter, C., Tyrchan, C., Engkvist, O., Papadopoulos, K., & Patronov, A. (2020). REINVENT 2.0: An AI tool for de novo drug design. *Journal of Chemical Information and Modeling*, *60*(12), 5918–5922. DOI: 10.1021/acs.jcim.0c00915 PMID: 33118816

Blunt, N. S., Camps, J., Crawford, O., Izsák, R., Leontica, S., Mirani, A., Moylett, A. E., Scivier, S. A., Sünderhauf, C., Schopf, P., Taylor, J. M., & Holzmann, N. (2022). A perspective on quantum computing for computational chemistry. *Journal of Chemical Theory and Computation*, *18*(12), 7001–7023. DOI: 10.1021/acs.jctc.2c00574 PMID: 36355616

Bonate, P. L. (2011). *Pharmacokinetic-Pharmacodynamic Modeling and Simulation* (2nd ed.). Springer. DOI: 10.1007/978-1-4419-9485-1

Boston Consulting Group (BCG). (2019). *Quantum computing in the life sciences: From hype to reality*. https://www.bcg.com/publications/2019/quantum-computing-transform-biopharma-research-development

Boulos, M. N. K. (2004). Towards evidence-based, GIS-driven national spatial health information infrastructure and surveillance services in the United Kingdom. *International Journal of Health Geographics*, *3*(1).

Boutilier, J. J., Chan, T. C., Ranjan, M., & Deo, S. (2021). Risk stratification for early detection of diabetes and hypertension in resource-limited settings: Machine learning analysis. *Journal of Medical Internet Research*, *23*(1), e20123. DOI: 10.2196/20123 PMID: 33475518

Bozorgi, P., Porter, D. E., Eberth, J. M., Eidson, J. P., & Karami, A. (2021). The leading neighborhood-level predictors of drug overdose: A mixed machine learning and spatial approach. *Drug and Alcohol Dependence*, *229*, 109143. DOI: 10.1016/j.drugalcdep.2021.109143 PMID: 34794060

Bradshaw, J., Kusner, M. J., Paige, B., Segler, M. H., & Hernández-Lobato, J. M. (2020). A generative model for electron paths. arXiv preprint arXiv:1805.10970. https://arxiv.org/abs/1805.10970

Brown, N., Fiscato, M., Segler, M. H., & Vaucher, A. C. (2018). GuacaMol: Benchmarking models for de novo molecular design. *Journal of Chemical Information and Modeling*, *59*(3), 1096–1108. DOI: 10.1021/acs.jcim.8b00839 PMID: 30887799

Brown, P., Tan, A.-C., El-Esawi, M. A., Liehr, T., Blanck, O., Gladue, D. P., Almeida, G. M. F., Cernava, T., Sorzano, C. O., Yeung, A. W. K., Engel, M. S., Chandrasekaran, A. R., Muth, T., Staege, M. S., Daulatabad, S. V., Widera, D., Zhang, J., Meule, A., Honjo, K., & Zhou, Y.RELISH Consortium. (2021). Large expert-curated database for benchmarking document similarity detection in biomedical literature search. *Database : The Journal of Biological Databases and Curation, 2019*, baz085. Advance online publication. DOI: 10.1093/database/baz085 PMID: 33326193

Brunton, S. L., Proctor, J. L., & Kutz, J. N. (2016). Discovering governing equations from data by sparse identification of nonlinear dynamical systems. *Proceedings of the National Academy of Sciences of the United States of America, 113*(15), 3932–3937. DOI: 10.1073/pnas.1517384113 PMID: 27035946

Cachata, D., Costa, M., Magalhães, T., & Gaspar, F. (2024). The Integration of Information Technology in the Management and Organization of Nursing Care in a Hospital Environment: A Scoping Review. *International Journal of Environmental Research and Public Health, 21*(8), 968. DOI: 10.3390/ijerph21080968 PMID: 39200579

Cao, Y., Romero, J., & Aspuru-Guzik, A. (2018). Potential of quantum computing for drug discovery. IBM Journal of Research and Development, 62(6), 6:1-6:20. DOI: 10.1147/JRD.2018.2888987

Cao, Y., Romero, J., Olson, J. P., Degroote, M., Johnson, P. D., Kieferová, M., Kivlichan, I. D., Menke, T., Peropadre, B., Sawaya, N. P. D., Sim, S., Veis, L., & Aspuru-Guzik, A. (2019). Quantum chemistry in the age of quantum computing. *Chemical Reviews, 119*(19), 10856–10915. DOI: 10.1021/acs.chemrev.8b00803 PMID: 31469277

Carracedo-Reboredo, P., Liñares-Blanco, J., Rodríguez-Fernández, N., Cedrón, F., Novoa, F. J., Carballal, A., Maojo, V., Pazos, A., & Fernandez-Lozano, C. (2021). A review on machine learning approaches and trends in drug discovery. *Computational and Structural Biotechnology Journal, 19*, 4538–4558. DOI: 10.1016/j.csbj.2021.08.011 PMID: 34471498

Cascone, S., Lamberti, G., Titomanlio, G., & Piazza, O. (2013). Pharmacokinetics of Remifentanil: A three-compartmental modeling approach. *Translational Medicine @ UniSa*, 18–22. PMID: 24251247

Castiello, C., Junghanns, P., Mergel, A., Jacob, C., Ducho, C., Valente, S., Rotili, D., Fioravanti, R., Zwergel, C., & Mai, A. (2023). GreenMedChem: The challenge in the next decade toward eco-friendly compounds and processes in drug design. *Green Chemistry, 25*(6), 2109–2169. DOI: 10.1039/D2GC03772F

Cattaneo, A., Vitali, A., Regazzoni, D., & Rizzi, C. (2024). A sustainable approach to telerehabilitation in Europe: Patients are ready, but caregivers are essential. *Studies in Health Technology and Informatics*. Advance online publication. DOI: 10.3233/SHTI240014 PMID: 38682507

Celebi, R., Uyar, H., Yasar, E., Gumus, O., Dikenelli, O., & Dumontier, M. (2019). Evaluation of knowledge graph embedding approaches for drug-drug interaction prediction in realistic settings. *BMC Bioinformatics*, *20*(1), 1–14. DOI: 10.1186/s12859-019-3284-5 PMID: 31852427

Centers for Medicare and Medicaid Services. (2021). *The Hospital Value-Based Purchasing (VBP)*. Program.

Chen, R. T. Q., Rubanova, Y., Bettencourt, J., & Duvenaud, D. (2018). *Neural ordinary differential equations*. In *Advances in Neural Information Processing Systems* (NeurIPS 2018), 31.

Chenais, G., Lagarde, E., & Gil-Jardiné, C. (2023, May 23). Artificial Intelligence in Emergency Medicine: Viewpoint of Current Applications and Foreseeable Opportunities and Challenges. *Journal of Medical Internet Research*, *25*, e40031. DOI: 10.2196/40031 PMID: 36972306

Chew, H. S. J., & Achananuparp, P. (2022). Perceptions and needs of artificial intelligence in health care to increase adoption: Scoping review. *Journal of Medical Internet Research*, *24*(1), e32939. DOI: 10.2196/32939 PMID: 35029538

Chithrananda, S., Grand, G., & Ramsundar, B. (2020). ChemBERTa: Large-scale self-supervised pretraining for molecular property prediction. arXiv preprint arXiv:2010.09885. https://arxiv.org/abs/2010.09885

Chodera, J., Lee, A. A., London, N., & von Delft, F. (2020). Crowdsourcing drug discovery for pandemics. *Nature Chemistry*, *12*(7), 581–581. DOI: 10.1038/s41557-020-0496-2 PMID: 32555379

Chong Yin, Siqi Liu, Fei Lyu, Jiahao Lu, Sune Darkner, Vincent Wai-Sun Wong, & Pong C. Yuen. (2024). XFibrosis: Explicit Vessel-Fiber Modeling for Fibrosis Staging from Liver Pathology Images. *Computer Vision and Pattern Recognition*, 11282–11291.

Choudhary, A., Harding, J. A., & Tiwari, M. K. (2019). Data mining in manufacturing: A review based on the kind of knowledge. *Journal of Intelligent Manufacturing*, *30*(4), 1393–1410. DOI: 10.1007/s10845-017-1318-0

Choudhury, C., Murugan, N. A., & Priyakumar, U. D. (2022). Structure-based drug repurposing: Traditional and advanced AI/ML-aided methods. *Drug Discovery Today, 27*(7), 1847–1861. DOI: 10.1016/j.drudis.2022.03.006 PMID: 35301148

Churpek, M. M., Yuen, T. C., & Edelson, D. P. (2013). Predicting clinical deterioration in the hospital: The impact of outcome selection. *Resuscitation, 84*(5), 564–568. DOI: 10.1016/j.resuscitation.2012.09.024 PMID: 23022075

Cockshott, I. D., Douglas, E. J., & Prys-Roberts, C. (1987). Pharmacokinetics of propofol during and after intravenous infusion in man. *British Journal of Anaesthesia, 59*, 941.

Consulting, L. E. K. (2024). *Quantum Computing in Biopharma: Future Prospects and Strategic.* https://www.lek.com/insights/hea/us/ei/quantum-computing-biopharma-future-prospects-and-strategic-insights

Cook, D., Brown, D., Alexander, R., March, R., Morgan, P., Satterthwaite, G., & Pangalos, M. N. (2014). Lessons learned from the fate of AstraZeneca's drug pipeline: A five-dimensional framework. *Nature Reviews. Drug Discovery, 13*(6), 419–431. DOI: 10.1038/nrd4309 PMID: 24833294

Cowie, M. R., Blomster, J. I., Curtis, L. H., Duclaux, S., Ford, I., Fritz, F., Goldman, S., Janmohamed, S., Kreuzer, J., Leenay, M., Michel, A., Ong, S., Pell, J. P., Southworth, M. R., Stough, W. G., Thoenes, M., Zannad, F., & Zalewski, A. (2017). Electronic health records to facilitate clinical research. *Clinical Research in Cardiology; Official Journal of the German Cardiac Society, 106*(1), 1–9. DOI: 10.1007/s00392-016-1025-6 PMID: 27557678

Cross, A., Bishop, L., Sheldon, S., Nation, P., & Gambetta, J. (2019). Validating quantum computers using randomized model circuits. *Physical Review. A, 100*(3), 032328. Advance online publication. DOI: 10.1103/PhysRevA.100.032328

Dabbah, S., Mishani, I., Davidov, Y., & Ben Ari, Z. (2025). Implementation of Machine Learning Algorithms to Screen for Advanced Liver Fibrosis in Metabolic Dysfunction-Associated Steatotic Liver Disease: An In-Depth Explanatory Analysis. *Digestion, 106*(3), 189–202. DOI: 10.1159/000542241

Dahlin, J. L., & Walters, M. A. (2014). The essential roles of chemistry in high-throughput screening triage. *Future Medicinal Chemistry, 6*(11), 1265–1290. DOI: 10.4155/fmc.14.60 PMID: 25163000

Danso, K. O., Asagba, P. O., Yarhere, I. E., Adumattah, P., & Amoaful, S. (2024). Implementing and Adopting EHR Systems in Developing Countries. *Ghana Journal of Nursing and Midwifery, 1*(4), 30–62. DOI: 10.69600/gjnmid.2024.v01.i04.30-62

Davenport, T. H., & Ronanki, R. (2018). Artificial intelligence for the real world. *Harvard Business Review*, *96*(1), 108–116.

Davenport, T., & Kalakota, R. (2019). The potential for artificial intelligence in healthcare. *Future Healthcare Journal*, *6*(2), 94–98. DOI: 10.7861/futurehosp.6-2-94 PMID: 31363513

De Cao, N., & Kipf, T. (2018). MolGAN: An implicit generative model for small molecular graphs. arXiv preprint arXiv:1805.11973. https://arxiv.org/abs/1805.11973

De Spiegeleer, B., & Wynendaele, E. (2025). Sustainability of drug discovery, development and use as embedded in European pharmaceutical policies. *Current Opinion in Green and Sustainable Chemistry*, *53*, 101028. DOI: 10.1016/j.cogsc.2025.101028

Delgadillo, J., Ali, S., Fleck, K., Agnew, C., Southgate, A., Parkhouse, L., Cohen, Z. D., DeRubeis, R. J., & Barkham, M. (2022). Stratified care vs stepped care for depression: A cluster randomized clinical trial. *JAMA Psychiatry*, *79*(2), 101–108. DOI: 10.1001/jamapsychiatry.2021.3539 PMID: 34878526

Denck, J., Ozkirimli, E., & Wang, K. (2023, September). Machine-learning-based adverse drug event prediction from observational health data: A review. *Drug Discovery Today*, *28*(9), 103715. DOI: 10.1016/j.drudis.2023.103715 PMID: 37467879

DesRoches, C. M., Campbell, E. G., Rao, S. R., Donelan, K., Ferris, T. G., Jha, A., Kaushal, R., Levy, D. E., Rosenbaum, S., Shields, A. E., & Blumenthal, D. (2008). Electronic health records in ambulatory care—A national survey of physicians. *The New England Journal of Medicine*, *359*(1), 50–60. DOI: 10.1056/NEJMsa0802005 PMID: 18565855

Destro, F., & Barolo, M. (2022). A review on the modernization of pharmaceutical development and manufacturing–Trends, perspectives, and the role of mathematical modeling. *International Journal of Pharmaceutics*, *620*, 121715. DOI: 10.1016/j.ijpharm.2022.121715 PMID: 35367580

Devgan, K., Sharma, S., Jangra, D., & Sharma, S. (2025). Artificial Intelligence-Enabled Apple Disease Monitoring System for environmental protection and resource conservation. In Advances in computational intelligence and robotics book series (pp. 271–300). https://doi.org/DOI: 10.4018/979-8-3373-3246-8.ch011

Devliyal, S., Goyal, H. R., & Sharma, S. (2024). ICDRET: A dynamic cyber risk estimation technique for intelligent Cyber-Physical Systems in PCS. *The Open Bioinformatics Journal*, *18*(1), e18750362380269. Advance online publication. DOI: 10.2174/0118750362380269250502062754

Devliyal, S., Sharma, S., & Goyal, H. R. (2024). EIAIMSPS: Edge inspired artificial intelligence-based multi stakeholders Personalized Security Mechanism in ICPS for PCS. *International Journal of Advanced Computer Science and Applications*, *15*(8). Advance online publication. DOI: 10.14569/IJACSA.2024.01508117

DiMasi, J. A., Grabowski, H. G., & Hansen, R. W. (2016). Innovation in the pharmaceutical industry: New estimates of R&D costs. *Journal of Health Economics*, *47*, 20–33. DOI: 10.1016/j.jhealeco.2016.01.012 PMID: 26928437

Dinh, A., Miertschin, S., Young, A., & Mohanty, S. D. (2019). A data-driven approach to predicting diabetes and cardiovascular disease with machine learning. *BMC Medical Informatics and Decision Making*, *19*(1), 211. Advance online publication. DOI: 10.1186/s12911-019-0918-5 PMID: 31694707

Dobson, C. M. (2004). Chemical space and biology. *Nature*, *432*(7019), 824–828. DOI: 10.1038/nature03192 PMID: 15602547

Douma, M. C., Rejeb, M. B., Zardoub, N., Braham, A., Chouchene, H., Bouallegue, O., & Latiri, H. S. (2024). Impact of Implementing Electronic Nursing Records on Quality and Safety Indicators in Care. *The Libyan Journal of Medicine*, *19*(1), 2421625. DOI: 10.1080/19932820.2024.2421625 PMID: 39570988

Duma, D., & Aringhieri, R. (2023). Real-time resource allocation in the emergency department: A case study. *Omega*, *117*, 102844. DOI: 10.1016/j.omega.2023.102844

Dunjko, V., & Briegel, H. J. (2018). Machine learning & artificial intelligence in the quantum domain: A review of recent progress. *Reports on Progress in Physics*, *81*(7), 074001. DOI: 10.1088/1361-6633/aab406 PMID: 29504942

Durairaj, M., Jayakumar, S., Karpagavalli, V., Maheswari, B. U., & Boopathi, S. (2023). Utilization of Digital Tools in the Indian Higher Education System During Health Crises. In *Multidisciplinary Approaches to Organizational Governance During Health Crises* (pp. 1–21). IGI Global. DOI: 10.4018/978-1-7998-9213-7.ch001

Dwivedi, Y. K., Hughes, L., Ismagilova, E., Aarts, G., Coombs, C., Crick, T., Duan, Y., Dwivedi, R., Edwards, J., Eirug, A., Galanos, V., Ilavarasan, P. V., Janssen, M., Jones, P., Kar, A. K., Kizgin, H., Kronemann, B., Lal, B., Lucini, B., & Williams, M. D. (2019). Artificial Intelligence (AI): Multidisciplinary perspectives on emerging challenges, opportunities, and agenda for research, practice and policy. *International Journal of Information Management*, *57*, 101994. DOI: 10.1016/j.ijinfomgt.2019.08.002

Edwards, C., Lai, T., Ros, K., Honke, G., & Ji, H. (2022). Translation between molecules and natural language. arXiv preprint arXiv:2204.11817. https://arxiv.org/abs/2204.11817 DOI: 10.18653/v1/2022.emnlp-main.26

Elton, D. C., Boukouvalas, Z., Fuge, M. D., & Chung, P. W. (2019). Deep learning for molecular design—A review of the state of the art. *Molecular Systems Design & Engineering*, *4*(4), 828–849. DOI: 10.1039/C9ME00039A

Ertl, P., & Schuffenhauer, A. (2009). Estimation of synthetic accessibility score of drug-like molecules based on molecular complexity and fragment contributions. *Journal of Cheminformatics*, *1*(1), 8. DOI: 10.1186/1758-2946-1-8 PMID: 20298526

Esteva, A., Robicquet, A., Ramsundar, B., Kuleshov, V., DePristo, M., Chou, K., Cui, C., Corrado, G., Thrun, S., & Dean, J. (2019). A guide to deep learning in healthcare. *Nature Medicine*, *25*(1), 24–29. DOI: 10.1038/s41591-018-0316-z PMID: 30617335

European Medicines Agency. (2023). *EMA Reflection Paper on Artificial Intelligence in Medicines Regulation.* https://www.ema.europa.eu

Fabian, B., Edlich, T., Gaspar, H., Segler, M., Meyers, J., Fiscato, M., & Ahmed, M. (2020). Molecular representation learning with language models and domain-relevant auxiliary tasks. arXiv preprint arXiv:2011.13230. https://arxiv.org/abs/2011.13230

Fatima, N., & Nayeem, N. (2016). Toxic effects as a result of herbal medicine intake. In InTech eBooks. DOI: 10.5772/64468

FDA. (2023). Emerging Technology Program. U.S. Food and Drug Administration. https://www.fda.gov/drugs/pharmaceutical-quality-resources/emerging-technology -program

Feng, C., Chen, H., Yuan, X., Sun, M., Chu, K., Liu, H., & Rui, M. (2019). Gene expression data based deep learning model for accurate prediction of Drug-Induced liver injury in advance. *Journal of Chemical Information and Modeling*, *59*(7), 3240–3250. DOI: 10.1021/acs.jcim.9b00143 PMID: 31188585

Fernandez, J. M., Choi, D., Ahmed, N., & Gupta, R. (2023). Hybrid data-driven and mechanistic modeling of propofol pharmacokinetics in three compartments using deep neural networks. *IFAC-PapersOnLine*, *56*(10), 850–857.

Finkelman, J. M., & Zhang, Y. (2022). The role of AI in pharmaceutical supply chain resilience. *The Journal of Supply Chain Management*, *58*(4), 9–21.

Fisher, C. K., Smith, A. M., & Walsh, J. R. (2021). Machine learning for comprehensive forecasting of Alzheimer's Disease progression. *Scientific Reports*, *11*(1), 1–13. DOI: 10.1038/s41598-021-99494-4 PMID: 33414495

Fourches, D., Muratov, E., & Tropsha, A. (2010). Trust, but verify: On the importance of chemical structure curation in cheminformatics and QSAR modeling research. *Journal of Chemical Information and Modeling*, *50*(7), 1189–1204. DOI: 10.1021/ci100176x PMID: 20572635

Fourkiotis, K. P., & Tsadiras, A. (2024). Applying Machine Learning and Statistical Forecasting Methods for Enhancing Pharmaceutical Sales Predictions. *Forecasting*, *6*(1), 170–186. DOI: 10.3390/forecast6010010

Fuller, A., Fan, Z., Day, C., & Barlow, C. (2020). Digital twin: Enabling technologies, challenges and open research. *IEEE Access : Practical Innovations, Open Solutions*, *8*, 108952–108971. DOI: 10.1109/ACCESS.2020.2998358

Gabrielsson, J., & Weiner, D. (2016). *Pharmacokinetic and Pharmacodynamic Data Analysis: Concepts and Applications* (5th ed.). CRC Press.

Gandu, Sravanthi, & Gandla, Kumaraswamy & Vaishnavi, M & Repudi, Lalitha. (. (2023). A review on implementation of automation in the pharmaceutical industries. *World Journal of Advanced Research and Reviews.*, *18*, 606–615. DOI: 10.30574/wjarr.2023.18.2.0858

Garg, S., Arora, K., Singh, S., & Nagarajan, K. (2024). Artificial Intelligence and Machine Learning in Drug Discovery and Development. In *Artificial Intelligence in the Age of Nanotechnology* (pp. 42–61). IGI Global.

Gartner. (2024). *Digital Twin Adoption in Pharma Manufacturing*. Gartner Research.

Gepts, E., Camu, F., Cockshott, I. D., & Douglas, E. J. (1987). Disposition of propofol administered as constant rate infusions in humans. *Anesthesia and Analgesia*, *66*(12), 1256–1263. DOI: 10.1213/00000539-198712000-00010 PMID: 3500657

Gerke, S., Minssen, T., & Cohen, G. (2020). Ethical and legal challenges of artificial intelligence-driven healthcare. In *Artificial Intelligence in Healthcare* (pp. 295–336). DOI: 10.1016/B978-0-12-818438-7.00012-5

Gerke, S., Minssen, T., & Cohen, G. (2020). Ethical and legal challenges of artificial intelligence-driven healthcare. *The Hastings Center Report*, *50*(1), 22–27. DOI: 10.1002/hast.1084

Gettman, D. (2023). Integration of Genomics and Artificial Intelligence in Pharmacy Practice: The Era of Predictive, Personalized Care. DOI: 10.13140/RG.2.2.31795.34086

Ginting, D. S., Dewi, W. N., & Lestari, W. (2024). Nurses' experiences using electronic medical record (EMR): A systematic review. *Malahayati International Journal of Nursing and Health Science, 7*(8), 976–983. DOI: 10.33024/minh.v7i8.625

Golas, S. B., Shibahara, T., Agboola, S., Otaki, H., Sato, J., Nakae, T., Hisamitsu, T., Kojima, G., Felsted, J., Kakarmath, S., Kvedar, J., & Jethwani, K. (2018). A machine learning model to predict the risk of 30-day readmissions in patients with heart failure: A retrospective analysis of electronic medical records data. *BMC Medical Informatics and Decision Making, 18*(1), 1–17. DOI: 10.1186/s12911-018-0620-z PMID: 29929496

Gómez-Bombarelli, R., Wei, J. N., Duvenaud, D., Hernández-Lobato, J. M., Sánchez-Lengeling, B., Sheberla, D., Aguilera-Iparraguirre, J., Hirzel, T. D., Adams, R. P., & Aspuru-Guzik, A. (2018). Automatic chemical design using a data-driven continuous representation of molecules. *ACS Central Science, 4*(2), 268–276. DOI: 10.1021/acscentsci.7b00572 PMID: 29532027

González Peña, O. I., López Zavala, M. Á., & Cabral Ruelas, H. (2021). Pharmaceuticals market, consumption trends and disease incidence are not driving the pharmaceutical research on water and wastewater. *International Journal of Environmental Research and Public Health, 18*(5), 2532. DOI: 10.3390/ijerph18052532 PMID: 33806343

Goodwin, G., Haddad, P., Ferrier, I., Aronson, J., Barnes, T., & Cipriani, A. Coghill, Fazel, S., Geddes, J., Grunze, H., Holmes, E., Howes, O., Hudson, S., Hunt, N., Jones, I., Macmillan, I., McAllister-Williams, H., Miklowitz, Morriss, R., & Young, A. (2016). Evidence-based guidelines for treating bipolar disorder: Revised third edition recommendations from the British Association for Psychopharmacology. Journal of Psychopharmacology, 30(6), 495–553.

Gopi, B., Sworna Kokila, M. L., Bibin, C. V., Sasikala, D., Howard, E., & Boopathi, S. (2024). Distributed Technologies Using AI/ML Techniques for Healthcare Applications. In *Advances in Human and Social Aspects of Technology* (pp. 375–396). IGI Global. DOI: 10.4018/979-8-3693-2569-8.ch019

Gossard, T. R., Trotti, L. M., Videnovic, A., & St Louis, E. K. (2021). Restless Legs Syndrome: Contemporary Diagnosis and Treatment. *Neurotherapeutics, 18*(1), <span class=”nowrap”>140-</span>155. DOI: 10.1007/s13311-021-01019-4

Gowri, N. V., Dwivedi, J. N., Krishnaveni, K., Boopathi, S., Palaniappan, M., & Medikondu, N. R. (2023). Experimental investigation and multi-objective optimization of eco-friendly near-dry electrical discharge machining of shape memory alloy using Cu/SiC/Gr composite electrode. *Environmental Science and Pollution Research International, 30*(49), 1–19. DOI: 10.1007/s11356-023-26983-6 PMID: 37126160

Goyal, P., & Malviya, R. (2023, October 4). Challenges and opportunities of big data analytics in healthcare. [Retraction in: Health Care Sci. 2025 Mar 25;4] [2] [:161. doi: 10.1002/hcs2.70006]. *Health Care Science, 2*(5), 328–338. DOI: 10.1002/hcs2.66 PMID: 38938583

Green, L. V. (2002–2003). How many hospital beds? *Inquiry : a Journal of Medical Care Organization, Provision and Financing, 39*(4), 400–412. DOI: 10.5034/inquiryjrnl_39.4.400 PMID: 12638714

Grisoni, F., Neuhaus, C. S., Gabernet, G., Müller, A. T., Hiss, J. A., & Schneider, G. (2020). Designing anticancer peptides by constructive machine learning. *ChemMedChem, 15*(4), 300–305. DOI: 10.1002/cmdc.201900599 PMID: 29679519

GSK. (2023). *Innovation and Automation Annual Report*. GlaxoSmithKline plc

Gude, S., & Gude, Y. S.GUDE. (2024). The synergy of artificial intelligence and machine learning in revolutionizing pharmaceutical regulatory affairs. *Translational and Regulatory Sciences, 6*(2), 37–45. DOI: 10.33611/trs.2024-005

Guimaraes, G. L., Sanchez-Lengeling, B., Outeiral, C., Farias, P. L. C., & Aspuru-Guzik, A. (2017). Objective-reinforced generative adversarial networks (ORGAN) for sequence generation models. arXiv preprint arXiv:1705.10843. https://arxiv.org/abs/1705.10843

Güleryüz, C., Sumrra, S. H., Hassan, A. U., Mohyuddin, A., Waheeb, A. S., Awad, M. A., Jalfan, A. R., Noreen, S., Kyhoiesh, H. A. K., & El Azab, I. H. (2025). A machine learning and DFT assisted analysis of benzodithiophene based organic dyes for possible photovoltaic applications. *Journal of Photochemistry and Photobiology A Chemistry, 460*, 116157. DOI: 10.1016/j.jphotochem.2024.116157

Gupta, A., & Sharma, S. (2024). Deep Learning Inspired Biomarker Diagnostic Enabled Heart Health Monitoring System for Cardiac Arrest Detection. In *2024 International Conference on Emerging Technologies and Innovation for Sustainability (EmergIN)*, 13–17. https://doi.org/DOI: 10.1109/EmergIN63207.2024.10960916

Gupta, R., Srivastava, D., Sahu, M., Tiwari, S., Ambasta, R. K., & Kumar, P. (2021). Artificial intelligence to deep learning: Machine intelligence approach for drug discovery. *Molecular Diversity, 25*(3), 1315–1360. DOI: 10.1007/s11030-021-10217-3 PMID: 33844136

Haber, P., Lintzeris, N., Proude, E., & Lopatko, O. (2009). Guidelines for the treatment of alcohol problems [Dataset]. In *PsycEXTRA Dataset.*

Hacker, P., Krestel, R., Grundmann, S., & Naumann, F. (2020). Explainable AI under contract and tort law: Legal incentives and technical challenges. *Artificial Intelligence and Law, 28*(4), 415–439. DOI: 10.1007/s10506-020-09260-6

Hansson, T., Oostenbrink, C., & van Gunsteren, W. (2002). Molecular dynamics simulations. *Current Opinion in Structural Biology, 12*(2), 190–196. DOI: 10.1016/S0959-440X(02)00308-1 PMID: 11959496

Hardebo, J. E., & Owman, C. (1980). Barrier mechanisms for neurotransmitter monoamines and their precursors at the blood-brain interface. *Annals of Neurology, 8*(1), <span class=”nowrap”>1-</span>31. DOI: 10.1002/ana.410080102

Harvey, H. B., & Gowda, V. (2021). Regulatory issues and challenges to artificial intelligence adoption. *Radiologia Clinica, 59*(6), 1075–1083. DOI: 10.1016/j.rcl.2021.07.007 PMID: 34689875

Hassan, T. M., Elmogy, M., & Sallam, E.-S. (2017). Diagnosis of Focal Liver Diseases Based on Deep Learning Technique for Ultrasound Images. *Arabian Journal for Science and Engineering, 42*(8), 3127–3140. DOI: 10.1007/s13369-016-2387-9

Heindel, G. A., & McIntyre, C. M. (2018). Contemporary challenges and novel strategies for health-system formulary management. *American Journal of Health-System Pharmacy, 75*(8), 556–560. DOI: 10.2146/ajhp170351 PMID: 29626005

He, J., Baxter, S. L., Xu, J., Xu, J., Zhou, X., & Zhang, K. (2019). The practical implementation of artificial intelligence technologies in medicine. *Nature Medicine, 25*(1), 30–36. DOI: 10.1038/s41591-018-0307-0 PMID: 30617336

Helm, J. M., Swiergosz, A. M., Haeberle, H. S., Karnuta, J. M., Schaffer, J. L., Krebs, V. E., & Ramkumar, P. N. (2020). Machine learning and artificial intelligence: Definitions, applications, and future directions. *Current Reviews in Musculoskeletal Medicine, 13*(1), 69–76. DOI: 10.1007/s12178-020-09600-8 PMID: 31983042

Hernández-Lobato, J. M., Houlsby, N., Ghahramani, Z., & Herbrich, R. (2014). *Probabilistic backpropagation for scalable learning of Bayesian neural networks.* In *Proceedings of the 32nd International Conference on Machine Learning* (ICML 2014), 1861–1869.

He, S., Barón, A., Munteanu, C. R., de Bilbao, B., Casañola-Martin, G. M., Chelu, M., Musuc, A. M., Bediaga, H., Ascencio, E., Castellanos-Rubio, I., Arrasate, S., Pazos, A., Insausti, M., Rasulev, B., & González-Díaz, H. (2025). Drug Release Nanoparticle System Design: Data Set Compilation and Machine Learning Modeling. *ACS Applied Materials & Interfaces*, *17*(3), 5290–5306. DOI: 10.1021/acsami.4c16800 PMID: 39800937

He, S., Guo, F., Zou, Q., & Ding, H. (2020). MRMD2.0: A Python tool for machine learning with feature ranking and reduction. *Current Bioinformatics*, *15*(10), 1213–1221. DOI: 10.2174/2212392XMTA2bMjko1

He, X., Zhao, Y., & Kumar, R. (2023). Transformer and LSTM hybrid model for depth-of-anesthesia prediction under propofol infusion. *IEEE Transactions on Biomedical Engineering*, *70*(7), 1980–1991.

Hill, N. R., Sandler, B., Mokgokong, R., Lister, S., Ward, T., Boyce, R., Farooqui, U., & Gordon, J. (2020). Cost-effectiveness of targeted screening for the identification of patients with atrial fibrillation: Evaluation of a machine learning risk prediction algorithm. *Journal of Medical Economics*, *23*(4), 386–393. DOI: 10.1080/13696998.2019.1706543 PMID: 31855091

Holloway, P. M., Willaime-Morawek, S., Siow, R., Barber, M., Owens, R. M., Sharma, A. D., Rowan, W., Hill, E., & Zagnoni, M. (2021). Advances in microfluidic in vitro systems for neurological disease modeling. *Journal of Neuroscience Research*, *99*(5), 1276–1307. DOI: 10.1002/jnr.24794 PMID: 33583054

Hoogeboom, E., Satorras, V. G., Vignac, C., & Welling, M. (2022). Equivariant diffusion for molecule generation in 3D. arXiv preprint arXiv:2203.17003. https://arxiv.org/abs/2203.17003

Hopkins, C., Surda, P., Walker, A., Wolf, A., Speth, M., Jacques, T., Hox, V., Van Gerven, L., Santamaria-Gadea, A., Segboer, C., Lourijsen, E., Turri-Zanoni, M., Huart, C., Rennie, C., Green, R., Society, N. S., Kelly, C., Knill, A., Lund, V., & Fokkens, W. (2021). EPOS 4 patients. *Rhinology*, *0*(0), 1–57. DOI: 10.4193/Rhin20.950 PMID: 34762718

Houssari, M., Boukhalfa, I., Henry, J., Mulder, P., Richard, V., Brakenhielm, E., Nili, R., Amet, D., Vidil, F., Beller, C. L., Pedard, M., Totoson, P., Demougeot, C., Salem, J., Germain, M., Hulot, J., Marie, C., Abudoureheman, A., Wuliya, Y., & Zhou, W. (2017). Discussed poster abstracts. *Fundamental & Clinical Pharmacology*, *31*(S1), 21–50. DOI: 10.1111/fcp.12272

Howard, S. T., Hursthouse, M. B., Lehmann, C. W., & Poyner, E. A. (1995). Experimental and theoretical determination of electronic properties in Ldopa. *Acta Crystallogr. B, 51*(3), <span class=”nowrap”>328-</span>337. DOI: 10.1107/S0108768194011407

Huang, Y., Pu, Q., Lan, W., Huang, C., & Zhong, C. (2025). SMDPG: Identifying Metabolite-Disease Associations via Optimized Negative Sampling and Sparse Graph Convolutional Network. *IEEE Transactions on Computational Biology and Bioinformatics*, 1–12. https://doi.org/DOI: 10.1109/TCBBIO.2025.3532256

Huang, K., Fu, T., Glass, L. M., Zitnik, M., Xiao, C., & Sun, J. (2020). DeepPurpose: A deep learning library for drug-target interaction prediction. *Bioinformatics (Oxford, England)*, *36*(22-23), 5545–5547. DOI: 10.1093/bioinformatics/btaa1005 PMID: 33275143

Hughes, J. P., Rees, S., Kalindjian, S. B., & Philpott, K. L. (2011). Principles of early drug discovery. *British Journal of Pharmacology*, *162*(6), 1239–1249. DOI: 10.1111/j.1476-5381.2010.01127.x PMID: 21091654

Hu, X., Sun, L., Zheng, R., Xia, X., Liu, M., Chen, W., Zhang, X., & Wang, C. (2024). Application of graph theory in liver research: A review. *Portal Hypertension & Cirrhosis*, *3*(4), 234–248. DOI: 10.1002/poh2.97

Hyo Jeong Ryu, Won ho Kang, Taeheon Kim, Jae Kyoung Kim, Kwang-Hee Shin, Jung-woo Chae, Hwi-yeol Yun. (2022). A compatibility evaluation between the physiologically based pharmacokinetic model and the compartmental PK model using the lumping method with real cases. *Frontiers in Pharmacology*, 13. PMID: 36034786

IDC (International Data Corporation). (2024). *Worldwide Global DataSphere Forecast*. Retrieved from https://www.idc.com

IDC Health Insights. (2024). *AI Control Towers in Pharma Supply Chains*. IDC Reports.

Irvin, J. A., Kondrich, A. A., Ko, M., Rajpurkar, P., Haghgoo, B., Landon, B. E., Phillips, R. L., Petterson, S., Ng, A. Y., & Basu, S. (2020). Incorporating machine learning and social determinants of health indicators into prospective risk adjustment for health plan payments. *BMC Public Health*, *20*(1), 1–10. DOI: 10.1186/s12889-020-08735-0 PMID: 32357871

Islam, T., Hussain, N., Islam, S., & Chakrabarty, A. (2018). Detecting Adverse Drug Reaction with Data Mining And Predicting its Severity With Machine Learning. In 2018 IEEE Region 10 Humanitarian Technology Conference (R10-HTC), 1–5. https://doi.org/.DOI: 10.1109/R10-HTC.2018.8629806

Ivanov, D., & Dolgui, A. (2020). Viability of intertwined supply networks: Extending the supply chain resilience angles towards survivability. *International Journal of Production Research*, *58*(10), 2904–2915. DOI: 10.1080/00207543.2020.1750727

Iyengar, K., Upadhyaya, G. K., Vaishya, R., & Jain, V. (2020). COVID-19 and applications of smartphone technology in the current pandemic. *Diabetes & Metabolic Syndrome*, *14*(5), 733–737. DOI: 10.1016/j.dsx.2020.05.033 PMID: 32497963

Jairoun, A. A., Al-Hemyari, S. S., Shahwan, M., Alkhoujah, S., El-Dahiyat, F., Jaber, A. A. S., & Zyoud, S. H. (2025a). Towards eco-friendly pharmaceuticals: Regulatory and policy approaches for sustainable medicines use. *Exploratory Research in Clinical and Social Pharmacy*, *17*, 100576. DOI: 10.1016/j.rcsop.2025.100576 PMID: 40026320

Jayaraman, A., & Olsen, B. (2024). Convergence of artificial intelligence, machine learning, cheminformatics, and polymer science in macromolecules. *Macromolecules*, *57*(16), 7685–7688. DOI: 10.1021/acs.macromol.4c01704

Jayatunga, M. K., Jung, S., & Chen, J. (2022). AI in small-molecule drug discovery: A coming wave. *Nature Reviews. Drug Discovery*, *21*(3), 175–176. DOI: 10.1038/d41573-022-00025-1 PMID: 35132242

Jazieh, A. R., & Kozlakidis, Z. (2020). Healthcare transformation in the post-coronavirus pandemic era. *Frontiers in Medicine*, *7*, 429. DOI: 10.3389/fmed.2020.00429 PMID: 32850915

Jiang, J., Ma, X., Ouyang, D., & Williams, R. O.III. (2022). Emerging artificial intelligence (AI) technologies used in the development of solid dosage forms. *Pharmaceutics*, *14*(11), 2257. DOI: 10.3390/pharmaceutics14112257 PMID: 36365076

Jin, W., Barzilay, R., & Jaakkola, T. (2020). Hierarchical graph-to-graph translation for molecules. arXiv preprint arXiv:1907.11223. https://arxiv.org/abs/1907.11223

Jumper, J., Evans, R., Pritzel, A., Green, T., Figurnov, M., Ronneberger, O., Tunyasuvunakool, K., Bates, R., Žídek, A., Potapenko, A., Bridgland, A., Meyer, C., Kohl, S. A. A., Ballard, A. J., Cowie, A., Romera-Paredes, B., Nikolov, S., Jain, R., Adler, J., & Hassabis, D. (2021). Highly accurate protein structure prediction with AlphaFold. *Nature*, *596*(7873), 583–589. DOI: 10.1038/s41586-021-03819-2 PMID: 34265844

Kadurin, A., Nikolenko, S., Khrabrov, K., Aliper, A., & Zhavoronkov, A. (2017). druGAN: An advanced generative adversarial autoencoder model for de novo generation of new molecules with desired molecular properties in silico. *Molecular Pharmaceutics*, *14*(9), 3098–3104. DOI: 10.1021/acs.molpharmaceut.7b00346 PMID: 28703000

Kamble, S. S., Gunasekaran, A., Gawankar, S. A., & Dhone, N. C. (2020). A performance measurement system for industry 4.0 enabled smart manufacturing system in SMMEs—A review and empirical investigation. *International Journal of Production Economics*, *229*, 107853. DOI: 10.1016/j.ijpe.2020.107853

Kankala, R. K., Xu, P.-Y., Chen, B.-Q., Wang, S.-B., & Chen, A.-Z. (2021). Supercritical fluid (SCF)-assisted fabrication of carrier-free drugs: An eco-friendly welcome to active pharmaceutical ingredients (APIs). *Advanced Drug Delivery Reviews*, *176*, 113846. DOI: 10.1016/j.addr.2021.113846 PMID: 34197896

Kapruwan, A., Sharma, S., & Goyal, H. R. (2025). ESCBR: Expert System Enabled Case-based Reasoning Approach in IDDCS for CIND. *Recent Patents on Engineering*, *19*. Advance online publication. DOI: 10.2174/0118722121336689250116074945

Kapruwan, A., Sharma, S., & Goyal, H. R. (2025a). iDDCS: Cervical intraepithelial neoplasia severity detection during vagina birth using artificial intelligence approach. *Multidisciplinary Science Journal*, *7*(8), 2025192. DOI: 10.31893/multiscience.2025192

Karpov, P., Godin, G., & Tetko, I. V. (2020). Transformer-CNN: Swiss knife for QSAR modeling and interpretation. *Journal of Cheminformatics*, *12*(1), 17. DOI: 10.1186/s13321-020-00423-w PMID: 33431004

Kartono, A., Anggraini, D., Wahyudi, S. T., Setiawan, A. A., & Irmansyah, . (2021). Study of Parameters Estimation of The Three-Compartment Pharmacokinetic Model using Particle Swarm Optimization Algorithm. *Journal of Physics: Conference Series*, *1805*(1), 012032. DOI: 10.1088/1742-6596/1805/1/012032

Katabarwa, A., Gratsea, K., Caesura, A., & Johnson, P. D. (2024). Early fault-tolerant quantum computing. *PFX Quantum : a Physical Review Journal*, *5*(2), 020101. DOI: 10.1103/PRXQuantum.5.020101

Kaul, A., Enslin, S., & Gross, T. (2020). Health AI: The state of play. *Deloitte Insights*. https://www2.deloitte.com

Kausik, S. K., Rashid, A. B., Baki, R. F., & Maktum, M. M. J. (2025). Machine learning algorithms for manufacturing quality assurance: A systematic review of performance metrics and applications. *Array (New York, N.Y.), 26*, 100393. DOI: 10.1016/j.array.2025.100393

Kexin Ding, Mu Zhou, Zichen Wang, Qiao Liu, Corey W. Arnold, Shaoting Zhang, & Dimitri N. Metaxas. (2022). Graph Convolutional Networks for Multi-modality Medical Imaging: Methods, Architectures, and Clinical Applications. *Electrical Engineering and Systems Science -Image and Video Processing, 3.*

Khadela, A., Popat, S., Ajabiya, J., Valu, D., Savale, S., & Chavda, V. P. (2023). AI, ML and other bioinformatics tools for preclinical and clinical development of drug products. *Bioinformatics Tools for Pharmaceutical Drug Product Development*, 255–284.

Kiogou, S. D., & Adam, T. J. (2023a). Clinical Data Repositories: Primary Sources of Drug-to-Drug Interaction Detection and Risk Assessment. *AMIA ... Annual Symposium Proceedings - AMIA Symposium. AMIA Symposium, 2022*, 625. https://pmc.ncbi.nlm.nih.gov/articles/PMC10148339/ PMID: 37128384

Kiran, A., Neerugatti, V., & Kumar, D. S. J. Somasekar, Santhosh Boddupalli, B. Sai Praneetha (2024), Revolutionizing cirrhosis liver disorder diagnosis: A deep learning approach with convolutional neural networks,V. Sharmila et al. (Eds), Challenges in Information, Communication and Computing Technology,449-454, Taylor & Francis Group

Kirkpatrick, T., Cockshott, I. D., Douglas, E. J., & Nimmo, W. S. (1988). Pharmacokinetics of propofol (Diprivan) in elderlv patients. *British Journal of Anaesthesia, 6O*, i46–i150. PMID: 3257879

Kitaev, A. Y. (2003). Fault-tolerant quantum computation by anyons. *Annals of Physics, 303*(1), 2–30. DOI: 10.1016/S0003-4916(02)00018-0

Klucken, J., Krüger, R., Schmidt, P., & Bloem, B. R. (2018). Management of Parkinson's disease 20 years from now: Towards digital health pathways. *Journal of Parkinson's Disease, 8*(s1), S85–S94. DOI: 10.3233/JPD-181519 PMID: 30584171

Knapp, B., Bardenet, R., Bernabeu, M. O., Bordas, R., Bruna, M., Calderhead, B., Cooper, J., Fletcher, A. G., Groen, D., Kuijper, B., Lewis, J., McInerny, G., Minssen, T., Osborne, J., Paulitschke, V., Pitt-Francis, J., Todoric, J., Yates, C. A., Gavaghan, D., & Deane, C. M. (2015). Ten simple rules for a successful cross-disciplinary collaboration. *PLoS Computational Biology, 11*(4), e1004214. DOI: 10.1371/journal.pcbi.1004214 PMID: 25928184

Kolluri, S., Lin, J., Liu, R., Zhang, Y., & Zhang, W. (2022). Machine learning and artificial intelligence in pharmaceutical research and development: A review. *The AAPS Journal*, *24*(1), 1–10. DOI: 10.1208/s12248-021-00644-3 PMID: 34984579

Komorowski, M., Celi, L. A., Badawi, O., Gordon, A. C., & Faisal, A. A. (2018). The Artificial Intelligence Clinician learns optimal treatment strategies for sepsis in intensive care. *Nature Medicine*, *24*(11), 1716–1720. DOI: 10.1038/s41591-018-0213-5 PMID: 30349085

Kopczyk, D. (2018). Quantum machine learning for data scientists. 10.48550/arXiv.1804.10068.

Koren, Y., van der Walt, J., & Eleveld, D. J. (2022). Symbolic regression for automated covariate modeling in pharmacokinetics: Application to a propofol three-compartment model. *CPT: Pharmacometrics & Systems Pharmacology*, *11*(12), 1441–1453.

Koshechkin, K. A., Lebedev, G. S., Fartushnyi, E. N., & Orlov, Y. L. (2022). Holistic approach for artificial intelligence implementation in pharmaceutical products lifecycle: A meta-analysis. *Applied Sciences (Basel, Switzerland)*, *12*(16), 8373. DOI: 10.3390/app12168373

Kumar, R., Jones, S., & Patel, N. (2024). Advances in automated anesthesia control: Integrating deep learning and control methods over three-compartment PK models. *Anesthesiology & Perioperative Science*, *5*(1), 34–49.

Kuo, T. T., Gabriel, R. A., Cidambi, K. R., & Ohno-Machado, L. (2020). EXpectation Propagation LOgistic REgRession on permissioned blockCHAIN (ExplorerChain): Decentralized privacy-preserving online healthcare analytics. *IEEE Journal of Biomedical and Health Informatics*, *24*(8), 2278–2287. DOI: 10.1109/JBHI.2020.2969648 PMID: 31841426

Layton, D. (2018). Developments and Future Directions of Prescription-Based Observational Cohort Pharmacovigilance. In Methods in pharmacology and toxicology (pp. 105–134). DOI: 10.1007/978-1-4939-8818-1_6

Leach, A. R. (2001). *Molecular modelling: Principles and applications* (2nd ed.). Pearson Education.

Lee, J., Bagheri, B., & Kao, H. A. (2015). A Cyber-Physical Systems Architecture for Industry 4.0-Based Manufacturing Systems. *Manufacturing Letters*, *3*, 18–23. DOI: 10.1016/j.mfglet.2014.12.001

Le, T. M., Vo, T. M., Pham, T. N., & Dao, S. V. T. (2020). A novel Wrapper–Based feature selection for early diabetes prediction enhanced with a metaheuristic. *IEEE Access : Practical Innovations, Open Solutions*, *9*, 7869–7884. DOI: 10.1109/ACCESS.2020.3047942

Li, Jian-qiang & Yu, F. & Deng, Genqiang & Luo, Chengwen & Ming, Zhong & Yan, Qiao. (2017). Industrial Internet: A Survey on the Enabling Technologies, Applications, and Challenges. IEEE Communications Surveys & Tutorials. PP. 1-1. .DOI: 10.1109/COMST.2017.2691349

Liang, Z., Zhang, S., Wei, A., Liu, Z., Wang, Y., Hu, H., Chen, W., & Qi, L. (2024). CylinGCN: Cylindrical structures segmentation in 3D biomedical optical imaging by a contour-based graph convolutional network. *Computerized Medical Imaging and Graphics*, *111*, 102316. DOI: 10.1016/j.compmedimag.2023.102316

Li, J., Fu, T., Song, H., Fan, J., Xiao, D., Lin, Y., Gu, Y., & Yang, J. (2024). Embedding-Alignment Fusion-Based Graph Convolution Network With Mixed Learning Strategy for 4D Medical Image Reconstruction. *IEEE Journal of Biomedical and Health Informatics*, *28*(5), 2916–2929. DOI: 10.1109/JBHI.2024.3365203

Li, J., Kong, M., Wang, D., Yang, Z., & Hao, X. (2022). Prediction of lncRNA–Disease Associations via Closest Node Weight Graphs of the Spatial Neighborhood Based on the Edge Attention Graph Convolutional Network. *Frontiers in Genetics*, *12*. Advance online publication. DOI: 10.3389/fgene.2021.808962

Li, S., Zhang, H., Holby, E. F., Zelenay, P., & Kort-Kamp, W. J. (2024). Machine learning-guided design, synthesis, and characterisation of atomically dispersed electrocatalysts. *Current Opinion in Electrochemistry*, *48*, 101578. DOI: 10.1016/j.coelec.2024.101578

Liu, W., Lu, P., & Zhou, J. (2025). Enhancing Disease-metabolite Associations Prediction with Weighted Graph Convolutional Networks Based on Community-driven Link Completion. *IEEE Transactions on Computational Biology and Bioinformatics*, 1–13. https://doi.org/DOI: 10.1109/TCBBIO.2025.3532644

Liu, D., Luo, Y., Zheng, J., Xu, H., Zhang, J., & Deng, L. (2021). GCNSDA: Predicting snoRNA-disease associations via graph convolutional network. *2021 IEEE International Conference on Bioinformatics and Biomedicine (BIBM)*, 183–188. https://doi.org/DOI: 10.1109/BIBM52615.2021.9669505

Liu, K., Sun, X., Jia, L., Ma, J., Xing, H., Wu, J., Gao, H., Sun, Y., Boulnois, F., & Fan, J. (2019). Chemi-Net: A Molecular Graph Convolutional Network for Accurate Drug Property Prediction. *International Journal of Molecular Sciences*, *20*(14), 3389. DOI: 10.3390/ijms20143389

Liu, Y., Chen, P. H. C., Krause, J., & Peng, L. (2019). How to read articles that use machine learning: Users' guides to the medical literature. *Journal of the American Medical Association*, *322*(18), 1806–1816. DOI: 10.1001/jama.2019.16489 PMID: 31714992

Liu, Y., Zhang, H., Chen, X., Wang, Q., & Li, M. (2024). Data-driven pharmacokinetic modeling for propofol using machine learning approaches in a three-compartment framework. *European Journal of Pharmaceutical Sciences*, *190*, 106464. DOI: 10.1016/j.ejps.2023.106464

Li, Y., Zhao, Y., Zhang, F., Liao, M., Yu, L., Chen, B., & Wang, Y. (2020). Liver segmentation from abdominal CT volumes based on level set and sparse shape composition. *Computer Methods and Programs in Biomedicine*, *195*, 105533. DOI: 10.1016/j.cmpb.2020.105533

Lou, B., & Wu, L. (2021). AI on drugs: Can artificial intelligence accelerate drug development? Evidence from a large-scale examination of bio-pharma firms. *Evidence from a Large-Scale Examination of Bio-Pharma Firms,(March 15, 2021). Management Information Systems Quarterly*, *45*(3), 1451–1482. DOI: 10.25300/MISQ/2021/16565

Low, L. A., Mummery, C., Berridge, B. R., Austin, C. P., & Tagle, D. A. (2021). Organs-on-chips: Into the next decade. *Nature Reviews. Drug Discovery*, *20*(5), 345–361. DOI: 10.1038/s41573-020-0079-3 PMID: 32913334

Lu, L., Zhang, J., Xie, Y., Gao, F., Xu, S., Wu, X., & Ye, Z. (2020). Wearable health devices in health care: Narrative systematic review. *JMIR mHealth and uHealth*, *8*(11), e18907. DOI: 10.2196/18907 PMID: 33164904

Lu, M., Yin, J., Zhu, Q., Lin, G., Mou, M., Liu, F., Pan, Z., You, N., Lian, X., Li, F., Zhang, H., Zheng, L., Zhang, W., Zhang, H., Shen, Z., Gu, Z., Li, H., & Zhu, F. (2023). Artificial intelligence in pharmaceutical sciences. *Engineering (Beijing)*, *27*, 37–69. DOI: 10.1016/j.eng.2023.01.014

Lundberg, S. M., & Lee, S. I. (2017). A unified approach to interpreting model predictions. *Advances in Neural Information Processing Systems*, *30*, 4765–4774.

Luo, S., Guan, J., Ma, J., & Peng, J. (2021). A 3D-based graph convolution network for predicting protein-ligand binding affinity. *bioRxiv*. DOI: 10.1101/2021.04.16.440230

Macarron, R., Banks, M. N., Bojanic, D., Burns, D. J., Cirovic, D. A., Garyantes, T., Green, D. V., Hertzberg, R. P., Janzen, W. P., Paslay, J. W., Schopfer, U., & Sittampalam, G. S. (2011). Impact of high-throughput screening in biomedical research. *Nature Reviews. Drug Discovery, 10*(3), 188–195. DOI: 10.1038/nrd3368 PMID: 21358738

Maguluri, L. P., Ananth, J., Hariram, S., Geetha, C., Bhaskar, A., & Boopathi, S. (2023). Smart Vehicle-Emissions Monitoring System Using Internet of Things (IoT). In *Handbook of Research on Safe Disposal Methods of Municipal Solid Wastes for a Sustainable Environment* (pp. 191–211). IGI Global.

Mak, K. K., & Pichika, M. R. (2019). Artificial intelligence in drug development: Present status and future prospects. *Drug Discovery Today, 24*(3), 773–780. DOI: 10.1016/j.drudis.2018.11.014 PMID: 30472429

Malathi, J., Kusha, K., Isaac, S., Ramesh, A., Rajendiran, M., & Boopathi, S. (2024). IoT-Enabled Remote Patient Monitoring for Chronic Disease Management and Cost Savings: Transforming Healthcare. In *Advances in Explainable AI Applications for Smart Cities* (pp. 371–388). IGI Global.

Marques, S. I., Sá, S. I., Carmo, H., Carvalho, F., & Silva, J. P. (2024). Pharmaceutical-mediated neuroimmune modulation in psychiatric/psychological adverse events. *Progress in Neuro-Psychopharmacology & Biological Psychiatry, 135*, 111114. DOI: 10.1016/j.pnpbp.2024.111114 PMID: 39111563

Martinelli, D. D. (2022). Generative machine learning for de novo drug discovery: A systematic review. *Computers in Biology and Medicine, 145*, 105403. DOI: 10.1016/j.compbiomed.2022.105403 PMID: 35339849

Maskus, K. E. (2012). *Private rights and public problems: The global economics of intellectual property in the digital age*. Peterson Institute for International Economics.

McKinsey & Company. (2023). *Quantum computing's potential in pharmaceuticals: A strategic perspective*. https://www.mckinsey.com/industries/life-sciences/our-insights/pharmas-digital-rx-quantum-computing-in-drug-research-and-development

Mervin, M. C., Moyle, W., Jones, C., Murfield, J., Draper, B., Beattie, E., Shum, D. H. K., O'Dwyer, S., & Thalib, L. (2018). The cost-effectiveness of using PARO, a therapeutic robotic seal, to reduce agitation and medication use in dementia: Findings from a cluster–randomized controlled trial. *Journal of the American Medical Directors Association, 19*(7), 619–622. DOI: 10.1016/j.jamda.2017.10.008 PMID: 29325922

Merz, K. M., Jr., & Roux, B. (Eds.). (2009). *Biological membranes: A molecular perspective from computation and experiment: Force field development and validation*. Birkhäuser. https://www.nbi.ku.dk/membranes/pdf/1996_HeimburgMarsh_BookChapter.pdf

Mieres-Perez, J., & Sanchez-Garcia, E. (2020). Quantum mechanics/molecular mechanics multiscale modeling of biomolecules. *Advances in Physical Organic Chemistry*, *54*, 65–112. DOI: 10.1016/bs.apoc.2020.08.002

Miotto, R., Wang, F., Wang, S., Jiang, X., & Dudley, J. T. (2018). Deep learning for healthcare: Review, opportunities and challenges. *Briefings in Bioinformatics*, *19*(6), 1236–1246. DOI: 10.1093/bib/bbx044 PMID: 28481991

Mishra, P., & Anand, S. (2022). Nanoceuticals as Theranostics Against Neurodegenerative Diseases. In *Role of Nutrients in Neurological Disorders* (pp. 263–279). Springer. DOI: 10.1007/978-981-16-8158-5_14

Mittelstadt, Brent & Allo, Patrick & Taddeo, Mariarosaria & Wachter, Sandra & Floridi, Luciano. (2016). The Ethics of Algorithms: Mapping the Debate. Big Data & Society.

Mohammadpour, A., Dolatabadi, M., Bontempi, E., & Shahsavani, E. (2025). Synthesis and characterisation of novel lignocellulosic biomass-derived activated carbon for dye removal: Machine learning optimization, mechanisms, and antibacterial properties. *Biomass and Bioenergy*, *192*, 107490. DOI: 10.1016/j.biombioe.2024.107490

Mori, Y., Kudo, S. E., East, J. E., Rastogi, A., Bretthauer, M., Misawa, M., Sekiguchi, M., Matsuda, T., Saito, Y., Ikematsu, H., Hotta, K., Ohtsuka, K., Kudo, T., & Mori, K. (2020). Cost savings in colonoscopy with artificial intelligence-aided polyp diagnosis: An add-on analysis of a clinical trial (with video). *Gastrointestinal Endoscopy*, *92*(4), 905–911. DOI: 10.1016/j.gie.2020.03.3759 PMID: 32240683

Morley, J., Machado, C. C., Burr, C., Cowls, J., Joshi, I., Taddeo, M., & Floridi, L. (2020). The ethics of AI in health care: A mapping review. *Social Science & Medicine*, *260*, 113172. DOI: 10.1016/j.socscimed.2020.113172 PMID: 32702587

Mubashir, T., Tahir, M. H., Mahmoud, M. H. H., Shafiq, Z., Ashraf, M., El Azab, I. H., & Janjua, M. R. S. A. (2023). Designing of symmetric and asymmetric small molecule acceptors for organic solar cells: A farmwork based on Machine learning, virtual screening, and structural analysis. *Journal of Photochemistry and Photobiology A Chemistry*, *444*, 114977. DOI: 10.1016/j.jphotochem.2023.114977

Mullard, A. (2016). Parsing clinical success rates. *Nature Reviews. Drug Discovery*, *15*(7), 447–447. DOI: 10.1038/nrd.2016.136 PMID: 27357012

Muniasamy, A. (2025b). Revolutionizing health monitoring: Integrating transformer models with multi-head attention for precise human activity recognition using wearable devices. *Technology and Health Care*, *31*(1), 395–409. DOI: 10.3233/THC-241064 PMID: 39269866

Muniasamy, A., & Asiri, F. (2025a). Advanced human activity recognition on wearables with multi-scale sparse attention. *Multimedia Tools and Applications*. Advance online publication. DOI: 10.1007/s11042-024-20475-6

Muralitharan, S., Nelson, W., Di, S., McGillion, M., Devereaux, P. J., Barr, N. G., & Petch, J. (2021). Machine learning-based early warning systems for clinical deterioration: Systematic scoping review. *Journal of Medical Internet Research*, *23*(2), e25187. DOI: 10.2196/25187 PMID: 33538696

Nakatsuka, T., Tateishi, R., Sato, M., Hashizume, N., & Kamada, A.. (2025). Deep learning and digital pathology powers prediction of HCC development in steatotic liver disease. *Hepatology (Baltimore, Md.)*, *81*(3), 976–989. DOI: 10.1097/HEP.0000000000000904

Nakov, N., Acevska, J., Brezovska, K., Kavrakovski, Z., & Dimitrovska, A. (2023). Green strategies toward eco-friendly HPLC methods in pharma analysis. In *High Performance Liquid Chromatography-Recent Advances and Applications*. IntechOpen. DOI: 10.5772/intechopen.110035

Nangia, A. K. (2024). Importance of Structural Databases, Molecular Pharmacophores, Supramolecular Heterosynthons, and Artificial Intelligence–Machine Learning–Neural Network Tools in Drug Discovery. *Crystal Growth & Design*, *24*(16), 6888–6910. DOI: 10.1021/acs.cgd.4c00422

Nassiri, K., & Akhloufi, M. A. (2024). Recent advances in large language models for healthcare. *BioMedInformatics*, *4*(2), 1097–1143. DOI: 10.3390/biomedinformatics4020062

Ngiam, K. Y., & Khor, I. W. (2019). Big data and machine learning algorithms for health-care delivery. *The Lancet. Oncology*, *20*(5), e262–e273. DOI: 10.1016/S1470-2045(19)30149-4 PMID: 31044724

Nichol, A. A., Batten, J. N., Halley, M. C., Axelrod, J. K., Sankar, P. L., & Cho, M. K. (2021). A typology of existing machine learning–based predictive analytic tools focused on reducing costs and improving quality in health care: Systematic search and content analysis. *Journal of Medical Internet Research*, *23*(6), e26391. DOI: 10.2196/26391 PMID: 34156338

Noor, S., AlQahtani, S. A., & Khan, S. (2025). Chronic liver disease detection using ranking and projection-based feature optimization with deep learning. *AIMS Bioengineering*, *12*(1), 50–68. DOI: 10.3934/bioeng.2025003

Novartis. (2023). *Technology Brief: Smart Manufacturing and Digital Twins*. Novartis AG.

O'Neill, J., Bartlett, J., & Mignone, J. (2007). Best practices in intercultural health.

Olivecrona, M., Blaschke, T., Engkvist, O., & Chen, H. (2017). Molecular de-novo design through deep reinforcement learning. *Journal of Cheminformatics*, *9*(1), 48. DOI: 10.1186/s13321-017-0235-x PMID: 29086083

Orchard, S., Al-Lazikani, B., Bryant, S., Clark, D., Calder, E., Dix, I., Engkvist, O., Forster, M., Gaulton, A., Gilson, M., Glen, R., Grigorov, M., Hammond-Kosack, K., Harland, L., Hopkins, A., Larminie, C., Lynch, N., Mann, R. K., Murray-Rust, P., & Hermjakob, H. (2011). Minimum information about a bioactive entity (MIABE). *Nature Reviews. Drug Discovery*, *10*(9), 661–669. DOI: 10.1038/nrd3503 PMID: 21878981

Oskin, M., Chong, F., & Chuang, I. L. (2002). A practical architecture for reliable quantum computers. *Computer*, *35*(1), 79–87. DOI: 10.1109/2.976922

Ovallath, S., & Sulthana, B. (2017). Levodopa: History and Therapeutic Applications. *Annals of Indian Academy of Neurology, 20*(3), <span class="nowrap">185-</span>189. DOI: 10.4103/aian.AIAN_241_17

Ozkizilcik, A., Williams, R., Tian, Z. R., Muresanu, D. F., Sharma, A., & Sharma, H. S. (2017). Synthesis of biocompatible titanate nanofibers for effective delivery of neuroprotective agents. In *Neurotrophic Factors: Methods and Protocols* (pp. 433–442). Springer.

Paananen, J., & Fortino, V. (2019). An omics perspective on drug target discovery platforms. *Briefings in Bioinformatics*, *21*(6), 1937–1953. DOI: 10.1093/bib/bbz122 PMID: 31774113

Pan, D., Lu, P., Wu, Y., Kang, L., Huang, F., Lin, K., & Yang, F. (2024). Prediction of multiple types of drug interactions based on multi-scale fusion and dual-view fusion. *Frontiers in Pharmacology*, *15*, 1354540. DOI: 10.3389/fphar.2024.1354540 PMID: 38434701

Parvatikar, P. P., Patil, S., Khaparkhuntikar, K., Patil, S., Singh, P. K., Sahana, R., Kulkarni, R. V., & Raghu, A. V. (2023). Artificial intelligence: Machine learning approach for screening large database and drug discovery. *Antiviral Research, 220*, 105740. DOI: 10.1016/j.antiviral.2023.105740 PMID: 37935248

Patel, V., & Shah, M. (2022). Artificial intelligence and machine learning in drug discovery and development. *Intelligent Medicine*, *2*(3), 134–140. DOI: 10.1016/j.imed.2021.10.001

Patil, A. D., Kasabe, P. J., & Dandge, P. B. (2022). Pharmaceutical and nutraceutical potential of natural bioactive pigment: Astaxanthin. *Natural Products and Bioprospecting*, *12*(1), 25. DOI: 10.1007/s13659-022-00347-y PMID: 35794254

Patil, R. S., Kulkarni, S. B., & Gaikwad, V. L. (2023). Artificial intelligence in pharmaceutical regulatory affairs. *Drug Discovery Today*, *28*(9), 103700. DOI: 10.1016/j.drudis.2023.103700 PMID: 37442291

Paul, D., ... (2010). Challenges and opportunities in drug discovery. *Nature Reviews Drug Discovery, 9*(3), 2 Abhijith, J., Adedoyin, A., Ambrosiano, J., Anisimov, P., Casper, W., Chennupati, G., Coffrin, C., Djidjev, H., Gunter, D., Karra, S., Lemons, N., Lin, S., Malyzhenkov, A., Mascarenas, D., Mniszewski, S., Nadiga, B., O'Malley, D., Oyen, D., Pakin, S., & Lokhov, A. (2018). *Quantum algorithm implementations for beginners* [Preprint]. arXiv. https://doi.org//arXiv.1804.03719DOI: 10.48550

Paul, D., Sanap, G., Shenoy, S., Kalyane, D., Kalia, K., & Tekade, R. K. (2021). Artificial intelligence in drug discovery and development. *Drug Discovery Today*, *26*(1), 80–93. DOI: 10.1016/j.drudis.2020.10.010 PMID: 33099022

Paul, D., Sanap, G., Shenoy, S., Kalyane, D., Kalia, K., & Tekade, R. K. (2021). Drug discovery in the age of big data: A systematic review. *Current Drug Targets*, *22*(5), 492–510. DOI: 10.2174/1389450122666210126163705

Paul, S. M., Mytelka, D. S., Dunwiddie, C. T., Persinger, C. C., Munos, B. H., Lindborg, S. R., & Schacht, A. L. (2010). How to improve R&D productivity: The pharmaceutical industry's grand challenge. *Nature Reviews. Drug Discovery*, *9*(3), 203–214. DOI: 10.1038/nrd3078 PMID: 20168317

Payal, Manju & Ananth Kumar, T. & Kumar K, Suresh. (2022). Integrating Natural language processing (NLP) and Machine learning Techniques for Healthcare Industries. .DOI: 10. 3030. 10.15680/IJIRCCE.2022.1005023l

Peixoto, D., Barbosa, A., Peixoto, H., Lopes, J., Guimarães, T., & Santos, M. (2022). Predictive analytics for hospital inpatient flow determination. *Procedia Computer Science*, *210*, 254–259. DOI: 10.1016/j.procs.2022.10.146

Peruzzo, A., McClean, J., Shadbolt, P., Yung, M. H., Zhou, X. Q., Love, P. J., Aspuru-Guzik, A., & O'Brien, J. L. (2014). A variational eigenvalue solver on a photonic quantum processor. *Nature Communications*, *5*(1), 4213. DOI: 10.1038/ncomms5213 PMID: 25055053

Pfizer. (2023). *Annual Sustainability and Innovation Report*. Pfizer Inc.

Pitchai, R., Guru, K. V., Gandhi, J. N., Komala, C. R., Kumar, J. R. D., & Boopathi, S. (2024). Fog Computing-Integrated ML-Based Framework and Solutions for Intelligent Systems: Digital Healthcare Applications. In *Technological Advancements in Data Processing for Next Generation Intelligent Systems* (pp. 196–224). IGI Global. DOI: 10.4018/979-8-3693-0968-1.ch008

Pogány, P., Arad, N., Genway, S., & Pickett, S. D. (2018). De novo molecule design by translating from reduced graphs to SMILES. *Journal of Chemical Information and Modeling*, *59*(3), 1136–1146. DOI: 10.1021/acs.jcim.8b00626 PMID: 30525594

Polypharmacy and Drug Adherence in Elderly Patients. (n.d.). Retrieved April 8, 2025, from https://www.uspharmacist.com/article/polypharmacy-and-drug-adherence-in-elderly-patients

Ponikowski, P., Voors, A. A., Anker, S. D., Bueno, H., Cleland, J. G. F., Coats, A. J. S., Falk, V., González-Juanatey, J. R., Harjola, V., Jankowska, E. A., Jessup, M., Linde, C., Nihoyannopoulos, P., Parissis, J. T., Pieske, B., Riley, J. P., Rosano, G. M. C., Ruilope, L. M., Ruschitzka, F., & Van Der Meer, P. (2016). 2016 ESC Guidelines for the diagnosis and treatment of acute and chronic heart failure. *European Heart Journal*, *37*(27), 2129–2200. DOI: 10.1093/eurheartj/ehw128 PMID: 27206819

Prabhakar, P., & Mamoni, B. (2021). Technical problems, regulatory and market challenges in bringing herbal drug into mainstream of modern medicinal practices. *Research Journal of Biotechnology*, *16*, 3.

Prabu, S., Senthilraja, R., Jayapoorani, S., & Arun, M. (2025). AI-Driven Predictive Maintenance for Smart Manufacturing Systems Using Digital Twin Technology. *International Journal of Computational and Experimental Science and Engineering.*, *11*. Advance online publication. DOI: 10.22399/ijcesen.1099

Purnamaningsih, S., Ismono, J., Utami, I., Parlindungan, V., & Hanifah, S. (2024). The Challenges of Data Privacy Laws in the Age of Big Data: Balancing Security, Privacy, and Innovation. *Join: Journal of Social Science.*, *1*(6), 455–465. DOI: 10.59613/gny8bq82

Rajkomar, A., Dean, J., & Kohane, I. (2019). Machine learning in medicine. *The New England Journal of Medicine*, *380*(14), 1347–1358. DOI: 10.1056/NEJMra1814259 PMID: 30943338

Ramezani, M., Takian, A., Bakhtiari, A., Rabiee, H. R., Ghazanfari, S., & Mostafavi, H. (2023). The application of artificial intelligence in health policy: A scoping review. *BMC Health Services Research*, *23*(1), 1416. DOI: 10.1186/s12913-023-10462-2 PMID: 38102620

Ramudu, K., Mohan, V. M., Jyothirmai, D., Prasad, D., Agrawal, R., & Boopathi, S. (2023). Machine Learning and Artificial Intelligence in Disease Prediction: Applications, Challenges, Limitations, Case Studies, and Future Directions. In *Contemporary Applications of Data Fusion for Advanced Healthcare Informatics* (pp. 297–318). IGI Global.

Ranjan, C., & Padhy, N. P. (2020). Quality control using artificial intelligence in pharmaceutical production. *Computers in Biology and Medicine*, *123*, 103877. DOI: 10.1016/j.compbiomed.2020.103877

Rasmussen, M., Pedersen, J., & Smith, L. (2024). A three-compartment population pharmacokinetic model for propofol in very-high-BMI patients: Weight descriptors and sex as covariates. *Acta Anaesthesiologica Scandinavica*, *68*(3), 210–221. DOI: 10.1111/j.1399-6576.1975.tb05243.x PMID: 1101602

Rawat, D., Sharma, S., & Bhadula, S. (2025). CT Imaging-Based Deep Learning System for Non-Small Cell Lung Cancer Detection and Classification. *International Journal of Advanced Computer Science and Applications*, *16*(5). Advance online publication. DOI: 10.14569/IJACSA.2025.0160561

Rawat, D., Sharma, S., & Bhadula, S. (2025b). Machine Vision Technique with Image Segmentation in Digital Diagnostic System for Lung Cancer Detection. In *2025 International Conference on Pervasive Computational Technologies (ICPCT)*, 35–40. https://doi.org/DOI: 10.1109/ICPCT64145.2025.10939214

Raza, M. A., Aziz, S., Noreen, M., Saeed, A., Anjum, I., Ahmed, M., & Raza, S. M. (2022). Artificial intelligence (AI) in pharmacy: An overview of innovations. *Innovations in Pharmacy*, *13*(2), 10–24926. DOI: 10.24926/iip.v13i2.4839 PMID: 36654703

Rebecca, B., Kumar, K. P. M., Padmini, S., Srivastava, B. K., Halder, S., & Boopathi, S. (2024). Convergence of Data Science-AI-Green Chemistry-Affordable Medicine: Transforming Drug Discovery. In *Handbook of Research on AI and ML for Intelligent Machines and Systems* (pp. 348–373). IGI Global.

Reiner, Z., Catapano, A. L., De Backer, G., Graham, I., Taskinen, M., Wiklund, O., Agewall, S., Alegria, E., Chapman, M. J., Durrington, P., Erdine, S., Halcox, J., Hobbs, R., Kjekshus, J., Filardi, P. P., Riccardi, G., Storey, R. F., Wood, D., Bax, J., & Zamorano, J. L. (2011). ESC/EAS Guidelines for the management of dyslipidaemias: The Task Force for the management of dyslipidaemias of the European Society of Cardiology (ESC) and the European Atherosclerosis Society (EAS). *European Heart Journal*, *32*(14), 1769–1818. DOI: 10.1093/eurheartj/ehr158 PMID: 21712404

Reker, D., Bernardes, G. J., & Rodrigues, T. (2019). Computational advances in combating colloidal aggregation in drug discovery. *Nature Chemistry*, *11*(5), 402–418. DOI: 10.1038/s41557-019-0234-9 PMID: 30988417

Reker, D., Hoyt, E. A., Bernardes, G. J., & Rodrigues, T. (2020). Adaptive optimization of chemical reactions with minimal experimental information. *Cell Reports. Physical Science*, *1*(10), 100247. DOI: 10.1016/j.xcrp.2020.100247

Rohani, N., & Eslahchi, C. (2019). Drug-Drug Interaction Predicting by Neural Network Using Integrated Similarity. *Scientific Reports 2019 9:1*, *9*(1), 1–11. DOI: 10.1038/s41598-019-50121-3

Rossi, J. G., Rojas-Perilla, N., Krois, J., & Schwendicke, F. (2022). Cost-effectiveness of artificial intelligence as a decision-support system applied to the detection and grading of melanoma, dental caries, and diabetic retinopathy. *JAMA Network Open*, *5*(3), e220269–e220269. DOI: 10.1001/jamanetworkopen.2022.0269 PMID: 35289862

Roux, G. L., Bruneau, C., Lelièvre, B., Deguigne, M. B., Turcant, A., Harry, P., & Boels, D. (2015). Recreational phenethylamine poisonings reported to a French poison control center. *Drug and Alcohol Dependence*, *154*, 46–53. DOI: 10.1016/j.drugalcdep.2015.05.048 PMID: 26205314

Rüßmann, M., Lorenz, M., Gerbert, P., Waldner, M., Justus, J., Engel, P., & Harnisch, M. (2015). Industry 4.0: The future of productivity and growth in manufacturing industries.

Saeed, F., Shiwlani, A., Umar, M., Jahangir, Z., Tahir, A., & Shiwlani, S. (2025). Hepatocellular Carcinoma Prediction in HCV Patients using Machine Learning and Deep Learning Techniques. *Jurnal Ilmiah Computer Science*, *3*(2), 120–134. https://doi.org/10.58602/jics.v3i2.48

Saggar, S., Mir, P. A., Kumar, N., Chawla, A., Uppal, J., & Kaur, A. (2022). Traditional and herbal medicines: Opportunities and challenges. *Pharmacognosy Research*, *14*(2), 107–114. DOI: 10.5530/pres.14.2.15

Sahu, A., Mishra, J., & Kushwaha, N. (2022). Artificial intelligence (AI) in drugs and pharmaceuticals. *Combinatorial Chemistry & High Throughput Screening, 25*(11), 1818–1837. DOI: 10.2174/1386207325666211207153943 PMID: 34875986

Salat, D., & Tolosa, E. (2013). Levodopa in the treatment of Parkinson's disease: Current status and new developments. *Journal of Parkinson's Disease, 3*(3), 255–269. DOI: 10.3233/JPD-130186 PMID: 23948989

Sangeetha, S. (2016). A study on problems and challenges faced by micro small and medium enterprises: A special reference to manufacturing sector in Coimbatore district. *International Journal of Academic Research and Development, 1*(9), 29–33.

Sangeetha, S., Suganya, P., Shanthini, S., Murthy, G. N. K., & Sathya, R. (2023). Crime Rate Prediction and Prevention: Unleashing the Power of Deep Learning. *Proceedings of the 4th International Conference on Smart Electronics and Communication, ICOSEC 2023*. https://doi.org/DOI: 10.1109/ICOSEC58147.2023.10276012

Sapkota, B., & Pariatamby, A. (2023). Pharmaceutical waste management system–Are the current techniques sustainable, eco-friendly and circular? A review. *Waste Management (New York, N.Y.), 168*, 83–97. DOI: 10.1016/j.wasman.2023.05.052 PMID: 37285639

Saravananathan, K., & Velmurugan, T. (2016). Analyzing Diabetic Data using Classification Algorithms in Data Mining. *Indian Journal of Science and Technology, 9*(43). Advance online publication. DOI: 10.17485/ijst/2016/v9i43/93874

Scalia, G., Grambow, C. A., Pernici, B., Li, Y. P., & Green, W. H. (2020). Evaluating scalable uncertainty estimation methods for deep learning-based molecular property prediction. *Journal of Chemical Information and Modeling, 60*(6), 2697–2717. DOI: 10.1021/acs.jcim.9b00975 PMID: 32243154

Scannell, J. W., Blanckley, A., Boldon, H., & Warrington, B. (2012). Diagnosing the decline in pharmaceutical R&D efficiency. *Nature Reviews. Drug Discovery, 11*(3), 191–200. DOI: 10.1038/nrd3681 PMID: 22378269

Scannell, J. W., & Bosley, J. (2016). When quality beats quantity: Decision theory, drug discovery, and the reproducibility crisis. *PLoS One, 11*(2), e0147215. DOI: 10.1371/journal.pone.0147215 PMID: 26863229

Schell, R. C., Allen, B., Goedel, W. C., Hallowell, B. D., Scagos, R., Li, Y., Krieger, M. S., Neill, D. B., Marshall, B. D. L., Cerda, M., & Ahern, J. (2021). Identifying predictors of opioid overdose death at a neighborhood level with machine learning. *American Journal of Epidemiology, 191*(3), 526–533. DOI: 10.1093/aje/kwab279 PMID: 35020782

Schlosshauer, M. (2007). *Decoherence and the quantum-to-classical transition.* Springer., DOI: 10.1007/978-3-540-35775-9

Schmidt, P., Biessmann, F., & Teubner, T. (2020). Transparency and trust in artificial intelligence systems. *Journal of Decision Systems*, *29*(4), 260–278. Advance online publication. DOI: 10.1080/12460125.2020.1819094

Schneider, G. (2018). Automating drug discovery. *Nature Reviews. Drug Discovery*, *17*(2), 97–113. DOI: 10.1038/nrd.2017.232 PMID: 29242609

Schot, J., & Steinmueller, W. E. (2018). Three frames for innovation policy: R&D, systems of innovation and transformative change. *Research Policy*, *47*(9), 1554–1567. DOI: 10.1016/j.respol.2018.08.011

Segal, C., Homza, A., Tu, R., & Xing, E. P. (2021). Leveraging multi-task learning to classify diseases from histology data: A comparison of deep learning architectures. arXiv preprint arXiv:2107.05984. https://arxiv.org/abs/2107.05984

Segler, M. H., Preuss, M., & Waller, M. P. (2018). Planning chemical syntheses with deep neural networks and symbolic AI. *Nature*, *555*(7698), 604–610. DOI: 10.1038/nature25978 PMID: 29595767

Selvaraj, C., Chandra, I., & Singh, S. K. (2022). Artificial intelligence and machine learning approaches for drug design: Challenges and opportunities for the pharmaceutical industries. *Molecular Diversity*, *26*(3), 1–21. DOI: 10.1007/s11030-021-10326-z PMID: 34686947

Selvaraj, K., & Subbian, S. (2023). Inter-Scale Amalgam Cluster Dense Graph Convolutional Network for Hepatocellular Carcinoma Detection. *International Journal of Intelligent Engineering and Systems*, *16*(6), 356–365.

Shafer, A., Doze, V. A., Shafer, S. L., & White, P. F. (1988). Pharmacokinetics and pharmacodynamics of propofol infusions during general anesthesia. *Anesthesiology*, *69*(3), 348–356. DOI: 10.1097/00000542-198809000-00011 PMID: 3261954

Shah, N. H., Milstein, A., & Bagley, S. C. (2019). Making machine learning models clinically useful. *Journal of the American Medical Association*, *322*(14), 1351–1352. DOI: 10.1001/jama.2019.10306 PMID: 31393527

Shaki, F., Amirkhanloo, M., Jahani, D., & Chahardori, M. (2024a). Artificial intelligence in pharmaceuticals: Exploring applications and legal challenges. *Pharmaceutical and Biomedical Research*, *10*(1), 1–10. DOI: 10.32598/PBR.10.1.1257.1

Shapiro, A. (2003). Monte Carlo sampling methods. In Sethi, S. P., Thompson, G. L., & Marti, K. (Eds.), *Handbooks in operations research and management science* (Vol. 10, pp. 353–425). Elsevier., DOI: 10.1016/S0927-0507(03)10006-0

Sharan, A. D., Schroeder, G. D., West, M. E., & Vaccaro, A. R. (2016). Understanding business models in health care. *Clinical Spine Surgery*, *29*(4), 158–160. DOI: 10.1097/BSD.0000000000000380 PMID: 27018909

Sharma, S., Tyagi, R., & Mohan, S. (2025). Blockchain-Based Security and Privacy in Digital Healthcare Recommender Systems. In In Healthcare Recommender Systems (pp. 221–237). https://doi.org/DOI: 10.1007/978-3-031-80056-6_10

Shinde, A., Pawar, D., & Sonawane, K. (2021). Automation in pharmaceutical sector by implementation of artificial intelligence platform: A way forward. *International Journal of Basic and Clinical Pharmacology*, *10*(7), 863–869. DOI: 10.18203/2319-2003.ijbcp20212387

Shor, P. W. (1996). Fault-tolerant quantum computation. In *Proceedings of 37th Conference on Foundations of Computer Science* (pp. 56–65). IEEE. DOI: 10.1109/SFCS.1996.548464

Simoens, S. (2009). Health economic assessment: A methodological primer. *International Journal of Environmental Research and Public Health*, *6*(12), 2950–2966. DOI: 10.3390/ijerph6122950 PMID: 20049237

Singh, R., Garg, R., Patel, N., & Braun, M. (2020).. . *Generative Adversarial Networks for Synthetic Defect Generation in Assembly and Test Manufacturing.*, *1-5*, 1–5. Advance online publication. DOI: 10.1109/ASMC49169.2020.9185242

Sivamaruthi, B. S., Nallasamy, P., Suganthy, N., Kesika, P., & Chaiyasut, C. (2022). Pharmaceutical and biomedical applications of starch-based drug delivery system: A review. *Journal of Drug Delivery Science and Technology*, *77*, 103890. DOI: 10.1016/j.jddst.2022.103890

Smith, A. L., Nguyen, P. T., & Banerjee, S. (2023). Deep reinforcement learning–based propofol dosing guided by three-compartment PK/PD simulations. *Journal of Clinical Pharmacology*, *63*(4), 367–379.

Staszak, M., Staszak, K., Wieszczycka, K., Bajek, A., Roszkowski, K., & Tylkowski, B. (2022). Machine learning in drug design: Use of artificial intelligence to explore the chemical structure–biological activity relationship. *Wiley Interdisciplinary Reviews. Computational Molecular Science*, *12*(2), e1568. DOI: 10.1002/wcms.1568

Stokes, J. M., Yang, K., Swanson, K., Jin, W., Cubillos-Ruiz, A., Donghia, N. M., MacNair, C. R., French, S., Carfrae, L. A., Bloom-Ackermann, Z., Tran, V. M., Chiappino-Pepe, A., Badran, A. H., Andrews, I. W., Chory, E. J., Church, G. M., Brown, E. D., Jaakkola, T. S., Barzilay, R., & Collins, J. J. (2020). A deep learning approach to antibiotic discovery. *Cell, 180*(4), 688–702. DOI: 10.1016/j.cell.2020.01.021 PMID: 32084340

Strome, T. L. (2020). *Healthcare Analytics for Quality and Performance Improvement* (2nd ed.). Wiley.

Subramanian, A., Narayan, R., Corsello, S. M., Peck, D. D., Natoli, T. E., Lu, X., Gould, J., Davis, J. F., Tubelli, A. A., Asiedu, J. K., Lahr, D. L., Hirschman, J. E., Liu, Z., Donahue, M., Julian, B., Khan, M., Wadden, D., Smith, I. C., Lam, D., & Golub, T. R. (2017). A next generation connectivity map: L1000 platform and the first 1,000,000 profiles. *Cell, 171*(6), 1437–1452. DOI: 10.1016/j.cell.2017.10.049 PMID: 29195078

Tackley, R. M., Lewis, G. T. R., Prys-Roberts, C., Boaden, R. W., Dixon, J., & Harvey, J. T. (1989). Computer-controlled infusion of propofol. *British Journal of Anaesthesia, 62*(1), 46–53. DOI: 10.1093/bja/62.1.46 PMID: 2783854

Tantawy, M. A., Weshahy, S. A., Wadie, M., & Rezk, M. R. (2021). Eco-friendly spectrophotometric methods for assessment of alfuzosin and solifenacin in their new pharmaceutical formulation; green profile evaluation via eco-scale and GAPI tools. *Current Pharmaceutical Analysis, 17*(8), 1093–1103. DOI: 10.2174/15734 12916999200730005740

Tasaka, Y., Tanaka, A., Yasunaga, D., Asakawa, T., Araki, H., & Tanaka, M. (2018). Potential drug-related problems detected by routine pharmaceutical interventions: Safety and economic contributions made by hospital pharmacists in Japan. *Journal of Pharmaceutical Health Care and Sciences, 4*(1), 33. DOI: 10.1186/s40780-018-0125-z PMID: 30564432

Teng, M., Singla, R., Yau, O., Lamoureux, D., Gupta, A., Hu, Z., Hu, R., Aissiou, A., Eaton, S., Hamm, C., Hu, S., Kelly, D., MacMillan, K. M., Malik, S., Mazzoli, V., Teng, Y. W., Laricheva, M., Jarus, T., & Field, T. S. (2022). Health care students' perspectives on artificial intelligence: Countrywide survey in Canada. *JMIR Medical Education, 8*(1), e33390. DOI: 10.2196/33390 PMID: 35099397

Theerthagiri, P. (2025), Liver disease classification using histogram-based gradient boosting classification tree with feature selection algorithm, *Biomedical Signal Processing and Control,* Volume 100, Part C,107102, ISSN 1746-8094, https://doi .org/10.1016/j.bspc.2024.107102

Thieme, A., Belgrave, D., & Doherty, G. (2020). Machine learning in mental health. *ACM Transactions on Computer-Human Interaction, 27*(5), 1–53. DOI: 10.1145/3398069

Thorlund, K., Dron, L., Park, J. J. H., Hsu, G., Forrest, J. I., & Mills, E. J. (2020). A real-time dashboard of clinical trials for COVID-19. *The Lancet. Digital Health, 2*(6), e286–e287. DOI: 10.1016/S2589-7500(20)30086-8 PMID: 32363333

Tian, J. (2022). A review of methodologies in detecting drug-drug interactions. *AIP Conference Proceedings, 2511*(1), 020022. Advance online publication. DOI: 10.1063/5.0094306

Tiwari, A., Behki, P., Kumar, V., & Mahajan, S. (2023). *MODERN HOSPITAL MANAGEMENT SYSTEM. Russell, S., & Norvig, P. (2021). Artificial Intelligence: A Modern Approach* (4th ed.). Pearson.

Topol, E. (2019). *Deep Medicine: How Artificial Intelligence Can Make Healthcare Human Again*. Basic Books.

Townshend, R. J., Eismann, S., Watkins, A. M., Rangan, R., Karelina, M., Das, R., & Dror, R. O. (2021). Geometric deep learning of RNA structure. *Science, 373*(6558), 1047–1051. DOI: 10.1126/science.abe5650 PMID: 34446608

Tricco, A. C. (1967). PRISMA extension for scoping reviews (PRISMA-ScR): Checklist and explanation. *Angewandte Chemie International Edition in English, 6*(11), 951.

Turner, H. C., Archer, R. A., Downey, L. E., Isaranuwatchai, W., Chalkidou, K., Jit, M., & Teerawattananon, Y. (2021). An introduction to the main types of economic evaluations used for informing priority setting and resource allocation in healthcare: Key features, uses, and limitations. *Frontiers in Public Health, 9*, 722927. DOI: 10.3389/fpubh.2021.722927 PMID: 34513790

UChicago Medicine. (2025). *AI Predictive Tool Enhances Patient Deterioration Detection*. Retrieved from https://www.uchicagomedicine.org

Udompap, P., Liu, K., Attia, I. Z., Canning, R. E., Benson, J. T., Therneau, T. M., Noseworthy, P. A., Friedman, P. A., Rattan, P., Ahn, J. C., Simonetto, D. A., Shah, V. H., Kamath, P. S., & Allen, A. M. (2025). Performance of AI-Enabled Electrocardiogram in the Prediction of Metabolic Dysfunction-Associated Steatotic Liver Disease. *Clinical Gastroenterology and Hepatology, 23*(4), 574–582.e3. DOI: 10.1016/j.cgh.2024.08.009

Upadhyaya, A. N., Saqib, A., Devi, J. V., Rallapalli, S., Sudha, S., & Boopathi, S. (2024). Implementation of the Internet of Things (IoT) in Remote Healthcare. In *Advances in Medical Technologies and Clinical Practice* (pp. 104–124). IGI Global. DOI: 10.4018/979-8-3693-1934-5.ch006

Vamathevan, J., Clark, D., Czodrowski, P., Dunham, I., Ferran, E., Lee, G., Li, B., Madabhushi, A., Shah, P., Spitzer, M., & Zhao, S. (2019). Applications of machine learning in drug discovery and development. *Nature Reviews. Drug Discovery*, *18*(6), 463–477. DOI: 10.1038/s41573-019-0024-5 PMID: 30976107

Vangeri, A. K., Bathrinath, S., Anand, M. C. J., Shanmugathai, M., Meenatchi, N., & Boopathi, S. (2024). Green Supply Chain Management in Eco-Friendly Sustainable Manufacturing Industries. In *Environmental Applications of Carbon-Based Materials* (pp. 253–287). IGI Global., DOI: 10.4018/979-8-3693-3625-0.ch010

Veltri, D., Kamath, U., & Shehu, A. (2018). Deep learning improves antimicrobial peptide recognition. *Bioinformatics (Oxford, England)*, *34*(16), 2740–2747. DOI: 10.1093/bioinformatics/bty179 PMID: 29590297

Verma, R., Christiana, M. B. V., Maheswari, M., Srinivasan, V., Patro, P., Dari, S. S., & Boopathi, S. (2024). Intelligent Physarum Solver for Profit Maximization in Oligopolistic Supply Chain Networks. In *AI and Machine Learning Impacts in Intelligent Supply Chain* (pp. 156–179). IGI Global. DOI: 10.4018/979-8-3693-1347-3.ch011

Vespoli, S., Mattera, G., Marchesano, M. G., Nele, L., & Guizzi, G. (2025). Adaptive manufacturing control with deep reinforcement learning for dynamic WIP management in Industry 4.0. *Computers & Industrial Engineering*, *202*, 110966. DOI: 10.1016/j.cie.2025.110966

Voermans, A. M., Mewes, J. C., Broyles, M. R., & Steuten, L. M. (2019). Cost-effectiveness analysis of a procalcitonin-guided decision algorithm for antibiotic stewardship using real-world US hospital data. *OMICS: A Journal of Integrative Biology*, *23*(10), 508–515. DOI: 10.1089/omi.2019.0113 PMID: 31509068

Voets, M. M., Veltman, J., Slump, C. H., Siesling, S., & Koffijberg, H. (2022). Systematic review of health economic evaluations focused on artificial intelligence in healthcare: The tortoise and the cheetah. *Value in Health*, *25*(3), 340–349. DOI: 10.1016/j.jval.2021.11.1362 PMID: 35227444

Voigt, P., & Von dem Bussche, A. (2017). The eu general data protection regulation (gdpr). *A practical guide, 1st ed., Cham: Springer International Publishing, 10*(3152676), 10-5555.

Von Wedel, P., & Hagist, C. (2020). Economic value of data and analytics for health care providers: Hermeneutic systematic literature review. *Journal of Medical Internet Research*, *22*(11), e23315. DOI: 10.2196/23315 PMID: 33206056

Vora, L. K., Gholap, A. D., Jetha, K., Thakur, R. R. S., Solanki, H. K., & Chavda, V. P. (2023a). Artificial intelligence in pharmaceutical technology and drug delivery design. *Pharmaceutics*, *15*(7), 1916. DOI: 10.3390/pharmaceutics15071916 PMID: 37514102

Vuyk, J., Engbers, F. H. M., Bum, A. G. L., Vletter, A. A., & Bovill, J. G. (1995). Performance of Computer-Controlled Infusion of Propofol: An Evaluation of Five Pharmacokinetic Parameter Sets. *Anesthesia and Analgesia*, *81*, 1275–1282. PMID: 7486116

Walter, Holmes. (2025). Integrating Federated Learning in Drug Development: Balancing Data Privacy and Predictive Accuracy.

Walters, W. P., & Barzilay, R. (2021). Applications of deep learning in molecule generation and molecular property prediction. *Accounts of Chemical Research*, *54*(2), 263–270. DOI: 10.1021/acs.accounts.0c00699 PMID: 33370107

Wang, T., Shao, W., Huang, Z., Tang, H., Zhang, J., Ding, Z., & Huang, K. (2021). MOGONET integrates multi-omics data using graph convolutional networks allowing patient classification and biomarker identification. *Nature Communications*, *12*(1), 3445. DOI: 10.1038/s41467-021-23774-w

Wang, X. V., & Wang, L. (2020). Digital twin-based WIP quality prediction for complicated product assembly. *Journal of Manufacturing Systems*, *56*, 262–271. DOI: 10.1016/j.jmsy.2020.06.004

Wan, Z., Sun, X., Li, Y., Chu, T., Hao, X., Cao, Y., & Zhang, P. (2025). Applications of Artificial Intelligence in Drug Repurposing. *Advancement of Science*, *12*(14), 2411325. DOI: 10.1002/advs.202411325 PMID: 40047357

Ward, P. J., Rock, P. J., Slavova, S., Young, A. M., Bunn, T. L., & Kavuluru, R. (2019). Enhancing timeliness of drug overdose mortality surveillance: A machine learning approach. *PLoS One*, *14*(10), e0223318. DOI: 10.1371/journal.pone.0223318 PMID: 31618226

Way, G. P., & Greene, C. S. (2018). Extracting a biologically relevant latent space from cancer transcriptomes with variational autoencoders. *Pacific Symposium on Biocomputing*, *23*, 80–91. DOI: 10.1142/9789813235533_0008 PMID: 29218871

Williams, K., Bilsland, E., Sparkes, A., Aubrey, W., Young, M., Soldatova, L. N., De Grave, K., Ramon, J., de Clare, M., Sirawaraporn, W., Oliver, S. G., & King, R. D. (2015). Cheaper faster drug development validated by the repositioning of drugs against neglected tropical diseases. *Journal of the Royal Society, Interface, 12*(104), 20141289. DOI: 10.1098/rsif.2014.1289 PMID: 25652463

Wolff, J., Pauling, J., Keck, A., & Baumbach, J. (2020). The economic impact of artificial intelligence in health care: Systematic review. *Journal of Medical Internet Research, 22*(2), e16866. DOI: 10.2196/16866 PMID: 32130134

World Health Organization. (2016). *Global Report on Diabetes*. World Health Organization.

Wu, Q., Chen, Y., & Feng, S. (2022). A convolutional neural network with self-attention for depth-of-anesthesia prediction under propofol anesthesia. *Computers in Biology and Medicine, 148*, 105801. DOI: 10.1016/j.compbiomed.2022.105801

Wu, Q., Han, J., Yan, Y., Kuo, Y.-H., & Shen, Z.-J. M. (2025). Reinforcement learning for healthcare operations management: Methodological framework, recent developments, and future research directions. *Health Care Management Science, 28*(2), 298–333. DOI: 10.1007/s10729-025-09699-6 PMID: 40202690

Wu, S., Roberts, K., Datta, S., Du, J., Ji, Z., Si, Y., Soni, S., Wang, Q., Wei, Q., Xiang, Y., Zhao, B., & Xu, H. (2020). Deep learning in clinical natural language processing: A methodical review. *Journal of the American Medical Informatics Association : JAMIA, 27*(3), 457–470. DOI: 10.1093/jamia/ocz200 PMID: 31794016

Wu, Z., Ramsundar, B., Feinberg, E. N., Gomes, J., Geniesse, C., Pappu, A. S., Leswing, K., & Pande, V. (2018). MoleculeNet: A benchmark for molecular machine learning. *Chemical Science (Cambridge), 9*(2), 513–530. DOI: 10.1039/C7SC02664A PMID: 29629118

Wyrembek, M., Baryannis, G., & Brintrup, A. (2025). Causal machine learning for supply chain risk prediction and intervention planning. *International Journal of Production Research*, 1–20. DOI: 10.1080/00207543.2025.2458121

Xie, Y., Nguyen, Q. D., Hamzah, H., Lim, G., Bellemo, V., Gunasekeran, D. V., Yip, M. Y. T., Qi Lee, X., Hsu, W., Li Lee, M., Tan, C. S., Tym Wong, H., Lamoureux, E. L., Tan, G. S. W., Wong, T. Y., Finkelstein, E. A., & Ting, D. S. (2020). Artificial intelligence for teleophthalmology-based diabetic retinopathy screening in a national programme: An economic analysis modelling study. *The Lancet. Digital Health, 2*(5), e240–e249. DOI: 10.1016/S2589-7500(20)30060-1 PMID: 33328056

Xiong, G., Wu, Z., Yi, J., Fu, L., Yang, Z., Hsieh, C., Yin, M., Zeng, X., Wu, C., Lu, A., Chen, X., Hou, T., & Cao, D. (2021). ADMETlab 2.0

Xue, J., Min, F., & Ma, F. (2020). Research on Diabetes Prediction Method based on Machine learning. *Journal of Physics: Conference Series, 1684*, 012062. DOI: 10.1088/1742-6596/1684/1/012062

Yang, B., Yang, Y., Wang, M., & Su, X. (2023). MRGCN: Cancer subtyping with multi-reconstruction graph convolutional network using full and partial multi-omics dataset. *Bioinformatics (Oxford, England), 39*(6). Advance online publication. DOI: 10.1093/bioinformatics/btad353

Yang, G., Zhang, J., Liu, Y., & Zhang, L. (2021). Artificial intelligence in manufacturing and maintenance: A review. *IEEE Access : Practical Innovations, Open Solutions, 9*, 123910–123931. DOI: 10.1109/ACCESS.2021.3111083

Yeager, D. S., Hanselman, P., Walton, G. M., Murray, J. S., Crosnoe, R., Muller, C., Tipton, E., Schneider, B., Hulleman, C. S., Hinojosa, C. P., Paunesku, D., Romero, C., Flint, K., Roberts, A., Trott, J., Iachan, R., Buontempo, J., Yang, S. M., Carvalho, C. M., & Dweck, C. S. (2019). A national experiment reveals where a growth mindset improves achievement. *Nature, 573*(7774), 364–369. DOI: 10.1038/s41586-019-1466-y PMID: 31391586

Young, J. C., Mitchell, C., & Redpath, S. M. (2020). Conservation Research, policy and practice. In *Cambridge University Press eBooks*.

Zhang, C., Zhang, Z., Zhang, F., Zeng, B., Liu, X., & Wang, L. (2024). A computational model for potential microbe–disease association detection based on improved graph convolutional networks and multi-channel autoencoders. *Frontiers in Microbiology, 15*. Advance online publication. DOI: 10.3389/fmicb.2024.1435408

Zhang, Y., Fan, M., Xu, Z., Jiang, Y., Ding, H., Li, Z., Shu, K., Zhao, M., Feng, G., Yong, K.-T., Dong, B., Zhu, W., & Xu, G. (2023). Machine-learning screening of luminogens with aggregation-induced emission characteristics for fluorescence imaging. *Journal of Nanobiotechnology, 21*(1), 107. DOI: 10.1186/s12951-023-01864-9 PMID: 36964565

Zhao, H., Li, X., Wang, Y., & Chen, L. (2024). LSTM-based real-time concentration tracking of propofol using a four-compartment PK/PD model in swine. *Frontiers in Medical Engineering, 10*, 112.

Zhao, J., Wang, J., & Anderson, N. (2024). Machine learning applications in forest and biomass supply chain management: A review. *International Journal of Forest Engineering, 35*(3), 371–380. DOI: 10.1080/14942119.2024.2380230

Zhao, X., Sun, Y., Zhang, R., Chen, Z., Hua, Y., Zhang, P., Guo, H., Cui, X., Huang, X., & Li, X. (2022). Machine learning modeling and insights into the structural characteristics of drug-induced neurotoxicity. *Journal of Chemical Information and Modeling*, *62*(23), 6035–6045. DOI: 10.1021/acs.jcim.2c01131 PMID: 36448818

Zhavoronkov, A., Ivanenkov, Y. A., Aliper, A., Veselov, M. S., Aladinskiy, V. A., Aladinskaya, A. V., & Zholus, A. (2019). Deep learning enables rapid identification of potent DDR1 kinase inhibitors. *Nature Biotechnology*, *37*(9), 1038–1040. DOI: 10.1038/s41587-019-0224-x PMID: 31477924

Zheng, C., Li, M., & Ding, J. (2021). Challenges and opportunities of nanomedicines in clinical translation. *Bio Integration*, *2*(2), 57. DOI: 10.15212/bioi-2021-0016

Zhou, L., Wang, N., Zhu, Z., Gao, H., Zhou, Y., & Fang, M. (2024). Identification of subtypes in digestive system tumors based on multi-omics data and graph convolutional network. *International Journal of Machine Learning and Cybernetics*, *15*(9), 3567–3577. https://doi.org/10.1007/s13042-024-02109-3

Zhuang, Z., & Barnard, A. S. (2024). Property Prediction for Complex Compounds Using Structure-Free Mendeleev Encoding and Machine Learning. *Journal of Chemical Information and Modeling*, *64*(24), 9205–9214. DOI: 10.1021/acs.jcim.4c01343 PMID: 39665625

Zinner, M., Dahlhausen, F., Boehme, P., Ehlers, J., Bieske, L., & Fehring, L. (2021). Quantum computing's potential for drug discovery: Early stage industry dynamics. *Drug Discovery Today*, *26*(7), 1680–1688. DOI: 10.1016/j.drudis.2021.06.003 PMID: 34119668

Zong, Z., Wang, H., & Lin, J. (2022). Clinical validation of a covariate-based propofol pharmacokinetic model under target-controlled infusion in surgery patients. *Journal of Clinical Anesthesia*, *80*, 110886.

About the Contributors

Anandhavalli Muniasamy is an Associate Professor in the Department of Computer Science at King Khalid University (KKU), Saudi Arabia. She holds a Ph.D. in Computer Science and Engineering from Sikkim Manipal University, India. Her primary research interests include data mining, data analytics, artificial intelligence (AI), soft computing, and data science, with a specific focus on machine learning and deep learning applications for advanced data analysis. She has an impressive academic and research portfolio, having published over 35 research articles in prestigious international journals and book chapters. She has actively participated in more than 30 national and international conferences, presenting her work on cutting-edge computational techniques and edited book publications. As a Principal Investigator and Co-Principal Investigator, she has led several university-funded research projectsand served as the Principal Investigator for a funded project supported by the All India Council for Technical Education (AICTE).In addition to her research contributions, Dr. Muniasamy has been a dedicated manuscript reviewer for leading international journals for over a decade and a Ph.D. thesis examiner for multiple universities. She has also been invited to deliver guest lectures and serves as an editorial board member for various renowned journals and conferences. She is an active member of professional organizations such as the International Association of Engineers (IAENG), the Computer Society of India (CSI), and the International Association of Computer Science and Information Technology (IACSIT). Her current research focuses on leveraging AI-driven techniques, particularly machine learning and deep learning, to solve complex problems in medical data analysis and deliver innovative solutions in her field. Affiliation: Department of Informatics and Computer Systems College of Computer Science Gregar Campus, King Khalid University Abha, Kingdom of Saudi Arabia. Email: anandhavalli@kku.edu.sa ; anandhavalli.dr@gmail.com

Gauthaman Karunakaran, Principal and Director of Government Pharmacy College, Sajong, Sikkim, is a distinguished academic and researcher with over 29 years of experience in teaching and research. Holding a PhD from Tamil Nadu Dr. MGR Medical University, he has an impressive research portfolio, including an h-index of 22, an i10-index of 33, and 2,139 citations with a ResearchGate score of 883. His accolades include the CSIR Young Scientist Award (Biology) in 2004, the AICTE Career Award for Young Teachers (2006), and the Sh. Mohamed Research Prize (Bahrain Research Day, 2018), among others. Dr. Karunakaran has held esteemed roles at institutions such as King Khalid University and the Himalayan Pharmacy Institute, contributing significantly to pharmacology and drug research. With 94 publications, five books, and 11 book chapters, his expertise spans pharmacovigilance, medical device monitoring, and curriculum development for pharmacy education in India and abroad.

***

Lovely Jacob A, Department of Chemistry Little Flower College (Autonomous), Guruvayur Thrissur Kerala Orchid Id: 0000-0001-5199-3856

Komal Bhardwaj is currently working at the Maharishi Markandeshwar Institute of Management, Maharishi Markandeshwar University as Assistant Professor of Finance. She has a rich experience of more than eight years of teaching in the field of management. She has a research experience in the areas of assets pricing, derivatives, option pricing and study on stock volatility. Her research interest includes consumer behaviour, investments, corporate governance, and assets liability management. She also worked as a Thesis supervisor for a program called upgrad-LJMU MBA at upgrade education private limited.

Harini Devendran is currently in her 5th year of MBBS at Mahsa University. She has a strong interest in AI in the medical field, robotics in surgery, and cardiology, particularly cardiovascular diseases and heart failure. Dr. Devendran has previously researched the prevalence of ADHD among medical students and the prevalence of VAP in ICU settings. She is also passionate about innovations such as telemedicine and wearable health technology to improve healthcare outcomes.

G. Sureshkumar is currently working as an Assistant Professor in the Department of Computer Science at Pondicherry University. He has more than 12 years of experience in teaching and researching. He completed his master's in Computer Science and Engineering from the College of Engineering Guindy of Anna University in 2006. He completed his Ph.D. in Computer Science and Engineering in

2014. He has published his research works in international journals and conferences. His research interests include Data Mining, Computational Intelligence, Information Retrieval, and Image processing.

Shwetha G K, Associate Professor, Department of Computer Science and Engineering, Vidyavardhaka College of Engineering, Mysuru, Karnataka.

Shruthi Anadhavalli Gathaman is a fifth-year MBBS student at Mahsa University, with a keen interest in integrating artificial intelligence into the medical field. She has contributed to significant research papers, including "Enhancing Medical Sector Efficiency: A Comprehensive Case Study Based on Data Visualization Tools for Business Applications" (DOI: 10.4018/979-8-3693-6537-3.ch011) and "Enhancing Business Applications in ENT Diseases Management Through Data Visualization" (DOI: 10.4018/979-8-3693-6537-3.ch010). Shruthi aims to leverage innovative technologies to improve healthcare delivery and patient outcomes.

K. Gowri, Department of Pharmacology, SRM College o Pharmacy, SRM Institute Of Science and Technology, Chengalpattu Tamilnadu

Deepak Gupta is a distinguished academician with over 20 years of teaching experience and expertise in Computer Science and Engineering. He holds a Ph.D. in Computer Engineering and has an extensive research portfolio, including many international journal papers, multiple conference proceedings, and several books. His research interests span machine learning, artificial intelligence, and data mining. Currently, Dr. Gupta serves as an Associate Professor and Academic Coordinator in the Department of Computer Science & Engineering at ITM Gwalior, MP, India. He has also contributed significantly to the field through patents and copyrights and actively engages as a reviewer, conference chair and editor.

Shahnazeer C K has 9 years of experience as an Assistant Professor in various Engineering Colleges in Kerala and 4 years of experience in Industry. She is a research scholar in Computer Science and Engineering, at Pondicherry University Karaikal Campus, Puducherry, India. Her qualifications include B.Tech in Information Technology from Government Engineering College Sreekrishnapuram Palakkad Kerala, India in 2006 and M.Tech in Information Technology from Anna University Coimbatore Tamil Nadu, India in 2010. Her research interests include Computational Intelligence and Cloud computing.

Rita Kadam is having 7 years of teaching and industrial experience. She is pursuing PHD in Reinforcement learning domain. Her Expertise in Java, Machine learning,Deep learning, Natural language Processing She has published 4 national international papers.

Simranjeet Kaur, a keen researcher working in the field of Pharmacology and pharmacy practice. currently working as an Assistant Professor at Faculty of pharmaceutical sciences, PCTE Group of institutes, Ludhiana,

Kaurish Murugesan is a final-year medical student at MAHSA University, Malaysia, with a keen focus on healthcare management and clinical leadership. His academic pursuits span emergency medicine, surgery, and patient care, with a particular interest in integrating business principles into healthcare to optimize patient outcomes and operational efficiency. Kaurish is passionate about healthcare policy and hospital administration, emphasizing the role of MBA principles in advancing medical practice. He has contributed to research, including studies on the prevalence of ventilator-associated diseases in ICU settings, reflecting his commitment to improving clinical and organizational standards in the healthcare sector.

Arshi Naim, is recognized among the top 2% of Global Scientists (Stanford University and Elsevier 2024). She is a distinguished scholar with a Ph.D. in Business Management and an MBA in Marketing. Her academic journey, rooted in excellence, began with First Class Honors in Economics from Aligarh Muslim University. As an e-learning expert and certified peer reviewer with Quality Matters, U.S., Dr. Naim has further enhanced her expertise with certificates in Digital Marketing and Social Media Analytics from Accenture, UK, and entrepreneurship from Harvard University. A prolific researcher, she has authored over 79 Scopus and Web of Science-indexed publications and penned more than 10 acclaimed books with prestigious publishers like Taylor & Francis, Nova Sciences and IGI Global. Her work seamlessly blends theory and practice, inspiring future generations of scholars. Through her commitment to mentoring doctoral students and her extensive contributions to global research, Dr. Naim continues to shape the landscape of academic excellence.

S Reshma, Associate Professor Department of Artificial Intelligence & Machine Learning, Dayananda Sagar College of Engineering, Bangalore

Jigar Rupani, School of Business and Management, Christ University, Bangalore Karnataka

S. Magesh is a distinguished academician and entrepreneur with multifaceted credentials in Engineering, Science, Arts, Administration, Technology, Linguistics, and Management. He began his academic career in 1999, advancing to Professor and Head of the Computer Science Department with 17 years in academia and 10 years in corporate roles. He has published 24 indexed journals, 2 patents, and 2 books. Magesh is currently performing research in Deep Learning at Dr. M.G.R. Educational and Research Institute, Chennai, India. His academic contributions have been recognized through publications in Web of Science, ESCI, SCOPUS, Springer, and Compendex.

Ajay Sharma is currently working as a Technical Consultant in UpGrad Education Pvt Ltd and is currently posted in the School of Computing at Lovely Professional University (LPU) Jalandhar Punjab. Before joining UpGrad, he worked as a junior research fellow in the Department of Biotechnology and Bioinformatics at Jaypee University of Information Technology Solan Himachal Pradesh. He has obtained his master's degree in Computer Science (Deep Learning) in the Domain of Biomedical Image Processing and a bachelor's degree in Bioinformatics from Shoolini University Himachal Pradesh. During his bachelor's, he got a certificate of merit. Mr. Ajay has completed his Computer Science Diploma from Lovely Professional University Jalandhar Punjab. During his bachelor's and master, he has presented, Demonstrated his work at different international conferences at AIIMS Rishikesh and PGIMER Chandigarh, IHBT Palampur.

Deepanshu Sharma is currently pursuing a Bachelor of Technology in Computer Science and Engineering with a specialization in Data Science (Artificial Intelligence and Machine Learning) from Lovely Professional University, Punjab, India. He specializes in deep learning, medical imaging, and computer vision. His recent work focuses on applying convolutional neural networks to the diagnosis of irreversible pulpitis using dental X-ray images. Deepanshu has actively contributed to AI-driven healthcare research and is passionate about leveraging artificial intelligence to enhance diagnostic accuracy and improve patient outcomes.

Sachin Sharma is currently working as a Professor, Amity School of Engineering and Technology, Amity University, Punjab, Mohali, India. He also worked as Associate Dean, International Affairs and Professor, Department of Computer Science and Engineering at Graphic Era Deemed to be University, Dehradun, Uttarakhand, India. He has experience of 15+ years in industry and academia. He is also Co-founder and Chief Technology officer (CTO) of IntelliNexus LLC, Arkansas, USA based company. He also worked as a Senior Systems Engineer at Belkin International, Inc., Irvine, California, USA. He received his Philosophy of Doctorate (Ph.D.) degree in Engineering Science and Systems specialization in Systems Engineering from University of Arkansas at Little Rock, USA with 4.0 out

4.0 GPA and M.S. degree in Systems engineering from University of Arkansas at Little Rock with 4.0 out 4.0 GPA. Dr. Sharma has authored/coauthored over 300+ publications in the form of books, patents, and papers in refereed journals and conference proceedings. He holds 100+ US, Indian and international patents in the area of IoT, wireless communication and AI. He has also served as a Guest Reviewer for several Special issues of IEEE/ACM Transactions. His research interests include 6G wireless communication networks, Cloud Computing, Artificial Intelligence, Quantum Computing, IoT, Vehicular ad hoc networking and Cyber security.

Shamneesh Sharma is currently serving as Senior Manager- Programs at upGrad Education Private Limited, Bangalore, India. and prior to this he was at iNurture Education Solution, Bangalore as Senior Faculty (Cloud Technology and Information Security) and deputed as Head in the Department of Computer Application, School of Computer Science & Engineering, Poornima University, Jaipur. He has worked as IT-Head and Associate Professor (CSE) at Alakh Prakash Goyal Shimla University, Shimla (H.P.). He has played a vital role in the implementation of New IT-Infrastructure, ERP System and Website Development along with its maintenance in the University. He is having more than 14 Years of academic and administrative experience in the field of Computer Science & Information Technology. He is B. Tech & M. Tech and Ph. D (Computer Science & Engineering). He has published more than 100 research manuscripts in various International & National journals & conferences. He has also presented papers in International and National conferences. He is a member of various International & National professional & academic bodies.

R. Sudhakar awarded B.E from Anna University, Chennai, M.Tech from DR.M.G.R University, Chennai and Ph.D in Computer Science and Engineering in 2017 from Anna University. At present he is working as an Associate professor in the Department of Computer Science & Engineering in Madanapalle Institute of Technology & Science, Madanapalle, Andhra Pradesh India. His research interests include Image Processing, Security in Wireless Adhoc Networks, IOT, Cloud Computing, Deep Learning.

Aishwarya Tipara has a work experience of 2 years in Sudha Engineering works as Production Manager.

Sujatha Vijayaraghavan is currently an Assistant Professor in the Mechatronics Engineering, SRM Institute of science and technology since 2019. She also worked as Associate Professor in Dept of Electronics and Instrumentation Engineering at Sri manakula vinayagar Engg college from June 2014-2019. She earned her doctorate in Instrumentation Engineering from the Faculty of Electrical Engineering,

Madras Institute of Technology, Anna University, Chennai in 2014. Her research concentrated on the "Design of Multivariable controllers using relay feedback responses". She also worked on Auto tuning of PID controllers. She pursued her Doctorate under the Guidance of Dr. Rames C. Panda, Senior Principal Scientist, Process Control laboratory, Department of Chemical Engineering, CSIR- Central Leather Research Institute (CLRI), Chennai. She is recipient of DST funded project as Senior Research Fellow 2010-2013.

Rajesh V. Argiddi, Associate Professor Department of Computer Science and Engineering, Walchand Institute of Technology, Solapur Solapur Maharashtra 413006

Mukesh Kumar Viswanathan is a final-year medical student at MAHSA University, Malaysia, with a keen interest in pediatric medicine and clinical research. He has contributed to studies on the prevalence of ADHD among medical students and the complications and preventive measures for safe blood transfusion in Malaysia. His pediatric-focused research interests include childhood obesity, neonatal jaundice management, vaccine hesitancy in parents, and early developmental screening, aiming to enhance child health outcomes through evidence-based approaches.

Index

A

AI in Drug Discovery 7, 31, 133, 145, 190
Artificial Intelligence 1, 2, 3, 5, 6, 8, 14, 17, 20, 22, 23, 24, 27, 28, 30, 31, 33, 35, 39, 44, 45, 48, 52, 54, 55, 56, 57, 68, 92, 94, 97, 99, 101, 102, 122, 125, 126, 145, 149, 153, 156, 157, 158, 162, 164, 167, 173, 181, 185, 190, 191, 192, 195, 196, 210, 211, 212, 213, 215, 216, 219, 221, 222, 228, 232, 233, 236, 240, 241, 243, 244, 251, 252, 253, 267, 268, 269, 270, 271, 277, 296, 297, 298, 300, 301, 314, 316, 324, 327, 329, 330, 332, 355, 372, 374, 375, 376, 377, 379, 382, 384, 385, 387, 394, 395, 418, 422

B

Big Data 22, 54, 93, 102, 158, 159, 162, 164, 165, 241, 242, 247, 248, 256, 257, 258, 271, 314, 394
Biodegradable Solvents 98, 99, 108, 110, 113, 118
Blood Concentration 333, 337, 350

C

Clinical Trial Optimization 14
Clinical Trials 1, 2, 3, 5, 6, 8, 9, 17, 18, 19, 20, 22, 24, 33, 34, 38, 41, 44, 51, 52, 54, 61, 63, 64, 67, 68, 90, 95, 102, 103, 106, 126, 129, 130, 139, 140, 146, 147, 245, 248, 249, 255, 315, 357, 359, 362, 366, 371, 377, 379, 381, 391, 393, 396, 408, 414, 415
Computer-Assisted Drug Design 1, 2, 3, 6, 20, 24

D

Data Analytics 2, 5, 24, 28, 102, 107, 158, 162, 165, 213, 237, 241, 248, 251, 256, 262, 271, 298, 314, 327
Digital Twins 4, 12, 113, 139, 146, 158, 160, 161, 162, 163, 164, 166, 167, 171, 174, 175, 177, 183, 186, 188, 191
Drug combinations 83, 234, 376, 383, 391, 409, 412, 413, 415, 416, 418
Drug Discovery 2, 3, 5, 6, 7, 8, 14, 18, 19, 20, 22, 23, 24, 29, 30, 31, 32, 33, 39, 40, 41, 42, 44, 51, 52, 54, 56, 59, 60, 61, 62, 63, 65, 66, 69, 70, 73, 74, 77, 78, 79, 80, 81, 82, 83, 84, 85, 86, 87, 88, 89, 90, 91, 93, 94, 101, 118, 119, 120, 122, 126, 130, 131, 132, 133, 140, 141, 145, 147, 150, 152, 153, 154, 156, 190, 196, 197, 211, 212, 240, 244, 251, 305, 395, 396, 416, 418
Drug Overdose 297, 298, 299, 301, 304, 305, 307, 314, 316, 324, 327, 328, 329, 331
Drug Polymer 195, 196, 199, 210, 213
Dynamic 3, 13, 64, 158, 162, 163, 170, 171, 189, 192, 217, 218, 220, 227, 229, 252, 274, 276, 297, 300, 301, 314, 315, 316, 324, 325, 327, 329, 331, 333, 334, 355, 379, 397, 417, 418

E

Electronic Health Records 3, 9, 28, 57, 140, 217, 225, 227, 234, 236, 247, 248, 249, 251, 252, 256, 258, 260, 263, 266, 267, 268, 271, 301, 305, 309, 314, 336, 357, 369, 372, 383, 387, 393, 394, 406, 417, 422
Estimation 60, 82, 151, 154, 183, 329, 333, 334, 335, 342, 345, 353, 358, 360, 374, 375, 376, 378, 381, 406
Ethical Challenges 27, 251

F

Formulary Design 215, 216, 218, 219, 220, 223, 226, 227, 228, 230, 232, 233, 234,

235, 236, 237, 238, 239, 244

G

Generative Artificial Intelligence 125, 329
graph networks 389, 390
Green Chemistry 97, 99, 100, 107, 108, 109, 110, 114, 118, 120, 122, 123

H

Healthcare Management 215
Healthcare Research 54, 247
Hospital Administration 215, 216, 218, 219, 220, 223, 224, 225, 226, 227, 228, 229, 230, 232, 235, 236, 237, 238, 239, 244, 260

I

Industry 4.0 157, 158, 162, 182, 186, 190, 191, 192, 193, 199

M

Machine Learning 3, 6, 9, 10, 13, 22, 23, 24, 27, 28, 49, 55, 56, 60, 61, 66, 68, 74, 78, 80, 81, 82, 83, 84, 88, 89, 90, 91, 92, 97, 99, 122, 145, 149, 151, 154, 155, 156, 158, 161, 162, 167, 168, 170, 173, 174, 175, 176, 181, 182, 186, 188, 190, 191, 193, 195, 196, 197, 198, 199, 210, 211, 212, 213, 215, 216, 217, 218, 224, 225, 226, 227, 231, 233, 234, 237, 240, 241, 242, 243, 244, 245, 258, 262, 267, 268, 269, 274, 276, 277, 281, 295, 297, 298, 300, 301, 302, 304, 305, 309, 310, 311, 314, 315, 325, 326, 328, 329, 330, 331, 333, 335, 342, 345, 346, 348, 349, 351, 352, 353, 354, 355, 358, 369, 370, 372, 377, 382, 386, 387, 393, 394, 395, 397, 405, 410, 414, 416, 420, 422
Machine Learning Algorithm 196, 311, 355
Machine Learning Model 225, 268
Medical Data 264, 271, 273, 274, 276, 277, 279, 282, 284, 285, 296
Modelling 5, 92, 270, 333, 334, 336, 339, 342, 370, 374, 376
Molecular Simulation 60, 82

N

Named Entity Recognition 357, 370, 383, 387, 390, 394, 395, 396, 401, 403, 405, 406, 414, 422
Nanotechnology 97, 98, 100, 101, 103, 118, 119, 211
Natural Language Processing 3, 4, 5, 8, 13, 28, 36, 39, 57, 131, 158, 172, 186, 193, 216, 225, 227, 230, 234, 242, 243, 245, 301, 314, 332, 367, 369, 375, 382, 387, 389, 395, 396, 398, 399, 404, 412, 414, 418, 422
Neurological Disorders 98, 101, 110, 118, 121, 407

P

Patient Feedback 230, 357, 369, 372, 378, 387
Patient Flow Optimization 223
Personalized Medicine 2, 49, 51, 74, 83, 89, 90, 95, 159, 215, 232, 234, 244, 245, 255, 274, 308, 391, 406, 414, 416
Pharmaceutical Industry 1, 2, 3, 4, 5, 6, 11, 14, 17, 20, 21, 22, 25, 27, 28, 44, 45, 48, 54, 60, 62, 89, 90, 93, 98, 107, 110, 126, 141, 143, 150, 158, 159, 160, 162, 167, 181, 186, 192, 213, 305, 329, 383, 398
Pharmaceutical Production 12, 22, 29, 99, 105, 110, 157, 159, 160, 161, 162, 163, 167, 168, 170, 176, 181, 183, 184, 185, 187, 193
Pharmaceutical R&D 61, 64, 102, 127, 130, 145, 147, 154, 182
Pharmaceutical Research 16, 28, 32, 50, 55, 59, 60, 62, 79, 90, 94, 98, 120, 126, 141, 156, 397
Pharmaceuticals 2, 16, 17, 18, 19, 20, 27, 31, 33, 35, 39, 47, 48, 50, 56, 92, 99, 105, 106, 107, 108, 111, 113, 114,

115, 118, 120, 123, 145, 159, 161, 162, 190, 196, 363
Pharmacokinetic Three Compartment Model 334
Pharmacovigilance 4, 18, 30, 38, 50, 52, 218, 219, 222, 255, 316, 327, 357, 358, 359, 360, 361, 362, 364, 366, 367, 369, 370, 371, 372, 374, 375, 377, 378, 379, 381, 382, 383, 385, 386, 387, 392, 394, 395, 396, 397, 405, 406, 409, 414, 416, 418, 419, 422
Precision Medicine 7, 49, 83, 139, 248, 406, 416, 417
Predictive Analytics 3, 4, 8, 10, 20, 24, 28, 38, 164, 167, 172, 186, 215, 219, 224, 227, 228, 229, 232, 236, 242, 244, 248, 255, 262, 275, 326, 414
Predictive Maintenance 11, 24, 34, 158, 165, 172, 173, 183, 186, 188, 191, 193, 227

Q

Quality Control 1, 2, 5, 6, 11, 12, 20, 22, 23, 24, 107, 134, 157, 159, 162, 165, 168, 172, 173, 178, 184, 186, 188, 197
Quantum Algorithms 61, 63, 72, 74, 76, 77, 78, 79, 80, 81, 82, 83, 85, 87, 89, 90, 95
Quantum Computing 59, 60, 61, 62, 63, 70, 71, 72, 73, 74, 76, 77, 78, 79, 80, 81, 82, 83, 85, 86, 87, 88, 89, 90, 91, 92, 93, 94, 95, 146, 150, 182
Quantum Machine Learning 74, 78, 80, 83, 84, 88, 89, 90, 91, 92, 182, 188

R

Regulatory Compliance 2, 4, 5, 11, 21, 25, 99, 110, 113, 157, 158, 159, 161, 164, 166, 173, 181, 186, 189, 193, 223, 261, 262, 265, 309, 383
Resource Allocation 38, 85, 159, 183, 215, 217, 219, 225, 226, 227, 228, 232, 233, 236, 239, 241, 244, 245, 250, 252, 269, 320
Response System 297, 301, 305, 307, 316, 320, 324, 327, 331
Robotics and Automation 162, 164, 170

S

Smart Manufacturing 157, 158, 159, 160, 161, 162, 163, 167, 168, 176, 180, 181, 185, 187, 188, 191, 192
Supply Chain Management 4, 5, 6, 20, 22, 122, 161, 198, 199, 213, 244, 245
Supply Chain Optimisation 196
Synthesis and Characterisation Analysis 196

V

visualization 16, 41, 88, 143, 394, 412, 413, 414, 415

www.ingramcontent.com/pod-product-compliance
Lightning Source LLC
LaVergne TN
LVHW062333300926
849161LV00007B/1673

* 9 7 9 8 3 3 7 3 2 0 4 3 4 *